The Nature of Su
the Goals of

The Nature of Suffering and the Goals of Nursing

Second Edition

Edited by
WILLIAM E. ROSA
and
BETTY R. FERRELL

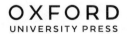

OXFORD
UNIVERSITY PRESS

Oxford University Press is a department of the University of Oxford. It furthers the University's objective of excellence in research, scholarship, and education by publishing worldwide. Oxford is a registered trade mark of Oxford University Press in the UK and certain other countries.

Published in the United States of America by Oxford University Press
198 Madison Avenue, New York, NY 10016, United States of America.

CIP data is on file at the Library of Congress

ISBN 978–0–19–766793–4

DOI: 10.1093/oso/9780197667934.001.0001

Printed by Sheridan Books, Inc., United States of America

Contents

Preface

Nessa Coyle

Although the nature of suffering and the goals of nursing have not fundamentally changed since the initial slim volume with that title (five chapters long), coauthored with Dr Betty Ferrell and influenced by the seminal work of Eric Cassell, was published in 2008, the depth of understanding of suffering with all of its complexities—and the interplay of the experience of suffering between patients, their families, and the nurse—has grown in maturity. This new and expanded volume—edited by Drs Betty Ferrell and William Rosa, 18 chapters long, and written by 31 nurse scholars—allows us to reflect on some of what we have learned over the intervening years. Our understanding of suffering has been both enriched and deepened.

Let Me Step Back for a Moment

In 1996 I wrote a chapter in a book on suffering edited by Dr. Betty Ferrell. The title of my chapter was "Suffering in the First Person," featuring glimpses of suffering through patient and family narratives—"I am more than my chart." The narratives were poignant—full of struggle, despair, strength, and courage. Those patients and families had so much to give and so much to teach and I had so much to learn. Years later in my PhD thesis I explored suffering through the lens of seven patients being cared for in an urban cancer center. These patients had expressed a desire that death would come soon. That the depth of their suffering had not been "heard" or "understood" was starkly evident in their words. Bearing witness to suffering has deeply affected me as a person and has been a gift to me. First-person narratives, being present in the face of suffering, and bearing witness to that suffering are the essence of nursing—it is what we do. Patients and their families are our teachers and always will be.

But in this age of rapid advances in science and evolving therapeutics, application of sophisticated technology in day-to-day patient care and multiple options to prolong life or to push inevitable death further and further away—or to end life at a time of one's choosing—may make listening, being present, and bearing witness more difficult. At the same time, medical uncertainty and health care disparities—all present in our complex multicultural societies—may complicate our interactions with patients and families and our ability to really "hear" what is being said and really "see" what is unfolding before us. There is also the pressure of time, increased caseloads, tasks to be completed, and extensive documentation to be done. Yet the nature of suffering continues to make itself known and the goals of nursing continue to be informed by the intent to comfort, accompany, and facilitate healing.

Nursing is not immune to the many changes in our society, health care systems, and delivery of care. New roles have evolved, with some advanced practice nurses taking on more of the traditional "medical" responsibilities and relying more and more on the "bedside" nurse to make sure the voice of the patient and family are both heard and honored—something may be lost through these transitions as well as something gained. A significant challenge is how to work as a team—a nursing team as well as an interdisciplinary team—with the voice of the patient and family and their values central to the care provided. As nurses of all educational preparations and specialties, we bring ourselves to these diverse situations: we listen and are present, we are silent, we offer both our training and ourselves, and we expect a great deal from both ourselves and others.

Nurses are not empty vessels able to absorb the suffering of others without an impact on their inner selves. One nurse who had been exposed to suffering over time while working in an intensive care unit and felt she could do little to alleviate it put it this way: "I continue to take care of my patients and give good physical care but I cannot be emotionally present anymore. I switch off emotionally—that's how I survive." The suffering of nurses and the impact of that suffering on patient well-being have at last been acknowledged.

We are all in this together—a diverse quilt of humanity, each part dependent on the other. We have different strengths and vulnerabilities; at times each of us needs a supportive hand or shoulder to lean on. Science and compassion go hand in hand—one alone is not sufficient.

Some final thoughts to provide a preamble or backdrop to what you will discover as you explore the chapters of this book. We bring ourselves to each patient and family interaction—our life histories, biases, personal hurts and struggles, and strengths. If we fail to recognize what is within us, we may fail to see what is in front of us. By helping others, we help ourselves. By working as a team, we help each other.

We need to be able to sit with uncertainty—with struggle, loss, and grief—to recognize it and learn from it. We need to be able to ground ourselves and learn "to be there in grief" but not swallowed up by it.

We need to be able to "still" our mind chatter, to calm our mind enough to listen, to tolerate silence, and to respect it as a space for others to fill. Every experience is unique and different. Make no assumptions about what you are about to hear—but listen with attention, curiosity, and acceptance.

And finally, we need to learn to forgive ourselves and move on. Sometimes you will feel like weeping; allow the tears to flow and the grief to pour out. We are all healers— wounded healers; we are both frail and strong.

Contributors

Elena Abascal, DNP, PMHNP-BC
Memorial Sloan Kettering Cancer Center
New York, NY, USA

Avery C. Bechthold, BSN, RN
University of Alabama at Birmingham
Birmingham, AL, USA

Teffin Benedict, MHA
The John A. Hartford Foundation
New York City, NY, USA

Amy Berman, BSN, RN, LHD (hon)
The John A. Hartford Foundation
New York, NY, USA

Janet Booth, MA, RN, NC-BC
Self-employed
CO, USA

Elizabeth G. Broden, PhD, RN
Dana-Farber Cancer Institute
Boston, MA, USA

Sheila Davis, DNP, ANP-BC, FAAN
Partners in Health
Boston, FL, USA

J. Nicholas Dionne-Odom, PhD, RN
University of Alabama at Birmingham
Birmingham, AL, USA

Christine R. Espina, DNP, RN
Western Washington University
Bellingham, WA, USA

Betty R. Ferrell, PhD, RN, MA, CHPN,
FAAN, FPCN
City of Hope
Duarte, CA, USA

Anessa Foxwell, MSN, ACHPN, FPCN
University of Pennsylvania
Philadelphia, PA, USA

Terry Fulmer, PhD, RN, FAAN
The John A. Hartford Foundation
New York, NY, USA

Tamryn F. Gray, PhD, RN, MSN, MPH
Harvard Medical School
Boston, MA, USA

Barbara A. Harris, PhD, RN
DePaul University
Chicago, IL, USA

Marc Julmisse, MPH, BSN, RN
Zanmi Lasante/Partners in Health Haiti
Boston, MA, USA

Mary Koithan, PhD, RN, CNS-BC, FAAN
Washington State University, College of
Nursing
Spokane, WA, USA

Mary Jo Kreitzer, PhD, RN, FAAN, FNAP
University of Minnesota
Minneapolis, MN, USA

Mark Lazenby, RN, PhD, FAAN
University of California
Irvine, CA, USA

Virginia Lee, PhD
McGill University Health Centre
Montreal, CA, USA

Blima Marcus, DNP, ANP-BC, RN, OCN
New York University Langone Health
New York, NY, USA

Frances T. McCarthy, MS, RNC-NIC, CPLC
Columbia University
New York City, NJ, USA

Kim Mooney-Doyle, PhD, RN, CPNP-AC
University of Pennsylvania
Philadelphia, PA, USA

Robin A. Narruhn, PhD, RN
Seattle University
Seattle, WA, USA

Katie E. Nelson, PhD, RN
Johns Hopkins University School of
Nursing
Baltimore, MD, USA

Judith A. Paice, PhD, RN, FAAN
Northwestern University; Feinberg School
of Medicine
Chicago, IL, USA

William E. Rosa, PhD, MBE, NP-BC,
FAANP, FAAN, FPCN
Memorial Sloan Kettering Cancer Center
New York, NY, USA

Cynda Hylton Rushton, PhD, RN, FAAN
Johns Hopkins University
Baltimore, MD, USA

Rumaysa Sharif, MPH
SUNY Downstate Health Sciences

University
New York, NY, USA

Alic G. Shook, PhD, RN
Seattle University
Seattle, WA, USA

Rebecca Slossberg,
MSG Candidate 2022, Intern
The John A. Hartford Foundation
New York, NY, USA

Elizabeth Johnston Taylor, PhD, RN,
FAAN
Loma Linda University
Loma Linda, CA, USA

Stephanie Van Hope, DNP, RN
Hope Holistic Wellness
Woodbourne, NY, USA

Renee Wisniewski, AGPCNP-BC,
ACHPN
Memorial Sloan Kettering Cancer Center
New York, NY, USA

1

The Nature of Suffering and the Practice of Nursing

Mark Lazenby

The Nature of Suffering

"To be human is to suffer," Betty Ferrell and Nessa Coyle wrote in this first volume of this book.[1]

Humans have long tried to understand—and explain—this fact of the human condition. The ancient Greek playwright Aeschylus tells us in a tragedy he wrote in the 5th century BCE, *Prometheus Bound*, that Zeus punished the Titan Prometheus with lifelong suffering for having stolen fire and given it to humans.[2] Before Prometheus's intervention, fire had only belonged to the gods. Zeus punished Prometheus by chaining him to a rock and sending an eagle to pluck out his liver during the day. At night, his liver regenerated, only for the eagle to return the next day to pluck it away again. Because Prometheus was half human, he felt the pain of the mortal wound inflicted by the eagle, but because he was half divine, he did not die from the wound. And when the eagle left for the night, Prometheus felt the pain of healing. Healing, itself, is often painful. Thus, Prometheus suffered without end. In 1618 AD, the Flemish painter Peter Paul Rubens depicted Prometheus's suffering in a piece now displayed at the Philadelphia Museum of Art (Figure 1.1).

In Aeschylus's play, Prometheus's never-ending punishment may have been at divine order, but Prometheus understood the experience in human, not divine, terms. Prometheus, after all, was as much human as divine. Humans, without fire, could not cook, warm themselves, see well at night, or fend off animals terrified of the chemical process of combustion. Indeed, Prometheus's sympathy for his fellow humans who did not have the essential element of fire led, in the end, to his inevitable suffering. It was as if Zeus said, "If you are going to show compassion for your fellow human, you will suffer as humans suffer." Prometheus's reply was that "suffering is a migrant bird that settles."[2]

Suffering, like death, is inevitable. The 20th-century philosopher Ludwig Wittgenstein remarked that death is "not an event in life; we do not live to experience death,"[3] though we all know, whether or not we like to admit it, that death shall one day come for us all. And we do experience others' deaths. Knowledge of death causes us to suffer.

Unlike us, however, Prometheus does not die. This is his divinity. In the myth, he is still, today, chained to the rock enduring the suffering of compassion for humanity. Some may say that Prometheus's physical pain is a sufficient cause of his suffering. It

Mark Lazenby, *The Nature of Suffering and the Practice of Nursing* In: *The Nature of Suffering and the Goals of Nursing.* Second Edition. Edited by: William E. Rosa and Betty R. Ferrell, Oxford University Press. © Oxford University Press 2023. DOI: 10.1093/oso/9780197667934.003.0001

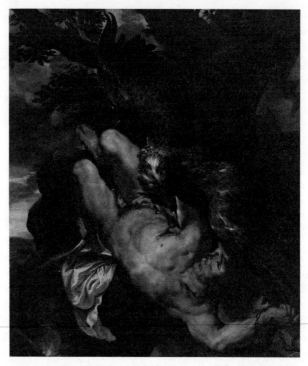

Figure 1.1 Prometheus bound.
Source: Rubens PP. *Prometheus Bound.* Philadelphia Museum of Art: Purchased with the W. P. Wilstach Fund, 1950, W1950-3-1. Photo by Alberto Otero Herranz, courtesy of the Prado Museum, 2015.

certainly is a part of it. But it is not the sum. Pain, as the contemporary essayist Elaine Scarry reminds us, has its etymological home in the Latin *poena*, which has the same root as the word for punishment.[4] Prometheus's punishment indeed brought physical pain, but Prometheus also bore the knowledge of the punishment that had been visited upon him for the good deed of giving humans fire. And he knew that his suffering would be constant. Rather than suffering from the knowledge of inevitable death, Prometheus suffers from his knowledge of the eagle's inevitable return.

Suffering, no matter the cause, is to be conscious of pain. It is to bear, to be put under, to carry, or to endure conscious awareness of pain. Suffering cuts to the core of what it means to be human: to have consciousness—awareness.

To be human is to be connected with other humans. It is through this connectedness that one has consciousness—awareness—of one's human destiny. Destiny is the shape of one's future and the future of the human community. Hope is predicated on an awareness of destiny, if only the hope for progeny or for the continuance of human history in the natural world. Events—such as war—that call into question the connectedness of humanity and the continuance of human history frighten us greatly, because they disrupt our sense of a future and, therefore, our sense of that which gives us hope. To be human is to have a sense of our world and our ability to shape the future— our destiny. Prometheus, chained to the rock, was helpless and hopeless: he could not flee or protect himself or have a hand in his future.

The possibilities of war today, given thermonuclear weaponry, threaten even the natural world with total destruction. The effects of greenhouse gases, effects brought about largely by our activity, also threaten the natural world. To be human is also to be harmonious with nature—to have an expectation of a future supported by the natural world. Prometheus and nature were no longer in harmony. Nature was red. And rather than a steppingstone to the heavens, the rock to which Prometheus was bound was a bed of torture.

The Hebrew scriptures also tackle the fundamental nature of human suffering as disconnection with humanity, one's own and that of others, and with nature. In this version, suffering originated when God banished Adam and Eve from Eden—the garden of eternal life where God himself walked in the cool of each day—for disobeying the divine command not to eat the fruit of the tree of knowledge. He exiled them to the desert, where God did not go and where they would one day die (Genesis 2:17). Adam and Eve's suffering, like Prometheus's, arose from their punishment, punishment that resulted in their being disconnected—helpless, hopeless, and inharmonious with nature. Theirs was a spiritual suffering.

When one, in the grip of suffering, is disconnected from others and from nature, one loses a sense of oneself in the human community and the natural order. Rather, one is trapped in oneself. The experience of suffering, because of its disconnecting interiority, cannot be shared with others. One cannot express suffering; one is caught in a wordless world. A wordless world is a meaningless world to which others do not have access.

In Case Exemplar 1.1, Beth, a patient newly diagnosed with life-limiting cancer, is trapped in her suffering. This suffering was, seemingly, at the hands of an external force that acted upon her to unjustly punish her: cancer. This language of giving agency to a seemingly external force, like cancer, is an attempt to exit the wordlessness of suffering. It is an attempt, Scarry says, to objectify one's suffering.[4]

Case Exemplar 1.1

Beth, a 47-year-old woman, recently saw her primary care provider for acute upper-left quadrant abdominal pain. A physical exam and laboratory and radiographic tests suggested the need for a transesophageal endoscopic biopsy of the pancreas, which revealed adenocarcinoma. A subsequent positron emission tomography scan revealed abdominal wall metastases. The primary tumor was deemed inoperable. Chemotherapy was started, but after one cycle, she was hospitalized for pancytopenia, abdominal pain, nausea and vomiting, laryngopharyngeal dysesthesias, fatigue, and symptoms of depression. The attending oncologist consulted with the palliative care service.

The palliative advanced practice nurse, Rosie, visited Beth in her hospital room. Rosie learned that Beth held an endowed professorship in early medieval English literature at the university to which the academic health center was attached. She had been happily married to a cancer biologist, also a university professor, for 21 years. They had two children, a 15-year-old daughter and an 11-year-old son. They loved hiking in the woods near their home with their two dogs, both huskies. Beth, in response to Rosie's question about her home life, adapted the lyrics to the Crosby, Stills, Nash, and Young song, "Our house is a very, very fine house ... with two dogs in the yard."[19] And then Beth blurted out in sobs, "I hate God."

Rosie sat with Beth in silence. She was simply present with—and for—Beth. After several minutes, Beth blurted out in as much a scream as she could muster, "What do you want me to say? F*** God! And I don't even believe in God."

Rosie clasped Beth's hands, looked into her eyes, and acknowledged her suffering. It was physical, Rosie said: her pain, nausea and vomiting, and fatigue were still uncontrolled. It was emotional: she was sad and lachrymose most of the day. But it was also spiritual, Rosie said to Beth: her anger came from her feeling as if she no longer had any control in her life. Feelings of helplessness and hopelessness are a human response to a life-limiting diagnosis of cancer, Rosie said. After some silence, Beth began speaking about the cancer as if it were an alien that inhabited her body with the sole purpose of killing her, of stealing her from her beloved husband and children, from her dogs, from the family hikes, and from the book she was writing—all for no good reason. Beth had lived a good and decent life. She was fit. She never smoked and drank only a little. She ate healthfully. This suffering was all too much, she said. "I don't know who I am anymore," Beth said to Rosie. "I'm not myself."

Rosie assessed Beth's physical symptoms and from that assessment worked with the palliative care team on a symptom management plan of care that the oncology team could follow.

Rosie also asked Beth whether she would be open to Rosie meeting her husband and children. The next day, they all met for 45 minutes. They told favorite stories, and then Rosie asked them if they had any questions about what was going on with their wife and mother. They talked openly about the cancer, the anticancer treatment, and the symptom management plan of care. "Will Mom be able to finish her book?" the daughter asked. Rosie said that she did not know but that perhaps they all could come up with a plan for how the book could be finished and published if Beth did not have enough time. Beth said that she had a colleague at another university with whom she was close and who could finish the book, if the colleague wanted to. They agreed to have another meeting in 2 days. At this meeting, Beth said to her husband and her children, "My body does not lie to me. I know I'm dying." Rosie then led them in thanking, forgiving, and expressing their love for each other.[20] After that meeting, Beth decided to end anticancer treatment and went home with hospice care. She died 5 days later.

When Beth's book came out in print a year later, Beth's husband sent it to Rosie at the hospital. Rosie found a picture tucked inside the jacket. It was of Beth in bed with her two huskies lying at her feet and her children next to her, each holding one of her hands. Rosie flipped to the first page and found an inscription: "You helped Beth live, even when she was dying."

Nurses may have encountered patients who have been dealt a heavy blow of a life-limiting diagnosis but who approach their diagnosis, and sometimes their physical pain, as the presence of wanted spiritual suffering. This is often true of people who believe in karma or in redemptive suffering. The contemporary psychologist Paul Bloom says that, for suffering to be wanted, suffering must have meaning.[5] That meaning is its object. However, unwanted suffering, as Beth's was, is objectless. There is no reason—no meaning—that justifies it. There is no point to it.

An object is external to language, to one's thinking, and hence, to one's mind. As such, the object is the referent. A referent is that to which one's words and thoughts point. It is essential that, when one talks (or thinks) about something, our words have referents—that they point to the object that gives words and thoughts meaning. However, when there is no object, there is nothing to point to outside us. One is then trapped in a wordless, meaningless world.

Suffering defies language. One can, of course, say that one suffers. This suffering can be because of pain, nausea and vomiting, grief, loss, separation, impending death, or compassion for others. But a cause is not a reason or a justification. Cancer, heart failure, end-stage kidney disease, sexual trauma, the wounds of war—these are causes. But they are not referents that supply the suffering with meaning.

Suffering, because it is inaccessible to language, leaves us groaning. It left Beth in the case exemplar making an utterance that did not make sense: she cursed a god in whom she did not believe. The Christian apostle Paul put this insight into the non-sensical utterances of suffering this way: "the spirit maketh intercessions for us with groanings which cannot be uttered" (Romans 8:26). Universally, groans and seemingly nonsensical utterances are attempts at supplying an object to—a referent for—unwanted, and hence objectless, suffering.

Objects connect us, as human subjects, to something outside us: to God, eternal life, wisdom, nature, loved ones, progeny, and so forth. Objectless suffering, on the contrary, creates an absolute split between one's reality and what would otherwise be the object if one's suffering could have an object. Objectless suffering alienates sufferers from God, from that which sufferers believe, from nature, from loved ones, from the future—even from sufferers' bodies. Objectless suffering creates a world in which sufferers suffer alone; sufferers find themselves in suffering-imposed solipsism. Their suffering is completely inaccessible to others. There is no object to which sufferers and others have the same access. Suffering alienates.

Suffering creates a split between sufferers and others. Sufferers have a complete grasp of their suffering, but others do not—cannot. Because of this inaccessibility, others may doubt sufferers. This is often the case when someone who by outward appearances has a good life but suffers from depression or anxiety, chronic fatigue or fibromyalgia, or migraine. What sufferers grasp—and hence easily know that they have—can be doubted and denied by others.

The importance of this insight about how suffering can be doubted by onlookers was made by a nurse-philosopher of the 20th and 21st centuries, Ruth McCorkle, who was also a symptom management researcher. Her experiences as an air force nurse during the Vietnam War led her to this insight.[6] In the planes that transported wounded and sometimes dying soldiers to hospitals, McCorkle witnessed soldiers' physical wounds, but their suffering, she said, was within. Even when they could talk, they groaned because they were in the solipsistic world of suffering, one she could not access but one she wanted to believe. She found that other health care providers often doubted soldiers' suffering. "It's not that bad of a wound. Why are you crying?" But she knew their crying was a wordless expression of suffering. Later, she worked with the psychiatrist Avery Weisman and psychologist William Worden who had, for patients diagnosed with cancer, given this wordless suffering a name: existential plight, a feeling of vulnerability, mood disturbance, and concerns about the future of one's existence.[7] When the face of death visits, one is trapped by its sight, as Prometheus was on the rock. Even if the face merely passes by, it causes suffering that defies language; it has no object. And others can easily deny that the sufferer has seen it.

Eric Cassel, in his foundational 1982 article in the *New England Journal of Medicine*, "The Nature of Suffering and the Goals of Medicine," defined suffering as "the state of severe distress associated with events that threaten the intactness of the person."[8] Suffering's objectlessness, its solipsism, and its alienation call into question the sufferer's personhood. It is not just that suffering resists language, but in so doing, it reverses sufferers to a prelingual state,[4] that is, to a stage in human development that is pre-sense, a stage in which we, as humans, do not create meaning, or at least cannot express meaning. As such, sufferers lose their ability to make sense of themselves and the world. This prelingual, pre-sense state is a state before personhood, a state in which sufferers cannot comprehend their existence. And in this state before personhood in which sufferers cannot comprehend their existence, sufferers lose the awareness that they are alive.

Others can respond to the prelingual groans of the sufferer who has lost awareness of aliveness with aversion—aversion not just at the crying soldier or the person who outwardly appears to have it all together but is depressed or anxious or in pain from no visible cause but also toward the person who is dying of a fungating breast tumor, for example. Even though the cause of her suffering is visible and the stench of the microbes infesting it smellable, it is not seeing and smelling the anatomical malady that elicits aversion as much as it is catching a glimpse and a whiff of the sufferer's loss of awareness of being alive. Humans naturally want to avert their gaze from death. After all, it is part of human nature to turn away from death—to flee from it—to preserve one's life. The objectlessness of death is abhorrent. Witnessing objectless suffering causes the observer to realize that death is the migrant bird that forgets to fly away.

To be human is to suffer: it is a fate all humans share. It involves the essence of being human. Suffering reverses sufferers to a wordless state of being. Wordlessness is meaninglessness. Suffering's meaninglessness, however, shows us the greatest source of suffering that is part and parcel of being human: death. In self-preservation, it is natural to avert one's gaze from death, for death ends human experience.

The Practice of Nursing

Nurses, however, cannot avert their gaze or turn away from sufferers. Nurses must be present, for presence, Ferrell and Coyle say, "is the essential task of nursing."[1]

Presence is not easy to define. There is no single nursing action that when complete can be checked off the to-do list as if to say, "I was present." Presence is not action per se. It is, rather, a state of being.[9] The origin of the English word "presence"—the Latin *praesentia*—suggests that it means to be at hand, to be there in the moment at the ready. Presence is, fundamentally, being in the presence *of* another person in a certain place at a certain time, not consumed with other tasks but rather *being*. "I am here," we say without words when we walk into the presence of someone who suffers. Being present—showing up—is the foundation of nursing presence, but there is more to it.

Presence includes an awareness of what we share with others. The contemporary feminist bioethicist Margaret Farley says that presence is "to find a location in human experience" where we "encounter the reality of ourselves and others."[10] When, as nurses, we are present to others who suffer, we encounter our common humanity. To be human, after all, is to be vulnerable to suffering. To be present to others who suffer is to overcome our urge to avert our gaze from them, in their prelingual, pre-sense state, a state in which they only have groans and writhing to express their suffering. When we show up to and do not avert our gaze from sufferers but rather are with them, we bring them out of their prelingual, pre-sense world—the world in which they are trapped, alone, without language—and usher them back into aliveness.

Nursing presence is being for the individual what the individual needs you to be for the individual to be alive.*

McCorkle understood the power of nursing presence. On one of the transport planes, a young, mortally wounded soldier, who was groaning from his wounds, asked McCorkle for his mother and his girlfriend. "Where are they?" he asked. He was terrified of not being alive and of the aloneness of his suffering. It was ostensibly a nonsensical question in that he was in a plane being transported from the battlefield in Southeast Asia to a hospital in Europe, and his family was in the United States. But his question arose from his suffering of being chained to the rock of death. McCorkle realized that he was terrified of his isolation. She held his hand and said, "I am here. I will not leave you." He died moments later. After this event and after her tour was complete, she returned to her studies and wrote a master's thesis on the effects of touch on the seriously ill.[11]

Touch, after all, is a bridge between living things when there are no words. Touch is the first step in giving words back to sufferers. Touch overcomes the aversion of death.

McCorkle went on to earn a PhD and afterward embarked on a career in palliative nursing, particularly of people diagnosed with life-limiting cancer. In the early 1970s she studied in the United Kingdom with Dame Cicely Saunders and the psychiatrist J. M. Hinton, who, in his 1963 article published in *QJM: An International Journal of Medicine*, pages 1–21, "The Physical and Mental Distress of the Dying,"[12] described a connection between dying patients' unrelieved physical distress and their mental distress. This relationship had been described only once before, by Sir William Osler in his Constable & Co., Ltd., 1906 book, *Science and Immortality*,[13] in which he described his observations of nearly 500 dying patients at Johns Hopkins University hospital and found a relationship between unrelieved physical distress and "mental apprehension." Following Osler and Hinton, McCorkle conducted a study in which she developed a scale that would, for the sufferer, name a physical symptom—its frequency, as it were—and the point at which the symptom became a burden the sufferer had to bear. She was interested in identifying the point at which untreated cancer-related symptoms pushed patients into the solipsistic wordless world of suffering. From this study came the McCorkle Symptom Distress Scale.[14] This scale, simple but profound in its truth, was the first of its kind by violating what was at the time considered to be psychometric protocol in which one did not mix the dimension of frequency (yes/no) with the dimension of a rating of (0 = Not at all distressing, 10 = Extremely distressing). Now, almost every symptom inventory uses such a mixed-dimension approach, for the approach gives the sufferer the chance to *name* the source and the burden of suffering. It ushers the sufferer out of the prelingual, pre-sense state of suffering and into the worded world of awareness of being alive.

Giving objectless suffering a name is not giving it a reason. There may never be a reason. And some people may not ever find meaning in their suffering, much less want to. But to say "This—this pain, these pins and needles I feel in my hands and feet, this nausea that I cannot shake—this is what is causing me not to feel like myself" is to give suffering a name. Naming the source of suffering, says Scarry, is to objectify it.[4] It is the case that by objectifying the referent of a person's physical suffering, that suffering becomes known to the one doing the assessment—the nurse. Now, both sufferer and nurse speak the same words; they both have the same object in view. The sufferer is no longer alone.

Of course, this object may be physical, but it may also be emotional, and it is always spiritual, in that it calls into question the intactness of the person. In the last article McCorkle wrote—which she wrote within a few weeks of her own death from an Agent Orange–related cancer[6]—she advocated for treating physical suffering first and then moving onto other sources of distress.[15] After all, as Ferrell and Coyle point out, physical "symptoms are experienced by *people*, not by bodily organs."[1] Just as it is difficult to concentrate when one feels physical distress, say, from hunger or tiredness, so too it is difficult to attend to spiritual distress when one is physically distressed.

The case exemplar illustrates this aspect of nursing presence. Rosie, the nurse, cared for Beth's physical distress first, which involved managing her physical symptoms; her emotional distress, which involved saying goodbye to her family; and finally her spiritual distress, which involved the helplessness and hopelessness of finishing her life's work, the book. By not averting her gaze from the suffering that tormented Beth, and then by assessing and addressing Beth's physical, emotional, and spiritual suffering, Rosie was for Beth what Beth needed Rosie to be to bring Beth back from suffering's reversion to a prelingual, pre-sense state to being aware of her aliveness, even as she was dying.

Nurses encounter suffering individuals when they are surrounded by other health care professionals, each treating a different aspect of the individual. In the complexity of our modern health care system, nurses provide "an intimate, personal encounter," Ferrell and Coyle say, an encounter in which the nurse becomes the "confidant, the vessel" of individuals' suffering "and the counselor for [their] spiritual distress."[1] The nurse touches the sufferer, assesses the sufferer, and then becomes the vessel of words that the sufferer no longer has. The nurse names, and thus objectifies, suffering. The nurse becomes life for sufferers who no longer have the strength within themselves for being alive.

This is the practice of nursing presence: it is overcoming aversion toward objectless suffering and being life for those whose suffering has caused them to question their very personhood.

The practice of nursing in response to suffering is not just for palliative care nurses. It is also for nurses who are the consciousness of aliveness for unhoused, hungry, and jobless individuals.[16] It is for environmental nursing, for the earth, which sustains all our lives, suffers from our destructive behaviors.[17] And it is for nurses themselves, who have provided care to unspeakable suffering during the SARS-CoV-2 pandemic.[18]

Being present to unspeakable suffering may cause nurses to suffer, in the same way that Prometheus's suffering was due to his sympathy for—his feeling with—the suffering of his fellow humans. Compassion is suffering with another. Nurses suffer. And it is for the nursing community to be present to each other in ways that only nurses can—that too is the practice of nursing.

Suffering is all around. "In every setting, across diseases, and in people of all ages," Ferrell and Coyle say, "suffering is part of being human." But they also say that being present to those who suffer—being life to those who need aliveness—"is the everyday work of nurses."[1]

Responses to Suffering

Unwanted suffering causes sufferers to regress to a prelingual state in which they lose senses of help and hope. Because of this prelingual state, sufferers cannot name the source of their suffering. Nurses can respond to this aspect of suffering with a thorough nursing assessment that allows sufferers to name their suffering's physical, emotional, and spiritual sources. This assessment brings sufferers out of the prelingual state and back into a state of words. The subsequent plan of care can restore sufferers' senses of help and hope. Because suffering always involves a challenge to sufferers' personhood, restoring senses of help and hope is restoring a sense of personhood. This is a spiritual response to suffering.

This spiritual response is the heart of nursing practice in the face of suffering. It is the response of touching the personhood of sufferers. By giving back words and senses of help and hope to sufferers, nurses connect sufferers with a sense of themselves, with connection to the human community, with nature, with that which they believe and that which they hold dear—from which suffering has alienated them. Connecting sufferers back to themselves is to connect them with being alive. This is nursing presence: to be for sufferers what they need to be alive.

Note

*   This sentence is a play on Virginia Henderson's definition of nursing as offered in her 1964 article "The Nature of Nursing," published in volume 64 of the *American Journal of Nursing*, pages 62–68.

References

1. Ferrell B, Coyle N. *The Nature of Suffering and the Goals of Nursing*. Oxford University Press; 2008.
2. Aeschylus, Scully J, Herington CJ. *Prometheus Bound*. Oxford University Press; 1975.
3. Wittgenstein L. *Tractatus Logico-Philosophicus*. Routledge & Kegan Paul; 1922:6.431.
4. Scarry E. *The Body in Pain: The Making and Unmaking of the World*. Oxford University Press; 1985.
5. Bloom P. *The Sweet Spot: The Pleasures of Suffering and the Search for Meaning*. ECCO, an imprint of HarperCollins Publishers; 2021.
6. Lazenby M. Assistance. In: Lazenby M. *Toward a Better World: The Social Significance of Nursing*. Oxford University Press; 2020:45–54.
7. Weisman AD, Worden JW. The existential plight in cancer: significance of the first 100 days. *Int J Psychiatry Med*. 1976;7(1):1–15. doi:10.2190/uq2g-ugv1-3ppc-6387
8. Cassel EJ. The nature of suffering and the goals of medicine. *N Engl J Med*. 1982;306(11):639–645. doi:10.1056/NEJM198203183061104
9. Lazenby M. Presence. In: Lazenby M. *Caring Matters Most: The Ethical Significance of Nursing*. Oxford University Press; 2017:65–69.
10. Farley M. *Compassionate Respect: A Feminist Approach to Medical Ethics and Other Questions*. Paulist Press; 2002.
11. McCorkle R. *The Effects of Touch on Seriously Ill Patients* [master's thesis]. College of Nursing in the Graduate School, University of Iowa; 1972.
12. McCorkle R, Young K. Development of a symptom distress scale. *Cancer Nurs*. 1978;1(5):373–378.
13. McCorkle R, Lazenby M. Adoption of universal psychosocial distress screening of cancer patients in low-resource settings is premature. *Cancer Nurs*. 2020;43(2):91–92. doi:10.1097/NCC.0000000000000658
14. Cavazos DM. Street nursing: teaching and improving community health [published online ahead of print, May 4, 2022]. *Hisp Health Care Int*. doi:10.1177/15404153221098958
15. Pollitt P, Sattler B, Butterfield PG, et al. Environmental nursing: leaders reflect on the 50th anniversary of Earth Day. *Public Health Nurs*. 2020;37(4):614–625. doi:10.1111/phn.12703
16. Hinton JM. The physical and menial distress of the dying. *QJM: An Intenational Journal of Medicine*. 1963;32(1):1–21.
17. Osler, W. *Science and Immortality*. A Constable & Complany Limited; 1906.
18. Dincer B, Inangil D. The effect of Emotional Freedom Techniques on nurses' stress, anxiety, and burnout levels during the COVID-19 pandemic: a randomized controlled trial. *Explore (NY)*. 2021;17(2):109–114. doi:10.1016/j.explore.2020.11.012
19. Crosby D, Stills S, Nash G, Young N. Our House. *Déjà Vu*. Atlantic; 1985.
20. Byock I. *The Four Things That Matter Most, 10th Anniversary Edition: A Book About Living*. Atria Books—Simon and Schuster; 2014.

2

Spiritual and Religious Perspectives About Suffering

Elizabeth Johnston Taylor

Spiritual and Religious Thinking About Suffering

Why? Why did this happen to me? Why now? Why do violence, pandemics, wars, disabling accidents, illness, and death happen? Why do humans suffer, especially when they have been good people? These "why?" questions are universal human questions that arise when tragedy or threat causes suffering. These questions may quickly lead to spiritual and religious (S/R) questions: Is there a Reality that ultimately influences or controls such suffering? Is this Reality evil or loving, or somehow both? If there is such a Reality, is it all-powerful, all-knowing, or always present to humans? If it exists, why does evil exist? Furthermore, is suffering somehow purposeful, prompting good outcomes?

Although these questions manifest in myriad ways, they are fundamentally spiritual and, sometimes, religious questions. That is, these questions reflect a search for meaning within a sacred context (spirituality), which may or may not involve religion (i.e., beliefs and practices that are formalized and experienced collectively to some extent).[1] Sometimes, S/R questions can be too deeply painful to express, or, for some, even too disturbing to consider. For example, maybe there isn't an all-powerful God. Or maybe Reality can no longer be experienced as loving. These beliefs could be too cognitively dissonant to recognize. Researchers have documented how experiencing such negative religious coping or S/R struggle does sometimes occur in response to difficult health-related contexts.[2–4] This S/R struggle can also be compounded when a person becomes aware that existent S/R beliefs are no longer comforting or believable. Thus, it is unsurprising that the S/R struggle is associated with poor mental health outcomes, such as depression.[5–8]

Conversely, however, persons experiencing suffering may also ask: Why not me? They may find that their S/R beliefs and practices provide a means for making sense of the suffering and for finding psychological comfort.[1] Their S/R beliefs contribute to a cognitive schema that affirms they are worthy, that their world is meaningful, and that the world is basically a good and safe place to exist. That is, their S/R provides the matrix for a healthful, functional worldview.[9] Indeed, Soenke and colleagues understood how religions, across time and cultures, provide humans with a "sacred armor" to buffer them from anxieties, including death anxiety.[10]

Whether S/R beliefs about suffering create inner struggle and discomfort or provide hope and comfort, they inherently provide a lens through which sufferers may

Elizabeth Johnston Taylor, *Spiritual and Religious Perspectives About Suffering* In: *The Nature of Suffering and the Goals of Nursing.* Second Edition. Edited by: William E. Rosa and Betty R. Ferrell, Oxford University Press. © Oxford University Press 2023. DOI: 10.1093/oso/9780197667934.003.0002 interpret their challenge. Given how S/R beliefs about suffering are integral to a response to illness, it is important for nurses to appreciate this dynamic and have some basic understanding about the diverse S/R beliefs related to suffering. Thus, this chapter will provide an overview of S/R beliefs related to suffering, especially focusing on the theological construct of theodicy. First, however, a model explaining the psychospiritual process guiding S/R thinking in response to suffering is reviewed. Given the process and outcomes presented, clinical implications for health care professionals are offered. This overview is influenced considerably by Western psychological and theological perspectives, which in turn are often influenced by Judeo-Christian worldviews. The struggles and benefits of ascribing S/R beliefs to suffering are illustrated by Susan, a nurse who has experienced physical, emotional, social, and spiritual suffering (see Case Exemplar 2.1).

Case Exemplar 2.1

Susan is a 64-year-old woman who lives with her faithful dog; her daughter and her daughter's partner live in a back house. Although she was raised nominally Christian and attended a Roman Catholic high school, Susan converted to Judaism in her 20s. She now participates daily in a Benedictine fellowship and attends a liberal Episcopal church weekly. As a "hyphenated" religious person, she participates in weekly Jewish and Christian worship services and meetings.

Susan cannot remember a time when she did not suffer with physical illness. Although she does not know how her mother's suspected Munchausen syndrome may contribute, she does know that her medical history is rich with multiple diagnoses. She presently lives with steroid-dependent asthma, immunodeficiency, severe rheumatoid arthritis and osteoarthritis (with resulting joint deformities), fibromyalgia, chronic pain, myopathy, hair loss, and dermatitis with prurigo nodules that itch and bleed. Thus, she lives with people saying things like "Your face is bigger than last time" and "Did you know you have a sore on your head?"

Susan's daily routine includes taking medications thrice a day, nebulizer treatments 3–4 times daily, physical therapy, cooking prepackaged meals, attending online meetings, and writing nursing education materials for her work. She also is seeing about 15 physicians and periodically goes to a health care facility for various tests or treatments. "I spend most of my life just trying to stay alive," Susan notes.

Given this context and its inherent losses (e.g., various physical functions, social roles, body image), Susan often finds herself asking, "Who am I?" Living with morbidities prompts her to also face her mortality. For example, she just completed a course on "ending well." Although death is not immanent, the course raised questions for her as to what religious tradition she wanted to die as.

Susan's religiosity has supported her to struggle with how to make sense of her suffering and transcend it. To quote Susan: "Going to church gives me strength and comfort. Connecting to people in my meetings also gives me support. Singing hymns and doing nature photography allows me to expand my world.... These activities keep me sane; they allow me to get to a bigger place—a place beyond my small world." Susan found comfort when her rabbi normalized her spiritual struggle and said it was "okay to kvetch with God." Books with prayers specifically for those with pain and loss have also been helpful to Susan.

How does Susan theologize about her suffering? "Some days I do it better than others.... Shit happens and keeps happening. I ask God if she has a plan; she's extremely quiet about it!

... When I was in high school, a well-meaning nun told me, 'God must really love you to give you so many crosses to bear.' Well, maybe God could start hating me?! ... Some would say suffering is to bring us closer to the suffering of Jesus; but no, it's not doing that for me. Now I think that God doesn't cause my suffering. God is with us cripples. She is a source of strength. She has work for me to do; in fact, I have a wordless knowing that I need to be doing the work I'm doing.... I have purpose."

When Suffering Challenges Spiritual/Religious Beliefs: The Process

One's social environment, including family (especially parents or parent figures), community, culture, and religion, heavily shapes a person's S/R beliefs.[11] But how does suffering impact these beliefs? Psychologist Crystal Park provides a theory about meaning making in response to trauma that is particularly relevant.[12] Park built on the notion of other psychologists who posit that everyone has a cognitive schema, or global meanings (i.e., beliefs and goals). People also instinctively assign meanings to traumatic situations; these traumas are explained by natural or by supernatural causes. For example, a person might explain cancer as being caused by pollution (a more proximal ascription) or by sin and other religious explanations (more distal ascriptions). When trauma occurs, if the situational meaning ascribed to a trauma is compatible with the global meanings held, no distress occurs. If, however, there is a discrepancy, there is a need to align the global and situational meanings. It is the misalignment of global and situational meanings that causes distress and the need to reconstruct satisfactory meaning.[12]

The process of reconstructing meaning involves managing intrusive rumination (inner dialogue) to reappraise the situation or reconstruct global meanings.[12] For example, if a pious patient prior to a cancer diagnosis believed that such a disease occurred only in persons who lived iniquitously, this patient would need to either change his ascribed meanings for the situation (e.g., to "genetics caused my cancer") or change his global meanings (e.g., "cancer can occur in anyone"). If the patient did not revise his cognitive schema, he might accept that he must be vile, which presumably would also cause inner distress. A team of Polish researchers examined how various types of inner dialogue mediated between S/R struggle and psychological well-being (PWB) among 143 Catholic undergraduate students. Ruminative inner dialogue was found to contribute to decreased PWB, whereas imagined supportive inner dialogue was linked with increased PWB.[13] Thus, examining the nature of one's inner dialogue may be therapeutic.

The successful reconstruction of meaning can be manifest not only in revised global or situational meanings but also in changed identities and perceptions of personal growth.[12,14] For example, cancer and trauma survivors often report renewed appreciation for their inner strength, increased spiritual awareness or faith and closeness to God, or heightened desire to help others.[15-17] S/R beliefs are integral to this process of posttraumatic growth. Typically, healthful S/R beliefs provide helpful situational meanings and contribute to such growth. Thus, illness can be a pivot point, an invitation to spiritual growth and inner transformation.[16]

To test Park's theory, Hall and colleagues interviewed 29 evangelical Christian patients about how they made meaning in response to a cancer diagnosis.[7] Using qualitative methods, they documented that one-third did experience distress because of a misalignment of global and situational meanings. The distress manifested in doubting God's justice, love, and existence, as well as in dismay from "unanswered" prayers. These doubts and questions about God were resolved with spiritual surrender, which included accepting that God is in control, having humility, and giving up the notion of a just world. Those who did not experience this distress appeared to be protected by an existent spiritual humility and confidence in God.[7]

In summary, Park's theory and the ensuing validating empirical evidence suggest that when situational and global meanings do not align, distress occurs. This suffering often necessitates reevaluation and reconstruction of S/R beliefs. Case exemplar Susan provides insight about this process of struggling to have satisfying global meaning. It appears that the global meanings provided to her during childhood and high school were unsatisfactory to her, prompting her journey to Judaism—a religion that respects struggling with God. As her illnesses have progressed and new losses occur, her question of "Who am I?" (or, "What goals can I pursue?" "What still identifies who I am?" "What is the meaning of my life?") reoccurs. Previous global meanings periodically are threatened by new situations. She (re)constructs global meaning by engaging with a plethora of S/R resources (e.g., prayer books, talking with clergy, joining a Benedictine fellowship, attending Christian and Jewish services weekly). This process supports her to search for satisfying S/R beliefs about suffering.

Spiritual/Religious Beliefs About Suffering

Humans need meaning systems, especially when they are suffering; S/R beliefs may provide these.[10] Thus, it is no surprise that 77% of over 35,000 US Americans surveyed in 2014 reported religion as *somewhat* or *very important in life*.[18] Over the past few decades, however, the number of those who do not affiliate with an organized religion has increased; presently, the US population is composed of 29% of these "Nones"— some of whom are "Dones" (i.e., done with institutionalized religion).[19] Nones, however, may self-report as spiritual. Indeed, 27% of American surveyed in 2017 acknowledged being *spiritual but not religious.* Only 18% in this same study identified as *neither religious nor spiritual.*[20] Regardless of whether an institutionalized religion functions as the "cultural arbiter of belief" for Nones, they still experience struggles of an S/R nature.[21,22]

What S/R beliefs do people ascribe to suffering? Because suffering is prevalent and human thought is diverse, it is natural that a variety of S/R beliefs about suffering exist. Often these beliefs are referred to as *theodicies*, or justifications for why an all-powerful (omnipotent) and all-knowing (omniscient) ultimate Other (typically, labeled as God) coexists with evil or whatever causes suffering.[23–25] Next, these theodicies and counterarguments for them are summarized. Given the centrality of God in theodical beliefs, it is beneficial to first consider some aspects of human thinking about God.

God

Although the certainty and nature of belief about God varied, 89% of Americans in the 2014 Pew survey believed in God.[18] Theories about how individuals come to know God—or understand their "God-image"—vary. The language of God-image connotes how humans know God as who they project God to be, by being the "image of God" and looking into the mirror.[11,26] For example, Jungian thinking (albeit oversimplified) suggests that as a person journeys toward individuation (a process of unraveling of the persona and ego-centeredness), they gain awareness of the individualized Self (an awareness of God within) and collective Self (the transpersonal core shared by all of humanity).[26] Hall and Fujikawa reviewed contemporary psychological literature about how people develop a God-image.[11] Regardless of whether considering Freudian, object relations, or attachment theories, the relationship one has with a parent figure is transferred to God. Thus, unless an idealized parent is substituted, one's perception of God will have parallels to one's perception of parents. In addition to the quality of one's early attachments, psychological needs, personality, culture, and contextual factors influence how one perceives and experiences God.[11]

The nature of God is examined in theodicies that wrestle not only with whether God is omnipotent and omniscient but also with whether God is impassible. That is, does the essence of God allow God to have feelings like humans? Some who suffer and accept that God is loving may wonder if God loves them specifically. Kopel et al. review various theological assertions in this regard and discuss how a nurse's interpretation will influence their response to a patient's suffering.[27] Process theologians argue that while God accompanies us in our suffering, God cannot impose power. Yet this raises the question, if God does not exert power to prevent evil, then is God responsible for it? Open and classical theists accept that God does experience emotion but vary in how they interpret this. Open theists emphasize the relationality of God—a passible and omnipotent God; classical theists recognize the limitations of human anthropomorphizing of God.[27]

Theodicies also raise the question of whether God, assumed to be loving, allows humans to have free will.[23,24,28,29] Does God indeed have the power to affect whether good or evil occurs? Or does love, by its inherent nature, preclude God from manipulating or controlling circumstances that cause suffering? Process theologians accept that God is neither omniscient nor omnipotent. Indeed, Macallan wrote, "no worse falsehood was ever perpetuated than that of the doctrine of omnipotence."[29(p40)] Others, however, view God as manifesting great love while restraining manipulative power. Of note here is a study of nearly 3,000 undergraduates that documented that a loving conceptualization of God was positively related to benevolent theodicies.[24] Thus, how one views God is central to how one ascribes global meanings or theodicies.

In addition to how one perceives God, it is helpful to observe how a person believes they are to relate to God when addressing a problem such as suffering. Phillips and colleagues proposed a descriptive theory for how humans relate to God during the process of religious coping.[30] They conjectured that a person could collaborate with God to cope (i.e., problem-solve in the context of relationship with God), self-direct their coping (i.e., problem-solve assuming God grants freedom to do so), or defer (i.e., abdicate control and completely give the problem-solving to God). Because the self-directing approach to coping proved conceptually unclear, further research revised the scale measuring it. Phillips et al. found that self-directed religious coping entailed two ways of viewing God: God as abandoning and God as supportive but nonintervening.[30] Considerable evidence of negative religious coping (e.g., God as abandoning, nonintervening, punishing) finds it consistently associated with maladaption.[3,5,6,30,31] Thus, both the conception of God and the conception of the nature of the God-human relationship are worth considering while caring for someone who suffers.

Theodicies

Several theodicies have been offered by theologians and philosophers over the past few centuries. Theodicies have been categorized in various ways, although the arguments behind them can overlap.[23,25,28,29] For this chapter, the following categorization is offered.

- *Punishment and warning theodicies* include thinking that bad things happen because humans have sinned or an individual has been bad; thus, they deserve consequences. It is assumed that there is a cause-and-effect relationship existing between sin and its consequences (e.g., if one does not obey God's laws of health, sickness can result). These theodicies include believing that evil is caused by an enemy, a dark force, or the demonic.
- The *free will defense theodicy* reasons that God created humans to have free will—to respond to and obey God's love and laws; God forcing obedience would be unloving and incongruent with God's nature.
- The *unreality of evil theodicies* posit that evil is an illusion; when seen from a larger, or divine, perspective, it has a different character or is insufficient to account for suffering. Another similar theodicy asserts that evil is a privation, a distortion of something intrinsically good (e.g., sickness is privation of health).
- The *evil is logically necessary theodicy* suggests that evil is necessary to demonstrate goodness (e.g., if everything were blue, we would not have color as a concept).

- *Teleological theodicies* propose that evil will be outweighed by good—ultimately. In the future, there will be harmony and perspective that provides meaning for current temporal sufferings (e.g., "When we get to Heaven, we'll see how all things worked together for good"). Another teleological theodicy proposes that evil brings out the moral, good qualities of humans; to gain these prized qualities, God created (or allowed) a world with evil. Thus, evil begets development of virtue, character, and spiritual growth—"soul making." Such theodicies likely assume that God is in complete control and there is some ultimate purpose of which we presently do not understand.
- The *God's power is limited theodicy*, espoused by process theologians, argues that God is finite and cannot be as omnipotent or omniscient as humans have often ascribed. This theodicy explains that God cannot control everything.
- The *no better world can exist theodicy* is the justification that Leibnitz, the originator of theodical discourse, proposed in the early 1700s. That is, evil does exist and God is good and omnipotent, but God had to choose the best option available.

Of course, theodicies cannot be proven. They are conjectures that ultimately cannot be refuted.[32] The humility that should result from this recognition will help nurses to approach their own and patients' theodicies with sensitivity.

Theodicies, nevertheless, prompt debates. Anti-theodicists argue that all theodicies are morally reprehensible. For example, how can a good God be portrayed as creating an "obstacle course" for soul making, when such a God seems sadistic? Or why does God need to be weakened by suggesting God is not omnipotent or omniscient to make God look still loving?[25] Franklin suggested that Leibnitz's "no better world can exist" theodicy is the only moral proposition. He concluded that "God and we are allies against suffering. Our suffering has meaning through its essential role in avoiding worse outcomes."[25(p575)] Thus, anti-theodicists remind that most theodicies can be refuted intellectually. Indeed, God cannot be objectively defended.[32]

Other theologians recognize the limitations of theodicies and stretch the discourse to accept that suffering is an invitation to delve more deeply into relationship—either with God or with others. After reviewing the existential theodicy of Kierkegaard, Slowikowski concluded that the goal of any theological excursion around suffering is to reconcile oneself to a good God, to seek the ultimate answers and meaning through faith, hope, and love.[32] Similarly, Sollereder accepts existing limitations of theodicies and argues for a compassionating theodicy where persons strive to oppose the corrosive effects of evil.[23] She believes theodicists are to recognize the sufferer as the expert theodicist and allow for lament, forgiveness, hospitality, and compassion in the presence of suffering.

It is helpful to have a cursory knowledge of the theological views about suffering from the perspective of various religious traditions. Box 2.1 synthesizes the religious interpretations of suffering written by theologians belonging to each tradition.[1] It should be expected, however, that persons even within the same culture or religion can hold differing theodicies. To illustrate, a study of chaplains (N = 298) from across the US validated that even these mostly Christian spiritual care experts' theodicies varied.[33] Indeed, case exemplar Susan illustrates with her pluralistic belief system how

Box 2.1 Selected World Religious Beliefs About Suffering: An Essentialized and Dangerously Simplified Overview

- **Atheist:** No supernatural force influences why events occur; science is relied upon for medical and psychological amelioration of suffering.
- **Buddhist:** Suffering occurs when humans project their desires outwardly, thinking that the world can fulfill these desires and make them happy. To escape suffering, one must understand the impermanence of earthly things, not identify self with these and seek them. Nurturing loving-kindness, ethical behavior, and equanimity can decrease suffering.
- **Christian**
  - **Baptist:** Whereas some will not link suffering to sin, others will. Some believe if they pray for a miracle, God will grant it.
  - **Christian Science:** Given the mind-body connection, negative thoughts and emotions cause suffering; spiritual-mindedness will bring healing.
  - **Jehovah's Witness:** Suffering results from individual and collective human sinfulness (i.e., disobeying God's laws and following Satan). Suffering can also occur because of being in the wrong place at the wrong time.
  - **Latter-day Saints:** Suffering is explained by nature and free will (individual or collective choices). We live in a "fallen world" and sickness and death are part of God's plan. However, God uses suffering to aid spiritual growth. Suffering allows preparation for eternal life.
  - **Orthodox Christians:** Whereas disease is explained scientifically, suffering is explained by a mind-body-spirit imbalance. Suffering will always bring about good, and this brings comfort.
  - **Pentecostalism:** Explanations for disease can include human sinfulness in a fallen world and divine punishment. Some believe that if they are right with God, there should be no suffering (because Jesus took human suffering upon himself); others believe that suffering indicates God's chastening them.
  - **Roman Catholic:** God does not will suffering but is present in it. Suffering was given value and meaning by Jesus's crucifixion.
- **Hindu:** Causes of suffering include negative mental state, imbalance of body elements, wrongful actions, evil "eye," and karma (bad actions committed in a previous life now affect one's current incarnation). Thus, suffering is a way to void past bad karma. Suffering also allows one to develop virtues.
- **Jewish:** Illness can occur because of lifestyle, genetics, and other reasons science explains. The duty of the Jew is to alleviate suffering. Suffering allows people to gain wisdom and communities to rally to provide care.
- **Modern Pagan:** Modern pagans generally reject teleological theodicy; some may accept karmic thinking. Suffering just happens, but the gods can provide support to cope.
- **Muslim:** Scientific explanations are accepted, as are beliefs that suffering allows one to worship God more and prepare them for Heaven. It can be a trial sent by God. If religious proscriptions observed do not remove the suffering, the suffering is accepted as God's will (i.e., "*in sha Allah*").
- **Sikh:** Suffering is inevitable in life, like a robe to wear. Spiritual causes include bad karma, forgetting God, and a mind-body-spirit imbalance. Suffering can be a means to strengthen their spiritual well-being.

Synthesized from Taylor EJ. *Religion: A Clinical Guide for Nurses.* Springer; 2012.

she as a Jew and Christian possesses global meanings that are presumably distinct from those of most observant Jews and Christians belonging to a single denomination. Unlike many Christians, Susan rejects that suffering is to bring us closer to the suffering of Jesus; unlike some Christians, Susan accepts that it is okay to kvetch with God. Like most theists, Susan finds comfort in her S/R beliefs.[24] Susan exemplifies the variation in S/R beliefs about suffering among humans.

Clinical Implications for Nurses

Some might assume that patients' deeply inward thoughts about the meaning of suffering are irrelevant to health care and that nurses have no business addressing them. After all, S/R perspectives are often private and invisible. Furthermore, if the topic were approached, might it unravel a garment that until now provided some protection and comfort? Are nurses capable of entering this "holy ground" without causing harm? Several arguments could deter consideration of a patient's S/R thinking about suffering. However, because there is so much evidence linking healthful S/R perspectives with adaptation, supporting it adds another "therapeutic" to nurses' capabilities.

Mounting empirical evidence also documents that S/R struggle (or negative religious coping) is associated with poor physical and psychological health outcomes for those who are physically well or ill, young or old.[4,8,34–36] For example, Ironson et al. found HIV disease progression slower among patients with a benevolent view of God compared with those who viewed God negatively (e.g., as punishing).[37] Pargament et al.'s findings from a longitudinal study of 596 older adults indicated that negative religious coping predicted increased mortality risk.[36] Tobin and Slatcher's analysis of religiosity and cortisol levels among 1,470 adults over 10 years led them to conclude that S/R struggle is a mechanism through which religiosity impacts health.[38] Several research teams have documented an association between S/R struggle and psychological distress (e.g., depression, anxiety, less life satisfaction).[5,6,34,35] Cowden et al. observed in a longitudinal study of persons with chronic illness (N = 302) that S/R struggle caused psychological distress and vice versa.[6] Thus, it behooves nurses to consider how a patient's global meanings—a psychospiritual rudder—steer the ship of health.

Based on their findings about the impact of S/R struggle, many of the researchers cited in the previous paragraph conclude that nurses ought to conduct an S/R screening. Indeed, while S/R struggle may be lower in some contexts (e.g., 30% among adolescents receiving a stem cell transplant[4]), it has been observed to be very high in some hospitalization contexts (e.g., 89% of adolescents admitted to a psychiatric unit[8]). This evidence supports screening for S/R distress. Box 2.2 offers selected questions (selected from or inspired by several sources[39–41]) for screening for S/R distress that can be used by any nurse. These questions may be appropriate at the time of admission or when a nurse is becoming acquainted with a patient who has a challenging situation. The assessment questions in Box 2.2 are more deeply probing questions when circumstances merit them and when the nurse is competent to ask them.

Box 2.2 Questions for Screening and Assessment of Spiritual/ Religious Beliefs About Suffering

---

For screening for spiritual distress:

- Do you struggle with the loss of meaning and joy in your life?
- Do you currently have what you would describe as religious or spiritual struggles?
- Are you at peace?
- Do you have any spiritual/religious concerns?
- Does your faith/beliefs provide you with all the strength and comfort that you need now?
- Is there a pain deep in your soul/being that is not physical?
- How are you … [dropping and softening the voice] inside?
- To what extent do you find life meaningful now, even amid the struggling/pain?

For further assessment:

- What purpose or meanings do you give to [the circumstance/s that caused suffering]?
- What are your beliefs about suffering? For example, what do you think might cause it?
- How are these beliefs helpful? Are any harmful?
- How did you learn these beliefs? (Follow-up questions could include: How did you learn this from your parents? From your community? From others you know who've suffered much?)
- (If belief in a divinity is expressed) How has the suffering affected the way you believe about and relate to God? (Substitute the patient's language for "God.") How do these beliefs affect the way you live with suffering?

Because S/R beliefs about suffering are so intimate, sacred, and potentially difficult to think and speak about, it is imperative that the nurse who broaches the topic have more than a beginner's level of competence. Indeed, harm could be done by a novice nurse who opens this "can of worms" and then leaves it exposed and unprotected. For instance, a nurse might avoid the S/R pain expressed using defense mechanisms (e.g., minimizing the patient's S/R pain or arguing with their thinking). This novice nurse might also approach the topic for hegemonic reasons or personal curiosity, rather than for a health-related reason. They might also insensitively impose the topic, without seeking some form of rapport and permission.[1,42] In contrast, respectful nurses who provide spiritually sensitive care improve patient satisfaction and well-being.[43]

When a nurse screens that S/R struggle exists and understands it to be impacting health, the following suggestions are offered so that the ensuing conversation can promote healing:

- Remember that revealing an S/R struggle is likely an incredibly difficult topic for a patient. It is challenging to admit such to oneself, never mind someone else. There is no need to problematize it, as it may even be a calling.[41] Thus, an attitude and posture of honoring the patient with an S/R struggle is paramount. Indeed, by modeling acceptance and compassion, the nurses can increase a patient's

self-acceptance and self-compassion. If God is known in relationship, such a therapeutic relationship will also allow a patient to experience God.
- While listening, note the patient's use of language.[42] Do they use "God" or some other term for the divine? (Notice how Susan used female pronouns for God.) What do they call their S/R struggle? Indeed, "struggle," "challenge," and "inner journey" are likely more comfortable terms than "negative coping," "spiritual distress," "existential crisis," and so forth. Of course, avoid theological jargon.[23,42]
- Use therapeutic communication skills. Remember to be nonjudgmental.[42] While it is easy to appreciate that giving negative responses to expressions of S/R struggle is harmful (e.g., "You really believe that?"), the nurse must also remember that praising the patient for their expressions of religiosity also is being judgmental and could prevent the patient from further authentic self-disclosure. For example, if a patient states, "I pray a lot" and the nurse responds, "Oh, that's so good!," the patient learns the nurse may not welcome an admission that praying is painful, as it brings to awareness doubt as to whether God is present. (A therapeutic response might be: "How is that for you?" or "What does prayer mean to you now as you live with this situation?" or "I'm guessing that maybe you pray more frequently now.")[41,42]

Allowing a person amid suffering to explore their inner S/R beliefs will allow them to gain insight, reflect, and self-correct if they find their beliefs unhelpful (i.e., their global and situational meanings misaligned). The nurse's role is to support and be a companion, not to fix or impose "right" beliefs.

Because most nurses are not spiritual care experts and because patients who are suffering and in S/R distress can benefit from expert spiritual care, a referral will likely be helpful. A referral to a board-certified chaplain is ideal if the resources are available, given lesser-trained chaplains (often volunteers) do not have the skills to address intense S/R struggle. Given that psychologists, psychiatrists, social workers, and other mental health therapists typically now are trained to respect patients' S/R needs, a referral to a mental health professional for S/R struggle may also be beneficial. Community clergy receive varying amounts of training in pastoral counseling and thus may or may not be skilled to address such inner pain. Spiritual directors, even laypersons trained in providing spiritual direction, will often have the spiritual and emotional stamina to bear witness to another's S/R struggle (see https://www.sdicompanions.org/find-a-spiritual-director-companion/). Thus, there are many resources with S/R expertise within and outside of the health care system; discussing options with a patient can encourage them to seek a spiritual care expert.

Conclusion

This chapter discussed S/R perspectives among persons who experience suffering. Many people who suffer find that their S/R beliefs provide comfort, guidance, hope, and meaning. For some, however, the meanings they have for the situation causing suffering do not align with their existing S/R beliefs; this then causes another layer of suffering, S/R struggle. While many learn that suffering produces increased spiritual awareness and growth (aspects of posttraumatic growth), the process of S/R struggle is distressing and associated with poor health outcomes. Thus, to fully understand a patient's experience of suffering, the nurse must seek to understand the S/R meanings ascribed and how these influence the patient's response to suffering. Implementing the clinical suggestions provided can help nurses to both support existing spiritual well-being and ameliorate S/R struggle.

References

1. Taylor EJ. *Religion: A Clinical Guide for Nurses*. Springer; 2012.
2. Gall TL, Bilodeau C. The role of positive and negative religious/spiritual coping in women's adjustment to breast cancer: a longitudinal study. *J Psychosoc Oncol*. 2020;38(1):103–117. doi:10.1080/07347332.2019.1641581
3. Pargament KI, Ano GG. Spiritual resources and struggles in coping with medical illness. *South Med J*. 2006;99(10):1161–1162. doi:10.1097/01.smj.0000242847.40214.b6
4. King SDW, Fitchett G, Murphy PE, et al. Religious/spiritual struggle in young adult hematopoietic cell transplant survivors. *J Adolesc Young Adult Oncol*. 2018;7(2):210–216. doi:10.1089/jayao.2017.0069
5. Ai AL, Carretta H. Depression in patients with heart diseases: gender differences and association of comorbidities, optimism, and spiritual struggle. *Int J Behav Med*. 2021;28(3):382–392. doi:10.1007/s12529-020-09915-3
6. Cowden RG, Pargament KI, Chen ZJ, et al. Religious/spiritual struggles and psychological distress: a test of three models in a longitudinal study of adults with chronic health conditions. *J Clin Psychol*. 2022;78(4):544–558. doi:10.1002/jclp.23232
7. Hall MEL, Shannonhouse L, Aten JD, McMartin J, Silverman E. Theodicy or not?: Spiritual struggles of evangelical cancer survivors. *J Psychol Theol*. 2019;47(4):259–277. doi:10.1177/0091647118807187
8. Leavitt-Alcántara S, Betz J, Medeiros Almeida D, et al. Religiosity and religious and spiritual struggle and their association to depression and anxiety among adolescents admitted to inpatient psychiatric units. *J Health Care Chaplain*. 2023;29(1):1–13. doi:10.1080/08854726.2022.2040227
9. Janoff-Bulman R. *Shattered Assumptions: Towards a New Psychology of Trauma*. Free Press; 2010.
10. Soenke M, Landau MJ, Greenberg J. Sacred armor: religion's role as a buffer against the anxieties of life and the fear of death. In: Pargament KI, Exline JJ, Jones JW, eds. *APA Handbook of Psychology, Religion, and Spirituality (Vol. 1): Context, Theory, and Research*. American Psychological Association; 2013:105–122.
11. Hall TW, Fujikawa AM. God-image and the sacred. In: Pargament KI, Exline JJ, Jones JW, eds. *APA Handbook of Psychology, Religion, and Spirituality (Vol. 1): Context, Theory, and Research*. American Psychological Association; 2013:277–292.
12. Park CL. Meaning making in the context of disasters. *J Clin Psychol*. 2016;72(12):1234–1246. doi:10.1002/jclp.22270
13. Zarzycka B, Puchalska-Wasyl MM. Can religious and spiritual struggle enhance well-being?: exploring the mediating effects of internal dialogues. *J Relig Health*. 2020;59(4):1897–1912. doi:10.1007/s10943-018-00755-w

14. Hart AC, Pargament KI, Grubbs JB, Exline JJ, Wilt JA. Predictors of self-reported growth following religious and spiritual struggles: exploring the role of wholeness. *Religions*. 2020;11(9):1–21. doi:10.3390/rel11090445

15. Kaur N, Porter B, LeardMann CA, Tobin LE, Lemus H, Luxton DD. Evaluation of a modified version of the Posttraumatic Growth Inventory-Short Form. *BMC Med Res Methodol*. 2017;17(1):69. doi:10.1186/s12874-017-0344-2

16. Balboni TA, Balboni MJ. The spiritual event of serious illness. *J Pain Symptom Manage*. 2018;56(5):816–822. doi:10.1016/j.jpainsymman.2018.05.018

17. Casellas-Grau A, Ochoa C, Ruini C. Psychological and clinical correlates of posttraumatic growth in cancer: a systematic and critical review. *Psychooncology*. 2017. doi:10.1002/pon.4426

18. Religious Landscape Study. Pew Research Center. Accessed April 17, 2022. https://www.pewresearch.org/religion/religious-landscape-study/

19. Smith G. About three-in-ten U.S. adults are now religiously unaffiliated. Pew Research Center. Published December 14, 2021. Accessed April 17, 2022. https://www.pewresearch.org/religion/2021/12/14/about-three-in-ten-u-s-adults-are-now-religiously-unaffiliated/

20. Lipka M, Gecewicz C. More Americans now say they're spiritual but not religious. Pew Research Center. Published September 6, 2017. Accessed April 17, 2022. https://www.pewresearch.org/fact-tank/2017/09/06/more-americans-now-say-theyre-spiritual-but-not-religious/

21. Mercadante LA. Spiritual struggles of nones and "spiritual but not religious" (SBNRs). *Religions*. 2020;11(10):1–16. doi:10.3390/rel11100513

22. van der Tempel J, Moodley R. Spontaneous mystical experience among atheists: meaning-making, psychological distress, and wellbeing. *Ment Health Relig Cult*. 2020;23(9):789–805. doi:10.1080/13674676.2020.1823349

23. Sollereder BN. Compassionate theodicy: a suggested truce between intellectual and practical theodicy. *Mod Theol*. 2021;37(2):382–395. doi:10.1111/moth.12688

24. Wilt JA, Exline JJ, Lindberg MJ, Park CL, Pargament KI. Theological beliefs about suffering and interactions with the divine. *Psycholog Relig Spiritual*. 2017;9(2):137–147. doi:10.1037/rel0000067

25. Franklin J. Antitheodicy and the grading of theodicies by moral offensiveness. *Sophia*. 2020;59(3):563–576. doi:10.1007/s11841-020-00765-w

26. Edinger EF. *The New God-Image: A Study of Jung's Key Letters Concerning the Evolution of the Western God-Image*. Chiron; 2015.

27. Kopel J, Babb FC, Hasker W, et al. Suffering and divine impassibility. *Proc (Bayl Univ Med Cent)*. 2022;35(1):139–141. doi:10.1080/08998280.2021.1981674

28. Rice R. *Suffering and the Search for Meaning: Contemporary Responses to the Problem of Pain*. InterVarsity Press; 2014.

29. Macallan BC. Getting off the omnibus: rejecting free will and soul-making responses to the problem of evil. *Open Theol*. 2020;6:35–42. doi:10.1515/opth-2020-0005

30. Phillips III RE, Lynn QK, Crossley CD, Pargament KI. Self-directing religious coping: a deistic god, abandoning god, or no god at all? *J Sci Study Relig*. 2004;43(3):409–418. doi:10.1111/j.1468-5906.2004.00243.x

31. Appel JE, Park CL, Wortmann JH, Schie HTV. Meaning violations, religious/spiritual struggles, and meaning in life in the face of stressful life events. *Int J Psychol Relig*. 2020;30(1):1–17. doi:10.1080/10508619.2019.1611127

32. Slowikowski A. Existential theodicy as a response to the limits of classic theodicy on the basis of Kierkegaard's religious writings. *Int J Syst Theol*. 2022;24(2):212–236. doi:10.1111/ijst.12554

33. Currier JM, Drescher KD, Nieuwsma JA, McCormick WH. Theodicies and professional quality of life in a nationally representative sample of chaplains in the veterans' health administration. *J Prevent Intervent Community*. 2017;45(4):286–296. doi:10.1080/10852352.2016.1197748

34. King SD, Fitchett G, Murphy PE, et al. Spiritual or religious struggle in hematopoietic cell transplant survivors. *Psychooncology*. 2017;26(2):270–277. doi:10.1002/pon.4029

35. Zarzycka B, Zietek P. Spiritual growth or decline and meaning-making as mediators of anxiety and satisfaction with life during religious struggle. *J Relig Health*. 2019;58(4):1072–1086. doi:10.1007/s10943-018-0598-y

36. Pargament KI, Koenig HG, Tarakeshwar N, Hahn J. Religious coping methods as predictors of psychological, physical and spiritual outcomes among medically ill elderly patients: a two-year longitudinal study. *J Health Psychol*. 2004;9(6):713–730. doi:10.1177/1359105304045366

37. Ironson G, Kremer H, Lucette A. Relationship between spiritual coping and survival in patients with HIV. *J Gen Intern Med*. 2016;31(9):1068–1076. doi:10.1007/s11606-016-3668-4

38. Tobin ET, Slatcher RB. Religious participation predicts diurnal cortisol profiles 10 years later via lower levels of religious struggle. *Health Psychol*. 2016;35(12):1356–1363. doi:10.1037/hea0000372

39. King SD, Fitchett G, Murphy PE, Pargament KI, Harrison DA, Loggers ET. Determining best methods to screen for religious/spiritual distress. *Support Care Cancer*. 2017;25(2):471–479. doi:10.1007/s00520-016-3425-6

40. Taylor EJ. Spiritual screening, history, and assessment. In: Ferrell B, Paice JA, eds. *Textbook of Palliative Nursing Care* 5ed. Oxford University Press; 2019:432–446.

41. Sandage SJ, Rupert D, Stavros GS, Devor NG. Relational spirituality in psychotherapy: healing suffering and promoting growth. American Psychological Association; 2020:chap Relational spirituality after the medical gaze (Chapter 1).

42. Taylor EJ. *What Do I Say? Talking with Patients About Spirituality*. Templeton Press; 2007.

43. Hodge DR, Sun F, Wolosin RJ. Hospitalized Asian patients and their spiritual needs: developing a model of spiritual care. *J Aging Health*. 2014;26(3):380–400. doi:10.1177/0898264313516995

3

Existential Suffering

Virginia Lee

With the accelerated pace of technology and medicine, the complexity of what it means to live and die has become increasingly complex in health care. Inherent to the work of nurses is the opportunity and obligation to accompany patients who may be facing a threat to life itself. Life-limiting illness and injury, personal adversity, and exposure to traumatic events can all trigger an unsolicited confrontation with one's mortality. Profound existential questions about life and death generally revolve around four major struggles: (1) the inevitability of *death* and the wish to live; (2) the meaninglessness of existence and the search for *purpose in life*; (3) awareness about the randomness of the universe and the fundamental need for *freedom* and choice; and (4) *existential isolation* and the need for connection.[1] The existential experience is relevant to many illnesses and other transformative life experiences[2-8] but has been historically prioritized in the cancer population.[9-11]

The variability and unpredictability of the human response to suffering and nurses' sense of moral responsibility can be daunting to effectively manage in the clinical setting. While nurses receive training in the areas of therapeutic communication and basic emotional support, specialized training in nursing curricula to alleviate crises of an existential nature is scant.[12] Nurses may often feel inadequately qualified to provide existential care for patients—an area of intervention that is conventionally delivered by trained psychotherapists.[13] The lack of safe and private spaces in acute care settings and the lack of time[14] for reflection further constrain nurses' abilities to respond, potentially leading to moral distress and a sense of professional helplessness.[15] However, when nurses are equipped with existential knowledge, the application of purposeful and timely compassionate caring practices is possible, leading to meaningful and rewarding work.[16] Identifying opportunities to provide existential care can be easily overlooked given the dynamic nature of existential experiences. Thus, the importance of having a theoretical perspective to guide the delivery of holistic and high-quality person-centered nursing care to alleviate existential distress and suffering cannot be overstated. A theoretical framework can orient the nurse to become more deliberate in the provision of existential care.

The purpose of this chapter is to situate existential suffering within a broader spectrum of the illness experience and to offer a reflection on the goals of nursing in the context of major life transitions due to life-limiting illness and other serious life events. To enable nurses to better understand, identify, and address the needs of patients with existential suffering, the concepts of mortality salience and existential health will be described. Nursing implications are provided, including suggestions for developing nursing-specific competencies. Clinical exemplars illustrate how nurses can respond to existential suffering in the clinical milieu.

Virginia Lee, *Existential Suffering* In: *The Nature of Suffering and the Goals of Nursing.* Second Edition. Edited by: William E. Rosa and Betty R. Ferrell, Oxford University Press. © Oxford University Press 2023. DOI: 10.1093/oso/9780197667934.003.0003

The Existential Experience

The impact of life-limiting illness and adversity can significantly unsettle beliefs about one's sense of self and one's understanding about their past, present, and future life. The existential experience refers to the widest range of existential needs, issues, concerns, and aspects of the patient experience, including existential suffering and health.[17] The literature generally centers around three key dimensions of the existential experience: (1) *coherence*: an understanding of the life lived and how the world works as explained by a uniquely personal global meaning system and life scheme; (2) *purpose in life*: a future-oriented view of one's life guided by short- and long-term goals and aspirations; and (3) *identity*: a belief that one's existence matters.[18]

Awareness of one's existence and the tension between life and death is not universally or inherently distressing.[19] Rather, events are considered neutral until appraised and imbued with meaning by the person experiencing them.[20] The meaning ascribed to any one event is uniquely influenced by one's history, values, beliefs, social background, and coping strategies and other personal and environmental factors.[21] For patients coping with major life transitions, responses will be varied as each person is unique, making prevalence of responses challenging to capture. For instance, prevalence of existential distress ranges from 13% to 50% among patients with cancer.[19,22] To understand existential suffering and intervene in a timely fashion, it is essential to appreciate the context of mortality salience and existential health.

Mortality Salience and Existential Health

Mortality salience is a shared social awareness about the inevitability and finality of one's eventual death.[23] Each person's developmental history, prior life challenges, resiliencies, and vulnerabilities will shape one's understanding and ability to cope when existential questions about life meaning and value are raised following a confrontation with mortality.[24] Terror management theory suggests that by adulthood, individuals become acutely aware of the ultimate existential absurdity—that humankind lives only to eventually die. To sustain a future-oriented worldview and pursuit of life goals, individuals engage in conscious as well as unconscious activities to avoid painful reminders of one's ultimate fate.[23]

A number of seminal theories describe the critical use of defense mechanisms to protect against death anxiety under everyday situations. Theorists posit that a global meaning system lays the foundation for a life scheme to assist individuals with creating a unique life philosophy and life framework to appraise, explain, understand, and make sense of daily life events and guide subsequent behaviors and actions.[20] Inherent in each global meaning system are individual beliefs and assumptions about the surrounding world, other people, and oneself.[25] An intact global meaning system is necessary to create a life scheme and build routines that confer a sense of predictability, control, and mastery as well as a sense of self-esteem, confidence, and self-efficacy to pursue short- and long-term goals. Terror management theory further suggests that spiritualty and religion, believing in an afterlife, creating legacy work, and/or the drive to contribute to something greater than oneself that will last beyond one's death may assuage the dis-ease associated with fear of nonexistence and annihilation.[23] Thus, under everyday life circumstances, a number of defense mechanisms are activated to buffer against death anxiety associated with the awareness of mortality. Such theoretical knowledge can provide nurses with a baseline understanding of existential health under nonthreatening conditions.

Existential Suffering

Unprecedented major life events such as illness, terrorist attacks, or natural disasters (whether lived or witnessed through exposure) can provoke existential distress and suffering. Existential distress and suffering not only embody an unwanted awareness of one's own mortality but also a perception of incomprehension so encompassing that the aforementioned defense mechanisms are overwhelmed and undermined, leading to the need to examine and redefine one's life philosophy, purpose in life, and identity.[18,20]

Although the two terms are sometimes used interchangeably in the literature, the term "existential distress" may be distinguished from "existential suffering." Existential *distress* is characterized by a temporary state of great physical or mental strain related to questions of coherence, meaning and purpose, and identity. Existential *suffering* is characterized by a conscious enduring and unrelenting state of distress that is linked to demoralization and includes a persistent loss of meaning and purpose in life, a perceived failure to meet one's own expectations and/or those of others, and a persistent failure to cope with life priorities or conditions that threaten the integrity of the self.[22,26] A state of demoralization may be seen in the patient with suicidal ideation or one who has expressed a desire for hastened death.[27] In practice, the clinical presentation of demoralization is difficult to recognize as it can occur independently from major depressive disorder[9,28] and in the absence of somatic symptoms and reduced functioning,[29] and can present with or without anhedonia or anxiety states.[30] Nurses play an important role in being present for the unfolding experience of the patient (Case Exemplar 3.1).

Case Exemplar 3.1

Marisa is meeting her patient, Lewis, a 33-year-old male with stage 4 colon cancer, for the first time. Lewis eagerly shows Marisa pictures of his 5-year-old daughter, Brianna. Recognizing Marisa's genuine presence, he opens up and shares that he is on medical leave from being a police officer, he has gone from being a competitive athlete to being completely deconditioned, and his wife left him after he received an ileostomy. He asks, "Why is this all happening to me? I can't bear to think of the future. Look what kind of a loser dad I turned out to be. I don't have a job. My wife left me just when I needed her most!" Marisa wasn't sure how to respond, but she paused. She asked Lewis, "What do your days look like for you now?" She followed with, "This sounds quite different from the life you had planned." She acknowledged the significant number of losses he had experienced in the past several months. She mostly listened and asked more exploratory questions, learning about what gave his life meaning and purpose. By the end of the shift with Lewis, she reflected, "I hear you. I can only imagine how hard it must be to not have the ability to plan the future with certainty. Listening to your story, I hear that despite all these challenges, you have so many strengths. And it is clear from your photos that you are a very important part of your daughter's life. Believe in your own ability to get through today, in small steps, to make it more manageable." Lewis replied, "Thank you. I'm going to be there for her when she graduates grades 1st, 2nd, 3rd grade heck, through high school and marriage! Thanks for caring. It means a lot to me."

At the time a nurse or other health care provider encounters a patient and/or family in crisis, the patient's existential experience may have already been altered by the life threat. A hallmark of existential distress and suffering is the awareness of being in a liminal state. The word "liminal," derived from the Latin word *limens*, means threshold. Liminal spaces are temporary passages or "neutral zones"[31] to allow a transition between the end of one space and the beginning of another. Individuals facing a life threat are forced out of a past comfortable life onto the unsettling threshold of a future life yet to be determined. Individuals in existential distress may report feeling destabilized, being unsure of one's grounding, and having lost their foothold. It is an in-between state of hovering, characterized by ambivalence and fluctuations in thoughts, mood, and feelings.

Bridges' transition model[31] offers one framework to understand existential liminality as the manifestation of a life scheme in transition.[32] A transition is an inner psychological process that individuals undergo to come to terms with new situations. Major life transitions typically begin with "endings," marked by a stark awareness of losses in the areas of life coherence (the perceived loss of a future that includes ruptured routines and shattered assumptions about justice, fairness, luck, and randomness), meaning (loss of life purpose, lost illusions of predictability and controllability), and value (loss of self-esteem and self-worth). A loss of temporal continuity can reveal deep fears about the distant future, and feelings of grief, hopelessness, helplessness, insecurity, and vulnerability can make it difficult to participate in everyday activities. Existential distress and suffering are characterized by a sense of disembodiment, disintegration, and disconnectedness (of being me yet not me).[33] Individuals may withdraw from social activities with family and friends.[33]

Attempts to redefine and reconstruct a global meaning system and life scheme have been referred to as a "search for meaning."[34] Contemplation to try to understand etiology, responsibility, and the impact on one's life situation is considered a normative response in the aftermath of traumatic experiences.[20] As individual's attempt to assimilate the stressor into an existing life scheme or to accommodate the stressor by altering the life scheme, fluctuations in mood and cognitive processing may resemble posttraumatic-like symptoms. Intrusive thoughts are commonly experienced in the form of ruminations, involuntary, recurrent, or distressing thoughts or dreams about the stressor event. To regulate against excessive emotional distress, individuals may engage in avoidant or distancing behaviors to deliberately suppress or keep threatening thoughts out of consciousness. Patients may describe feeling emotionally numb or actively redirect conversations away from the stressor event. The oscillation between the desire to process the impact of the stressor event and to repel reminders of the stressor is a distinguishing characteristic of the dialectical coping involved in the search for meaning.[17]

The search for meaning is generally portrayed as an in-between phase when answers are not yet readily available to fully grasp and understand how to live with the existential paradox (e.g., "Am I living or dying?") following a confrontation with one's mortality. Attempts to process and integrate the reality of the stressor event through reflection of the past, present, and future are emotionally and intellectually taxing. The loss of former life routines, inability to accomplish daily tasks, dashed goals, increasing symptom burden, and increasing dependence may lead to regrets and a lamented life.[2-8] The loss of personal liberty and freedom as a consequence of newly imposed limitations and restrictions can lead to frustration, anger, social isolation, and diminished feelings of self-efficacy, self-esteem, and self-worth.[2-8]

Theoretically, existential suffering can be alleviated by helping individuals to reconstruct a global meaning system and intact life scheme.[9,10,20] Numerous references in the literature allude to getting back to a "new normal," which suggests a successful integration of the stressor into a readjusted and redefined life scheme.[35] A postadversity global meaning system may have qualitatively changed new values and beliefs are adopted. The preexisting life scheme may have shifted to accept a more vulnerable self living in an uncertain world. Although individuals may or may not rely less on death-avoidant coping mechanisms, a reasonable return to meaningful life activities is possible. Having confronted the possibility of one's own death, some individuals may emerge from this search for meaning feeling a sense of personal growth and a stronger sense of agency and clarity about what matters most. This phenomenon, called post-traumatic growth, includes a new appreciation of living in the present moment, seeking and cultivating meaningful relationships with significant others, and an openness to welcoming new possibilities.[36] See Case Exemplar 3.2 for a case that illustrates the role of meaning making in alleviating existential suffering and fostering connection within important relationships.

Case Exemplar 3.2

Genevieve is working the evening shift and checks in on Mr. Beauchemin's tracheotomy. She smiles and says, "Mr. Beauchemin, you did very well this week! You went through a lot after 3 months on a ventilator in the ICU. The team is amazed at your progress and we think you will soon breathe on your own and then we will remove the breathing tube. The plan is for you to go home next week." To her surprise, Mr. Beauchemin starts crying. He shakes his head and says, "Why go home?! My wife is not there anymore. I'm all alone." Genevieve encourages him to share what he means by being all alone. She learns that his wife was diagnosed with advanced dementia and was hospitalized for safety reasons and is unable to return home. They have been married for 61 years, and he is not able to see his two children very often. "I feel like I'm in jail. I can't eat what I want, when I want. I can't drive where I want to go. I don't have much time left. I want to live my last days the way I want—with my wife in my own home." As he started to talk about his life, Genevieve highlighted his sense of resilience, resourcefulness, and sense of humor that used to win friends in the community. It was clear he felt some shame around his increasing dependency related to his illness. Genevieve made a referral to the social worker to inquire about the possibility of his being placed with his wife in a residence. For the rest of her week, Genevieve aimed to learn more about his life through reminiscence and introduced the idea of working on a legacy project to offer his wife and his children a meaningful opportunity for connection while apart. As Genevieve reassured him that she would look forward to hearing about his life, he said with a grin that he'll have to think about the best stories to share with her.

Responses to Suffering

Knowledge Can Guide Existential Care

Deeply rooted in the origins of nursing practice is the prevention of illness or injury, promotion of health, alleviation of suffering, and promotion of a dignified death.[37] Nursing is about understanding the human condition in all its complexity, to support patients to make sense of life events and to assist patients to make choices that can affect all aspects of their health.[21] Whether the nurse-patient encounter is a single moment or a series of regularly planned interactions over a longer period of time, nurses have a responsibility to provide holistic care for the patient that includes existential competency. This becomes increasingly important in attempting to understand how the patient's view of self amid health and illness is evolving and what signs of distress may be present.

An enhanced awareness of the full spectrum of the existential experience allows nurses to reconceptualize, label, and give value to everyday nursing actions, thus helping them to understand the gravity and importance of expressing empathy, demonstrating a caring presence, and showing a genuine interest in knowing the patient in their full humanity. Such knowledge can assist nurses to deliver more purposeful interventions to manage existential suffering in spite of the challenges that may exist in clinical settings. Existential suffering may be interpreted as the inability to reconcile a new life scheme that sees only limited options and results in feelings of entrapment and isolation in the old life scheme. The goal of nursing in the alleviation of existential suffering is aimed at understanding the subjective world of the patient, to assist in the exploration of new perspectives and choices, to assist in the search for meaning and purpose in life, and to offer a sense of connection to convey that the patient—and all of the feelings and thoughts they have surrounding their current sense of identity—matters throughout transitions.

The importance of defining nursing competencies to alleviate existential distress and suffering is particularly important where there is a lack of continuity among nurses and when instrumental task workloads pose significant challenges to initiating existential discussions in the clinical environment.[38] Existential competencies can define how to apply the existential knowledge and skills and provide direction for nurses to identify and act when an opportunity arises to explore the patient's existential experience. Adopting a nursing approach that includes the concept of cocreation, defined as a joint process of sharing knowledge, attentive listening, and exploration of different perspectives, can build confidence and contribute to a sense of preparedness when addressing the existential needs of patients.[39] Keeping appraised of the literature, debriefing with colleagues, role playing, and seeking out meaning making and other communication skills-building approaches can facilitate existential competencies, buffer moral distress, and increase job satisfaction. An openness to initiate and receive existential discussions with patients during routine care can build a repertoire of learning moments that can gradually foster more ease and less helplessness when addressing existential concerns in practice.[40]

The development of good existential competency begins with letting go of preconceived notions that existential issues only occur with advanced illness or at end of life. Each nurse-patient encounter offers an opportunity to explore and assess the patient's perception of the impact and severity of the stressor event at that moment. The uniqueness of existential concerns is that these concerns may not be proportionate to the amount of physical pain experienced, can occur in the presence of joy or in the absence of depression, and can occur in the absence of physical symptoms.[29,30] A patient in existential distress may still be able to laugh and enjoy the moment but may be unable to look forward to a future. Existential concerns may not necessarily be captured by conventional measures of distress screening.[42] For example, individuals living with early-stage life-limiting disease such as cancer, end-stage renal disease, or heart failure may also harbor unexpressed emotions and struggle with their reflections about functional changes and altered life goals for the future. Such concerns may be inadvertently overlooked if current measures of distress screening based on level of disease burden or later stages of illness are used.[43] Similarly, while the end of cancer treatment may seem like a pivotal moment for celebration, some patients may only begin to process their situation at the completion of treatment and feel bereft upon facing the loss of familiar facets of their pretrauma lives and identities.[44] Conversely, patients diagnosed with advanced cancer may not express expected levels of heightened distress if they perceive their life to be intact and well lived.

Facilitating disclosure about existential concerns and uncovering existential suffering are common challenges in the clinical setting. Rarely are existential concerns disclosed explicitly as "existential" by patients. Rather, existential matters may be implicit, subtle, indirect utterances embedded during routine day-to-day conversations.[38,40,41,44,45] The multidimensional nature of the existential experience means that existential suffering may frequently be entangled in myriad everyday routine events and underlying existential messages can be found embedded within patients' questions, stories, and day-to-day conversations. Patients may convey existential concerns with discomfort, hesitance, or ambivalence not only in the choice of language used ("It's sad because there was nothing to do about it") but also in terms of body language (stuttering, speaking rapidly, whispering, using a low voice, sitting uneasily, gazing away).[41] Patients may downgrade or display little emotion or interject smiling or laughter during serious conversations about illness that would be expected to engender existential issues during routine hospital consultations.[38] Existential concerns may be couched in questions about biomedical terms, test results, statistics, prognostication, and treatment options.[38,41] Existential matters or concerns are often conflated with religion or spirituality. By asking open-ended questions, gathering more information, observing, listening, and attending to the cues communicated by the patient, nurses can approach each encounter as an opportunity to learn about who this human being is and better understand how they see the world within the context of their social, cultural, and health narratives. Nurses can establish supportive conditions for the patient to explore their own situation and come to understand how they explain their current and potential future circumstances.

Well-timed nursing interventions in response to existential distress can be spontaneous or purposeful. Existential competency means that the nurse will sense when to focus on an existential concern or experience when an opportunity spontaneously presents. An openness to listen for existential cues while completing instrumental tasks or other activities of clinical practice reduces the chances of being caught off guard or missing an opening to have a meaningful conversation with a patient. Nurses can hone their skills to become more attuned to the subtle signals embedded in patient stories that may be emanating from the patient. The hallmarks of existential anxiety can be manifested in patient expressions that refer to uncertainty and the difficulty of facing the unknowable, noticing losses and change, conceding the lack of control over choices, feeling a loss of dignity, feeling alone, noticing changes in the quality of friendships and relationships with others, or feeling that life is meaningless. Given that nursing has the highest proportion of direct patient-facing time among all disciplines, it is highly likely that a nurse will be present for these pivotal moments of sharing in day-to-day conversations. Therefore, a nurse's preparation for engaging in these exchanges is critical to holistic care delivery and to the alleviation of both anticipatory and palpable existential suffering.

Existential competency also means that the nurse can plan to set aside time to purposefully conduct an existential assessment when caring for individuals at higher risk for existential suffering. Research in an oncology context suggests that patients who are female, single, experiencing high symptom burden, have a low social network,[26,30] have an intolerance to uncertainty or tend to use avoidant coping behaviors,[46] or engage in self-blame[19] may be at higher risk of existential distress. It has been suggested that when emotional responses appear disproportionate to loss or when physical symptoms are unremitting, existential distress may be at play. Nurses can apply their existential knowledge to consider whether and to what extent the patient's life scheme or global meaning system had been impacted by the stressor event, whether the patient has access to adequate coping resources, and whether the integrity of the patient had been impacted to successfully meet the demands of the life threat.

The oscillation between existential health and existential suffering is another hallmark of the existential experience.[17] Individuals may display discomfort or hesitation to directly explore concerns of an existential nature, or the intensity of the existential suffering may defy the ability to communicate through language. Following exposure to life-limiting situations, patients often process their situation by reviewing and taking stock of their life (to rebuild an intact life scheme that makes sense), by adjusting their life goals and priorities (to redefine their purpose in life), and to redefine their identity and who they are (to preserve self-esteem). The role of the nurse is to facilitate a climate of openness and reinstate a sense of security in the patient, who may then share and sort through the entanglement of physical, emotional, relational, spiritual, and existential suffering.[40] Nurses can play an important role in these situations by educating and normalizing the ebb and flow of cognitive processing of highly stressful events. In these instances, nurses can consider offering patients alternate means for expression including art therapy,[51] music therapy,[52] and reflective journals.[53] Complementary therapies can acknowledge patients' suffering, potentially reveal a deeper perspective and understanding into the patient experience, and offer solace when suffering must be endured. Sorting through existential dilemmas will take time and will likely not be resolved in one encounter. Nurses can normalize that there is no predetermined time frame to process major life transitions and help patients anticipate the changes relative to their cognitive, social, and emotional states during the transition toward healing.

As frontline health providers, nurses are ideally suited to provide the continued presence, knowledge, and agency to structure optimal conditions for existential care. The environmental conditions to optimally address existential suffering include ensuring that basic symptom relief and physiological needs are satisfied. Although low symptom burden may or may not be associated with existential distress, high symptom burden is consistently associated with existential distress, demoralization, and death anxiety.[47,48] Without proper symptom management, higher-level needs for transcendence and meaning will be harder to fulfill. Referral to social services and humanitarian assistance programs can be coordinated to meet specific needs such as food, transportation, rent, and utilities. Once the basic physiological, safety, and security needs are adequately addressed, there may be more openness to have existentially oriented conversations about the goals of care, belonging, and fulfillment in the context of existential distress. Proffering a safe space or an "emotional container" to hold the suffering can help set the environment to further confront what is at the core of the suffering.[39,40] Demonstrating compassionate care by establishing and continually building trust, employing respect and consideration in behavior and demeanor, and seeking to know the person are all key elements of such a container.[49]

Gauging the patient's readiness and willingness to engage in conversations about existential issues is another competency to achieve more meaningful and productive discussions. The complexity of broaching end-of-life conversations between patients, family members, and health care providers was described in a qualitative study that examined how health care providers initiated conversations about death and dying with patients at risk of dying from heart failure.[50] Changes in the patient's clinical status, direct queries from the patient, and organizational policy were identified as facilitative triggers to initiate, plan, and hold conversations. Yet, the powerful emotions that were evoked by such conversations about death and dying were perceived as evasive maneuvers by the patient to avoid, deter, or stifle conversations from going further. Conversations regarding death and dying were perceived as awkward and out of context in a curative setting and often led to conversations about "death without dying."[50]

Supporting existentially difficult conversations in practice implies that nurses must convey an openness to receive and hold the patient's pain and suffering while being responsive to the patient's cues to engage in deeper reflection. Patients must feel secure enough in the nurse-patient relationship to expose their feelings of despair and desolation. Small gestures take on more significance for patients in existential distress. For example, addressing a patient by name, establishing eye contact, or remembering a personal detail about the patient can acknowledge the patient's existence, convey a sense of connection and communicate that their being in the world is significant, and buffer a sense of isolation. Conversely, results from a study of medical oncology nurses highlighted the importance of self-awareness to discern when the nurse's own temptation to console patients at the end of life may clash with the patients' lack of readiness to "tear off the protective scab of denial."[40] The study recommended that nurses ask patients for their permission to explore more sensitive topics and exercise sensitivity to avoid being too forthright when patients may not yet be ready to confront their fears.

Many patients deal with existential questions in terms of living and not just in terms of dying.[54] Nurses frequently inquire about everyday life routines that may have appeared superficial in the life before the life threat. However, what may have been previously considered a mundane activity of daily living may shift in significance and assume a different meaning following the confrontation with one's mortality. The longing for familiar life routines may suddenly signify a powerful foothold for maintaining one's self-esteem or perceiving the world as secure, predictable, and controllable.[33,54] In this context, nursing strategies to "know the patient" that may come intuitively should be reframed as a purposeful nursing intervention. Informal, naturally occurring nurse-patient exchanges often include stories and updates about the patient's life at home, work, and school and in the community. Such conversations about everyday routines offer rich sources of information to increase the nurse's understanding of the patient's sense of coherence, life scheme, meaning, and purpose in life. These conversations offer nonthreatening windows of opportunity to explore the patient's global meaning system and life scheme. Patients reported feeling more open and willing to discuss matters of an existential nature with nurses more than other health care professionals.[55] In fact, some authors have suggested that existential anxiety and distress may reflect a normative adaptive response to a major life transition, and referral to specialized health care providers should be reserved for more unrelenting existential suffering.[42] Taking the time to listen and know the patient and understand their joys, preferences, stressors, hopes, and challenges in light of a dramatically changed life context is an important nursing intervention that can reinstate feelings of connectedness and self-worth in a patient in existential distress.

The life review approach to elicit existential concerns has implications for nurses in the clinical setting. The life review is a critical and transversal element across the majority of the existential interventions. Systematic reviews and meta-analyses document the effectiveness of existential, meaning-oriented interventions.[56] When nurses encounter patients, it is important to remember they have a historical background of other pivotal life events. Conversations that aim to review and take stock of the life already lived or contemplate a life that may not come to fruition is a daunting endeavor for the patient and can create significant existential distress. To successfully establish a deep connection with one patient at a time and understand what may potentially help each reengage in a new normal is an acquired competency. Establishing a nurse-patient connection is a key nursing intervention. Research has shown that patients' perceiving a strong connection to at least one health care provider can make a difference to buffer the sense of disconnectedness in the midst of existential distress.[57] The medical chart is only one source of data to get to know the patient. Each person's history and background offer a rich compendium of information to understand how the stressor event fits into the patient's life scheme. It is important to recognize that healing conversations need not always focus on end-of-life discussions per se. Creative and novel approaches can be tried to elicit the arc of one's life story. A stance of genuine curiosity can be incorporated into a more holistic evaluation of the nature of the existential distress. Eliciting an understanding of each individual's life story can help nurses understand which dimension of the existential experience is threatened from the patient's perspective and help cocreate strategies to maintain the integrity of this particular patient.

The role of the nurse is to regularly check in, ask permission to delve deeper, and respect the patient's pace to move in and out of conversations about everyday living and to explore more profound existential dimensions when appropriate. Nursing assessments can explore different aspects of the existential experience, including the following: (1) Sense of coherence: Asking open-ended questions to explore a patient's understanding or expectations of their situation may reveal passing expressions of surprise, shock, and uncertainty. Asking questions that seek to understand how the patient views their current life situation against a backdrop or timeline of their life may lead to patient reflections about not knowing what to expect or adopting a wait-and-see attitude. These may signal that there is an existential shift and a renegotiation of a life philosophy or life scheme.[58] (2) Goals and purpose in life: Patient conversations may allude to a sense of urgency to complete unfinished business or an acute awareness of time as a dwindling and finite resource. This topic of time can open opportunities to further explore what matters most in the present moment and shape discussions about treatment preferences and goals of care.[58] (3) Identity: Personal stories, dreams, and aspirations about family, school, career, social commitments, and legacy can reveal a lot about the individual's identity and narrative of how they see their future self.[44] Statements that allude to being a burden on others can suggest existential concerns that link self-worth to the need of being functional, active contributors to family and society. (4) Isolation: Stories about changing social dynamics with family, friends, or colleagues are a frequent concern expressed by patients following severe life-threatening situations. Difficulty sustaining relationships or self-imposed withdrawal from friends or social networks requires an assessment to discern the need for accompaniment during a normative transition or referral for more specialized care. (5) Freedom and choice: Patients have been reported to prefer receiving experimental treatments that they knew they may not benefit from as a way to avoid the fear of the unknown and avoid confronting the helplessness of not being in treatment. The nurse's role is considered paramount in conversations with patients about how to manage life with respect to different treatment options.[55]

Conclusion

This chapter sought to provide relevant theoretical knowledge to understand existential distress and suffering within the broader spectrum of the existential experience under everyday life circumstances. While the challenges of supporting existential distress and suffering may seem imposing and elusive, it appears that the fundamental skills needed to begin to address and alleviate existential distress are entirely within nurses' scope of practice and competencies. The tools necessary to address existential distress and suffering are part of the very essence and foundation of nursing. Deep, cocreated relationships between the nurse and the patient are essential to understand, assess, and manage existential suffering. Nursing actions to alleviate existential distress are characterized by knowing the patient, establishing trust, setting aside time, being attentive, and being responsive to the dialectical nature of existential concerns. Having a genuine sense of curiosity to learn about the background of who this person has been, who they are in this moment, and who they are becoming[39] is key to discovering the elements that matter most at that moment for the patient. Considering the high acceptability by patients for nurse-led psychological support[59] and the rich existential experiences found in day-to-day nurse-patient interactions,[41,45,50,54,58] nurses play a crucial role in the alleviation of existential distress and suffering.

References

1. Yalom ID. *Existential Psychotherapy*. Basic Books; 1980.
2. Bolton LE, Seymour J, Gardiner C. Existential suffering in the day to day lives of those living with palliative care needs arising from chronic obstructive pulmonary disease (COPD): a systematic integrative literature review. *Palliat Med*. 2022;36(4):567–580. doi:10.1177/02692163221074539
3. Schulz VM, Crombeen AM, Marshall D, et al. Beyond simple planning: existential dimensions of conversations with patients at risk of dying from heart failure. *J Pain Symptom Manag*. 2017;54(5):637–644.
4. Andersen AH, Assing Hvidt E, Huniche L, Hvidt NC, Roessler KK. Why we suffer? Existential challenges of patients with chronic illness: a Kierkegaardian inspired interpretative phenomenological analysis. *J Humanist Psychol*. 2021:1–28. doi:10.1177/00221678211002439
5. Høgsnes L, Norbergh KG, Melin-Johansson C. "Being in between": nurses' experiences when caring for individuals with dementia and encountering family caregivers' existential life situations. *Res Gerontol Nurs*. 2019;12(2):91–98. doi:10.3928/19404921-20190207-01
6. Pinel EC, Helm PJ, Yawger GC, Long AE, Scharnetzki L. Feeling out of (existential) place: existential isolation and nonnormative group membership. *Group Process Intergroup Relat*. 2022;25(4):990–1010. doi:10.1177/1368430221999084
7. Tsai K, Chang PJ, Mathew AJ, et al. Exploring spirituality of elders relocating into long-term care facilities. *Open J Occupat Ther*. 2022;10(2):1–11. doi.org/10.15453/2168-6408.1959
8. Davidov J, Russo-Netzer P. Exploring the phenomenological structure of existential anxiety as lived through transformative life experiences. *Anxiety Stress Coping*. 2022;35(2):232–247. doi.org/ 10.1080/10615806.2021.1921162
9. Vehling S, Philipp R. Existential distress and meaning-focused interventions in cancer survivorship. *Curr Opin Support Palliat Care*. 2018;12(1):46–51. doi:10.1097/SPC.0000000000000324

10. Lichtenthal WG, Roberts KE, Pessin H, Applebaum A, Breitbart W. Meaning-centered psychotherapy and cancer: finding meaning in the face of suffering. *Psychiatric Times.* 2020;37(8):23–25.

11. Rosa WE, Chochinov HM, Coyle N, Hadler RA, Breitbart WS. Attending to the existential experience in oncology: dignity and meaning amid awareness of death. *J Clin Oncol Global Oncol.* 2022;8:e2200038. doi:10.1200/GO.22.00038

12. Alavi NM, Hosseini F. Educating the existential view to nurses in cancer care: a review. *Iran J Nurs Midwifery Res.* 2019;24(4):243–250. doi:10.4103/ijnmr.IJNMR_108_18

13. Breitbart WS, Lichtenthal WG, Applebaum AJ. Meaning-centered psychotherapy. In: Steel JL, Carr BI, eds. *Psychological Aspects of Cancer.* Springer; 2022:399–409. doi.org/10.1007/978-3-030-85702-8_23

14. Carr TJ. Facing existential realities: exploring barriers and challenges to spiritual nursing care. *Qual Health Res.* 2010;20(10):1379–1392. doi:10.1177/1049732310372377

15. Lagerdahl A, Scalpello A, Brown M, et al. Nurses' attitudes and beliefs around exploring the existential concerns of people with cancer. *Cancer Nurs Practice.* Published May 25, 2022. Accessed June 15, 2022. doi:10.7748/cnp.2022.e1805

16. Hoeve YT, Brouwer J, Roodbol PF, Kunnen S. The importance of contextual, relational and cognitive factors for novice nurses' emotional state and affective commitment to the profession. A multilevel study. *J Adv Nurs.* 2018;74:2082–2093.

17. Tarbi E, Meghani S. Existential experience in adults with advanced cancer: a concept analysis. *Nurs Outlook.* 2019;67(5):540–557. doi:10.1016/j.outlook.2019.03.006

18. George LS, Park CL. Do violations of global beliefs and goals drive distress and meaning making following life stressors? *Illness Crisis Loss.* 2022;30(3):378–395. doi:10.1177/1054137320958344

19. Bovero A, Sedghi NA, Opezzo M, et al. Dignity-related existential distress in end of life cancer patients: prevalence, underlying factors, and associated coping strategies. *Psychooncology.* 2018;27:2631–2637.

20. Park CL. Making sense of the meaning literature: an integrative review of meaning making and its effects on adjustment to stressful life events. *Psychol Bull.* 2010;136(2):257–301.

21. Gottlieb LN, Gottlieb B. Strengths-based nursing: a process for implementing a philosophy into practice. *J Fam Nurs.* 2017;23(3):319–340. doi:10.1177/1074840717717731

22. Vehling S, Kissane DW. Existential distress in cancer: alleviating suffering from fundamental loss and change. *Psychooncology.* 2018;27:2525–2530.

23. Rhodes N. Terror management theory: mortality salience. In: Bulck J, ed. *The International Encyclopedia of Media Psychology.* John-Wiley & Sons, ILonc; September 9, 2020. Accessed June 15, 2022. doi.org/10.1002/9781119011071.iemp0127

24. Lo C. A developmental perspective on existential distress and adaptation to advanced disease. *Psychooncology.* 2018;27(11):2657–2660. doi:10.1002/pon.4767

25. van Bruggen, V, Klooster PM, van der Aa N, Smith AJ, et al. Structural validity of the World Assumption Scale. *J Trauma Stress.* 2018;31:816–825. https://doi.org/10.1002/jts.22348

26. Bovero A, Botto R, Adriano B, Opezzo M, Tesio V, Torta R. Exploring demoralization in end-of-life cancer patients: prevalence, latent dimensions, and associations with other psychosocial variables. *Palliat Support Care.* 2019;17(5):596–603. doi:10.1017/S1478951519000191

27. Kolva E, Hoffecker L, Cox-Martin E. Suicidal ideation in patients with cancer: a systematic review of prevalence, risk factors, intervention and assessment. *Palliat Support Care.* 2020;18(2):206–219. doi:10.1017/S1478951519000610

28. Nanni MG, Caruso R, Travado L, et al. Relationship of demoralization with anxiety, depression, and quality of life: a Southern European study of Italian and Portuguese cancer patients. *Psychooncology.* 2018;27:2616–2622.

29. Kious BM, Battin MP. Suffering and the completed life. *Am J Bioeth*. 2022;22(2):62–64.
30. Bobevski I, Kissane DW, Vehling S, McKenzie DP, Glaesmer H, Mehnert A. Latent class analysis differentiation of adjustment disorder and demoralization, more severe depressive and anxiety disorders, and aromatic symptoms in patient with cancer. *Psychooncology*. 2018;27:2623–2630.
31. Bridges W. *Transitions: Making Sense of Life's Changes*. Lifelong Books; 2019.
32. Haverland JA. Life in transition: using reflection and gratitude to discover hope, optimism, and resilience. *Character Transitions*. 2021;7:10–24.
33. Missel M, Bergenholtz H, Beck M, Donsel PO, Simonÿ C. Understanding existential anxiety and the soothing nature of nostalgia in life with incurable esophageal cancer: a phenomenological hermeneutical investigation of patient narratives. *Cancer Nurs*. 2022;45(1):E291–E298. doi:10.1097/NCC.0000000000000916
34. Quinn B. Role of the body in cancer, sense-making and the search for meaning. *Cancer Nurs Practice*. 2020;19(4):24–30. doi.org/10.7748/cnp.2020.e1703
35. Baker P, Beesley H, Fletcher I, Ablett J, Holcombe C, Salmon P. "Getting back to normal" or "a new type of normal"?: A qualitative study of patients' responses to the existential threat of cancer. *Eur J Cancer Care*. 2016;25:180–189. doi:10.1111/ecc.12274
36. Davis CG, Porter JE. Pathways to growth following trauma and loss. In: Snyder CR, Lopez J, Edwards LM, Marques SC, eds. *The Oxford Handbook of Positive Psychology*. Oxford University Press; 2021:919–927.
37. Nightingale N. *Notes on Nursing: What It Is and What It Is Not*. Harrison; 1860.
38. Ikander T, Dieperink KB, Hansen O, Raunkiær M. Patient, family caregiver, and nurse involvement in end-of-life discussions during palliative chemotherapy: a phenomenological hermeneutic study. *J Fam Nurs*. 2022;28(1):31–42. doi:10.1177/10748407211046308
39. Hemberg J, Bergdahl E. Dealing with ethical and existential issues at end of life through co-creation. *Nurs Ethics*. 2020;27(4):1012–1031.
40. Tornøe KA, Danbolt LJ, Kvigne K, Sørlie V. The challenge of consolation: nurses' experiences with spiritual and existential care for the dying—a phenomenological hermeneutical study. *BMC Nurs*. 2015;14:62. doi:10.1186/s12912-015-0114-6
41. Larsen BH, Lundeby T, Gerwing J, Gulbrandsen P, Førde R. "Eh—what type of cells are these—flourishing in the liver?": cancer patients' disclosure of existential concerns in routine hospital consultations. *Patient Educ Couns*. 2019;105(7):2019–2026.
42. Bai M. Psychological response to the diagnosis of advanced cancer: a systematic review. *Ann Behav Med*. 2022;56(2):125–136. doi.org/10.1093/abm/kaab068
43. Steinhauser KE, Stechuchak KM, Ramos K, Winger J, Tulsky JA, Olsen MK. Current measures of distress may not account for what's most important in existential care interventions: results of the outlook trial. *Palliat Support Care*. 2020;18(6):648–657. doi:10.1017/S1478951520001170
44. Currin-McCulloch J, Kaushik S, Jones B. "When will I feel normal?": disorienting grief responses among young adults with advanced cancer. *Cancer Nurs*. 2022;45(2):E355–E363. doi:10.1097/NCC.0000000000000977
45. Tarbi EC. "If it's the time, it's the time": existential communication in naturally-occurring palliative care conversations with individuals with advanced cancer, their families, and clinicians. *Patient Educ Couns*. 2021;104(12):2963–2968. doi.org/10.1016/j.pec.2021.04.040
46. Lebel S, Maheu C, Tomei C, et al. Towards the validation of a new, blended theoretical model of fear of cancer recurrence. *Psychooncology*. 2018;27(11):2594–2601. doi:10.1002/pon.4880
47. An E, Lo C, Hales S, Zimmermann C, Rodin G. Demoralization and death anxiety in advanced cancer. *Psychooncology*. 2018;27:2566–2572. https://doi.org/10.1002/pon.4843

48. Rantanen P, Chochinov HM, Emanuel LL, et al. Existential quality of life and associated factors in cancer patients receiving palliative care. *J Pain Symptom Manag.* 2022;63(1):61–70. doi:10.1016/j.jpainsymman.2021.07.016

49. Sinclair S, McClement S, Raffin-Bouchal S, et al. Compassion in health care: an empirical model. *J Pain Symptom Manag.* 2016;51(2):193–203. doi:10.1016/j.jpainsymman.2015.10.009

50. Schulz VM, Crombeen AM, Marshall D, Shadd J, LaDonna KA, Lingard L. Beyond simple planning: existential dimensions of conversations with patients at risk of dying from heart failure. *J Pain Symptom Manag.* 2017;54(5):637–644. doi:10.1016/j.jpainsymman.2017.07.041

51. Reilly RC, Lee V, Laux K, Robitaille A. Creating doorways: finding meaning and growth through art therapy in the face of life-threatening illness. *Public Health (Elsevier).* 2021;198:245–251. doi:10.1016/j.puhe.2021.07.004

52. Engelbrecht R, Bhar S, Ciorciari J. Planting the SEED: a model to describe the functions of music in reminiscence therapy. *Complement Ther Clin Pract.* 2021;44. doi:10.1016/j.ctcp.2021.101441

53. Banerjee M, Hegde S, Thippeswamy H, Kulkarni GB, Rao N. In search of the "self": holistic rehabilitation in restoring cognition and recovering the "self" following traumatic brain injury: a case report. *Neurorehabilitation.* 2021;48(2):231–242. doi:10.3233/NRE-208017

54. Salander P. "Spirituality" hardly facilitates our understanding of existential distress—but "everyday life" might. *Psychooncology.* 2018;27:2654–2656. https://doi-org.proxy3.library.mcgill.ca/10.1002/pon.4784

55. Gregersen TA, Birkelund R, Wolderslund M, Dahl Steffensen K, Ammentorp J. Patients' experiences of the decision-making process for clinical trial participation. *Nurs Health Sci.* 2022;24(1):65–72. https://doi.org/10.1111/nhs.12933

56. Terao Takeshi T, Moriaki S. The present state of existential interventions within palliative care. *Front Psychiatry.* 2022;12:811612. doi.10.3389/fpsyt.2021.811612

57. Jewett PI, Vogel RI, Galchutt P, et al. Associations between a sense of connection and existential and psychosocial outcomes in gynecologic and breast cancer survivors. *Support Care Cancer.* 2022;30(4):3329–3336. doi:10.1007/s00520-021-06784-8

58. Tarbi EC, Gramling R, Bradway C, Broden EG, Meghani SH. "I had a lot more planned": the existential dimensions of prognosis communication with adults with advanced cancer. *J Palliat Med.* 2021;24(10):1443–1454. doi:10.1089/jpm.2020.0696

59. Brebach R, Sharpe L, Costa DSJ, Rhodes P, Butow P. Psychological interventions targeting distress for cancer patients: a meta-analytic study investigating uptake and adherence. *Psychooncology.* 2016;25:882–890.

4

Pain and Suffering

Judith A. Paice and Betty R. Ferrell

Introduction

The terms "pain" and "suffering" are so closely associated that they are often used in unison: "The patient is experiencing great pain and suffering." While many factors contribute to the experience of suffering, the presence of pain is often viewed as a central cause and even considered synonymous with suffering. Pain is described with words such as horrendous, unbearable, uncontrollable, unimaginable, extreme, and agonizing. The language of pain is an indicator of the deep psychological and existential dimensions of this physical sensation.

From the earliest exploration of the human experience of pain, scientists have acknowledged that it is more than a neurologic event. The disciplines of nursing, medicine, psychology, and psychiatry as well as basic scientists have described the complex, intense response to this physiologic event.[1-4] Since the 1960s with the advent of the hospice movement, pain has been recognized by pioneers such as Dame Cicely Saunders as a "whole person" experience, "total pain," and "a bio-psycho-social" phenomenon. Psychiatrists including Victor Frankl and Harvey Chochinov have extended this inquiry by studying the meaning of suffering and transcendence associated with serious illness.

Nurses, as the professionals most often present across all settings of care, provide attention to pain and suffering in daily practice.[5] Nurses assess the underlying cause of pain, administer medications, provide nonpharmacologic and complementary therapies, and evaluate the patient's response. Nurses also bear witness to pain and its associated suffering through presence, listening, and silence. The call-bell request of "I need my pain medication" is often a real message of "I am suffering" and a plea for a compassionate presence.

Figure 4.1 captures this whole-person experience of pain and the overlapping dimensions of physical, psychological, social, and spiritual well-being impacted by pain. The experiences of pain and suffering are distinct yet closely interwoven into the daily lives of people living with pain.

Pain and Physical Well-Being

People experiencing chronic painful syndromes, such as low back pain, and life-threatening illness, such as widespread cancers with extensive bone metastasis, provide models of the association of pain with overall physical well-being. Pain is often

Judith A. Paice and Betty R. Ferrell, *Pain and Suffering* In: *The Nature of Suffering and the Goals of Nursing*. Second Edition.
Edited by: William E. Rosa and Betty R. Ferrell, Oxford University Press. © Oxford University Press 2023.
DOI: 10.1093/oso/9780197667934.003.0004

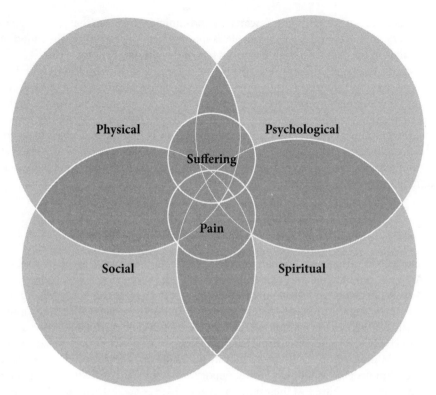

Figure 4.1 Integration of the Ferrell quality-of-life model with the concepts of pain and suffering.

accompanied by numerous other symptoms; for example, the patient who takes opioids for pain associated with a pancreatic tumor often then experiences opioid-induced nausea and constipation. The relief of pain can cause new sources of discomfort and significantly add to suffering.[6]

On a daily basis patients with pain associated with serious illness negotiate the balance of pain relief and the price of pain relief. For example, an elderly man with late-stage prostate cancer and pain associated with bone metastases may limit his use of pain medications in order to avoid becoming lethargic so that he can drive to visit his father each day in a nursing home. His compromised pain relief increases his physical pain and suffering but his choice supports his existential need to "be a good man" and "a good son." Upon deeper listening to this man's pain treatment choices, the nurse caring for him also learns of his even deeper angst, and suffering, as he recognizes that he may die and leave his father alone.

Patients often describe the development of pain as a pivotal point in their illness. They frequently share how they lived and coped with a chronic or serious illness "until the pain began." Central to this experience is often that pain led to decreased function, informing a loss of independence, isolation, depression, increased burden on caregivers, and the beginning of a "downward spiral." A very common theme in the literature and our work as nurse researchers and clinicians has been that pain is a constant reminder of the illness and a relentless source of fear for the future. The suffering attributed to the pain is often an unspoken fear of the ultimate concern: death.

Patients repeatedly describe their pain as a key source of their suffering, and they also share a sense of betrayal by their own bodies as the pain "takes over" their life. For many people, pain may have been the first symptom they experienced that led to the initial diagnosis of a life-threatening illness. The "headache" is actually a brain tumor and the shooting pain from the back to hip may be the beginning of decades of severe rheumatoid disease altering all life plans, changing roles, dependence, intimacy, and meaning in life. Across many diagnoses, there is a frequent association of pain with diminished quality of life and a loss of control.

Pain and Its Impact on Social Well-Being

The negative consequences of pain on social health and well-being are extensive, affecting not only the person with pain but also their loved ones, nurses, other professional caregivers, and the community. People with chronic pain experience great losses, including a shrinking social sphere. Being unable to work or gather with family and friends increases isolation and reduces the support and nurturing gained from these activities. Families often experience impaired social health as they take on more responsibilities within the home previously performed by the person in pain. Their worlds diminish too as they have fewer opportunities for social activities. Loved ones often remark they have lost their partner to pain. Nurses and other professionals experience moral distress at witnessing pain and suffering. And our communities lose the benefits of productive members of society when people in pain or their caregivers can no longer work.

Suffering becomes a shared experience as family members witness pain and as they often feel inadequate in their attempts to provide pain relief. Caregivers of patients at the end of life often derive great meaning from their ability to diminish the patient's pain, or, conversely, they may suffer immensely if they are unable to relieve the patient's pain. These feelings extend into bereavement and caregivers often voice the experience as a key aspect of their grief.[7]

People in Pain

One in five people describe having chronic pain, with close to 7.4% reporting high-impact pain.[8] High-impact pain is defined as pain that limits life or work activities and has negative social consequences. Pain can lead to reduced productivity at work, missed days on the job, and even loss of employment. Financial stress ensues, along with feelings of shame or embarrassment, all contributing to further isolation and diminished social well-being.[9] Unemployment can be particularly disastrous for the person in pain as health care insurance may be tied to one's job.

Because pain is more prevalent in older age, elderly adults are more likely to experience significant pain.[8] Living with chronic pain as an older adult restricts activities of daily living and limits access to the world and people around them.[10] The resultant loneliness and isolation, along with a sense that health care professionals do not believe them or have few treatment options, lead them to suffer in silence.[11]

Family

Family members take on new responsibilities when a loved one becomes disabled by pain.[12] These obligations often include increased time spent in doing household chores and greater responsibility in coordinating their loved one's medical care.[13] Many partners report changes in their own employment while having to carry out this new caregiver role.[14] While responsibilities increase, intimacy may decrease. Severe pain hinders sexual activity, and medications used to treat pain can reduce libido and performance. At a time when greater connection is needed, sexual satisfaction and intimacy for both patient and partner are diminished.

Professionals

Nurses are constant witnesses to patients' pain. Moral distress ensues when nurses perceive they are unable to provide adequate relief, particularly when they know better pain control is possible.[15] Some nurses respond to this distress through avoidance behaviors, such as declining to acknowledge or assess the patient's pain by focusing on other tasks. They may spend less time with the patient or use communication that limits the patient's report of pain, such as "It cannot be that bad." Other examples of avoidance include reluctance to contact the prescribing provider for modifications in the medication regimen. And while some nurses may become hardened or avoid managing the pain, others become so distressed that they change jobs or leave the profession. The moral distress associated with observing pain and suffering is often cited as a key reason for nurses' distress.[16,17]

Community

The health of communities is greatly affected by the social effects of unrelieved pain. Pain strains communities through lost productivity when those in pain work fewer hours or are unable to work at all. Medical costs increase. Volunteerism declines for patients and their loved ones. And unfortunately, the most vulnerable, disadvantaged populations and communities are the most deeply affected. Chronic pain is strongly associated with high disability, low educational level, manual occupations, and economic difficulty.[18,19] These factors are also more common in communities predominantly composed of Black, Indigenous, and People of Color (BIPOC). Chronic pain is similarly more prevalent in rural communities, settings already lacking adequate access to health care and other resources.[8]

Because moderate to severe chronic pain is often treated with opioids, lack of early attention to safety issues to mitigate misuse and diversion can lead to inappropriate access of these medications within the community.[20,21] These patterns have sparked the substance use disorder epidemic and confusion about prescribing practices in clinical, scholarly, and policy settings. Although currently fueled primarily by illicit fentanyl and other substances rather than prescription opioids, this epidemic has exploded, with more than 100,000 deaths in the United States during 1 year.[22] The devastating effect on communities includes loss of lives and widespread grief, an increase in the number of children without parents, diminished social connections, lost productivity, and strained community resources. Efforts to mitigate the epidemic have had unintended consequences. The number of opioid-related deaths continues to grow despite a marked decrease in opioid prescribing overall, including for those with cancer. This reduction is associated with an increase in pain-related emergency admissions and hospitalizations.[23] And as with chronic pain, disadvantaged communities are greatly affected by the epidemic and efforts to mitigate these opioid-related deaths, including those serving BIPOC and rural settings.

Pain and Its Impact on Psychological Well-Being

Social health and psychological well-being are inextricable. The social isolation associated with pain contributes to loneliness, depression, and other negative emotions, and these psychological effects impair social health. Pain is defined as "an unpleasant sensory and emotional experience," which illustrates the fundamental contribution of psychological elements to this phenomenon.[24] As a result, the consequences of chronic pain on psychological health are significant. Studies consistently demonstrate that people with chronic pain report higher levels of depression, anxiety, somatization, anger, and impaired emotional functioning.[25,26]

These negative emotions make it more difficult for people to cope with chronic pain. Exacerbating coping difficulties is the effect of pain and anxiety on sleep, further reducing energy levels and inhibiting exercise. All of these interact to worsen pain and psychological health, leading to what is often referred to as the "chronic pain cycle." Interdisciplinary pain programs aim to treat anxiety, manage sleep disorders, improve activity, and enhance coping skills.

People with poorly understood pain syndromes, such as fibromyalgia, experience additional psychological stress as their reports of pain may not be believed by professionals or their loved ones. People with serious illness face another emotional challenge—uncertainty. Those who have been diagnosed with cancer often report the constant stress of not knowing "when the other shoe will drop."[27] Since pain is often an early warning sign of cancer, any report of pain is then perceived as an indication the cancer has recurred.

A related response is catastrophizing, in which the individual in pain tends to magnify the intensity, feels helpless, and ruminates endlessly about the pain. This has been described in acute and chronic pain, as well as in many underlying etiologies (including arthritis, back pain, cancer, fibromyalgia, interstitial cystitis, musculoskeletal pain syndromes, pelvic pain, and sickle cell pain).[28] In experiments using painful stimuli in healthy volunteers, having control over the stimulation reduced the suffering component of the painful experience.[29] In another study of experimental pain, suffering, but not pain intensity, was associated with fear of pain.[30] All of these findings support the complexity of psychological responses to pain and reinforce the need to address psychological well-being and health in those experiencing pain.

While psychological needs are addressed by many professionals including psychologists, psychiatrists, and social workers, nurses also play a critical role in assessing and responding to psychological concerns and the resulting impact on suffering. Mindful presence, deep listening, and empathic verbal and nonverbal communication skills are essential as nurses assess psychological well-being and plan interventions for psychological symptoms. The ability to illicit the patient's story, be present as they describe the psychological effects of pain, and respond with compassion are at the center of nursing practice.

Pain and Spiritual/Existential Well-Being

Clinicians and researchers have recognized the strong association of pain with psychological symptoms such as anxiety, depression, and fear.[31,32] Pain is also described as an existential experience, associated with questioning God or a higher power. The question of "why me?" by those living with serious illness often extends to "and why must I be in pain?"

Living with severe pain may lead the person to wish for death.[33] People living with chronic pain may confide in the nurse their deepest feelings of being exhausted from living with pain and being "ready for this to end." Nurses are often engaged in intimate conversations as patients living with serious illness and pain speak of seeking forgiveness for life events and regrets. Hospice and palliative care teams assess existential and spiritual concerns and help the patient obtain spiritual care from chaplains, but this is also a responsibility of all members of the team.

Responding to suffering is by no means limited to hospice and palliative care. Nurses in neonatal intensive care units, emergency departments, nursing homes, dialysis centers, rehabilitation clinics, and every setting of care encounter suffering in their daily practice.[34]

The multiple dimensions of pain and suffering also often reflect culturally based values and traditions. The expression of pain, ranging from silence or stoicism to loud moaning or wailing, is often reflective of culturally based norms of communication, roles, and beliefs.

Pain is often the constant reminder of the seriousness of the illness, such as in the case of a diabetic whose peripheral neuropathy creates a constant awareness of an illness that will likely progress and further impact daily life. Pain is frequently associated with recognition of mortality, such as in the case of a woman living with ovarian cancer and whose abdominal pain is the trigger for paralyzing fear that the cancer is spreading.[35,36]

Case Exemplars 4.1 and 4.2 illustrate the intersection between pain and suffering. Pain and suffering are often linked: assessment and treatment share certain commonalities, and effective relief can lead to improved quality of life.

Case Exemplar 4.1

Pain Relief with Ongoing Suffering

Nan Henry is a 75-year-old woman with pancreatic cancer who was initially seen for severe right upper quadrant pain. After undergoing a celiac plexus block, she reported that the pain was completely relieved. However, the oncology nurse noted that Nan appeared to continue to be distressed and was often tearful. As the nurse used quiet presence and open-ended questioning, Nan revealed that because of her physical decline, she and her husband had to move in with her daughter and son-in-law and their small children. Although she valued the time with her very energetic grandchildren, she greatly missed being in her own home and being with her friends in her old neighborhood. She hated having to use a walker and her loss of independence. Nan's husband had early dementia and she felt great stress having to provide care for him. Her anxiety escalated and she slept poorly. She feared death and the future felt "like a black hole." She felt betrayed by her body and abandoned by God.

The oncology nurse had already begun providing generalist-level palliative care by eliciting Nan's worries and fears with compassion. She also realized that because Nan's suffering was complex, she would require more specialized care and consulted the palliative care team. Through the work of the entire team—nurses, physicians, chaplains, and social work—Nan was able to describe her values and goals with team members. Nan's anxiety and sleeplessness were addressed. The team guided her to identify spiritual beliefs and rituals that might bring her strength. She learned to accept her strengths and forgive her faults. Through this work, Nan became less anxious and began to slowly realize the things that brought meaning to her life. She engaged in life review and began to compose letters to her family to share at important future events in their lives, such as graduations and birthdays. This work did not negate the fact that Nan has a serious illness that will lead to her death, yet it allowed her the dignity and peace to appreciate the sacredness of her life.

Case Exemplar 4.2

Relief of Suffering Despite Ongoing Pain

Felipe Gonzalez had a great job in construction. He enjoyed the work, the collegiality on the job site, and the income, especially with lots of overtime pay. At age 45, he was at the prime of his life and proud that he was able to provide for his wife and three teenage children. Everything changed when he suffered an injury on the job resulting in severe, chronic back pain. He was told surgery was not indicated, his medications were ineffective, and after numerous visits to specialists, he gave up on any hope of relief. He could no longer work or be physically active and his wife reported that he spent most of the day on the couch drinking beer. Although initially supportive, his wife grew weary of his inactivity, his drinking, his anger, and her increased workload. She felt he was a stranger, no longer the man she had married. Their children felt the increased tension; over time they spent less time at home and their grades in school suffered. Felipe feared his life was disintegrating and his family was falling apart, yet he felt powerless to make a change.

After presenting him with an ultimatum that she would leave him if he did not get help, Felipe went to his primary care clinic. The nurse practitioner suggested an interdisciplinary pain clinic composed of physicians, nurses, physical and occupational therapists, psychologists, dieticians, and others. Felipe was skeptical but reluctantly agreed to try this approach as nothing else had worked. After thorough evaluation, Felipe developed short- and long-term goals with the team. He underwent extensive physical and occupational therapy, which initially worsened his pain. Ready to give up at times, he stuck with the program and gradually, over time, he noted it was a little easier to move without severe worsening of the back pain. He learned healthy eating techniques and how to recognize stress eating that was adding weight to his frame. The psychologists offered strategies to assist with optimal coping and learning to live despite pain. His wife attended sessions designed to foster family growth and healing. The team helped him meet his long-term goal to return to work by referring him for work training opportunities that would provide skills for a job that did not require physical labor.

At the end of the program, Felipe observed with wonder that although he still had pain, he felt more energy, was able to move, and was more optimistic about the future. He was no longer suffering.

Treatment of Pain and Suffering

As both pain and suffering affect all aspects of the person's quality of life, successful relief must include comprehensive assessment followed by interdisciplinary care. The core components of pain assessment have been well described and align with the quality-of-life model—physical, psychological, social, and spiritual components. Physical aspects of pain assessment are well known to nurses and include location, quality, intensity, and frequency, along with factors that alleviate or aggravate the pain. Less attention has been paid to the assessment of the other components of the model. Probing questions may include: How does this pain affect your ability to be with family and friends or to participate in the activities you enjoy? In what way does the pain influence your mood? What gives you strength throughout this experience? Does pain test this strength or your spirit? The insightful nurse will incorporate these responses to build a wholistic approach to pain relief, integrating the interdisciplinary team.

Despite the fact that relief of suffering is the goal of palliative care,[37] the assessment of suffering is less well established. Part of this absence of attention is due to a lack of a universally accepted definition of suffering or an established framework for this phenomenon. Suffering is defined as distress that occurs when a person's whole-ness is threatened, disrupted, or injured (Cassell).[38] Suffering, alone or occurring in the presence of pain, is a subjective, negative affective experience.[39] Although pain and suffering are distinct, both are subjective experiences that are often interrelated. Similar to pain, suffering incorporates physical, psychological, social, and spiritual dimensions.

The assessment of pain and suffering drives appropriate management and is guided by the quality-of-life model. Physical measures may include interventions to address pain and other symptoms, including pharmacology, physical therapy, heat or cold, and massage, along with invasive procedures. Attention to psycho-logic factors starts with believing the person's report of pain and dismissing con-cerns that it is "all in their head." Counseling, coaching, and mindfulness address the aspects of pain and suffering that relate to psychological factors. Social variables can be attended to through interventions designed to return the person to their so-cial settings, ranging from returning to work to simply being able to be with family and loved ones; rehabilitation, retraining, and other support services encourage these efforts. The spiritual domain is addressed through inquiry, counseling, prayer, legacy making, and other efforts to enhance resilience, provide purpose, and sup-port transcendence.

Responses to Suffering

The compassionate nurse will respond to pain and suffering with presence, inviting the individual to share their experiences. Listening, and using strong communication techniques that gently elicit thoughtful replies, is truly the core of nursing assessment. The insightful nurse will consider the whole person and all the domains that may con-tribute to pain and suffering: physical, psychological, social, and spiritual. Nurses pro-vide reassurance that the patient's reports are believed and taken seriously and the team will attend to their pain and suffering. Reframing the meaning of the patient's distress is especially important when patients or their loved ones view pain and suf-fering as punishment, weakness, or a result of some failing. Nurses deliver many of the interventions designed to relieve pain and suffering or they are primary sources of referrals to their colleagues to provide these services. Nurses also bring the team to-gether to ensure continuity throughout the course of care.

Nurses amplify the voices of those in pain and suffering through their clinical expertise, patient advocacy, interdisciplinary collaboration, and leadership. Nurses are uniquely prepared, and well positioned, to address pain and suffering. Nurses are the most trusted of all health care professionals and have the most contact with patients. Nurses have a moral responsibility to not only address the pain and suf-fering of each individual in their care but also advocate for vulnerable populations, such as disadvantaged communities, uninsured individuals, children, the elderly, those with substance use disorder, and the disabled. These are populations that have traditionally received inadequate attention and treatment of pain due to mispercep-tions and stigma.

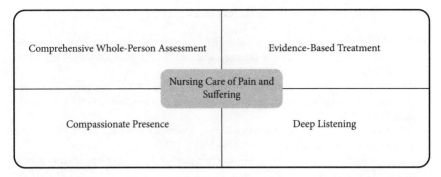

Figure 4.2 Nursing care of pain and suffering.

Amid pain and suffering, nurses need to carefully examine their own purpose to remain whole and fully present. Nurses need the courage to acknowledge the loss and grief inherent in caring for people who are in pain and suffering and continue their own ongoing healing. Building personal awareness through self-reflection and the support of colleagues will help nurses find balance and meaning as they bear witness to intense pain and suffering.

Figure 4.2 illustrates the dimensions of nursing care of people in pain. Nurses expertly apply comprehensive whole-person assessment to determine the cause of the pain and its impact on the person experiencing it. Nurses apply evidence-based practice as they deliver care, including patient teaching and support and pharmacologic and integrative therapies. They also provide compassionate presence and deep listening as essential skills to address pain and suffering.

Conclusion

Pain and suffering are all too common in our contemporary health care systems, particularly amid the growing global burden of chronic illnesses. The complexities of our current organizations often leave patients feeling lost and uncared for at a deeply vulnerable time in their lives. The unintended consequences of efforts to mitigate the epidemic of substance-related deaths have created challenges in accessing pain treatment along with profound stigma, affecting all patients, but particularly damaging for disadvantaged communities. Thoughtful nurses begin the healing process with their presence in the face of pain and suffering, listening to and eliciting the patient's story. Empathy and skill are crucial so that people who are in pain and suffering feel heard and valued. Compassion is essential but, without knowledge about the current evidence of effective therapies, is insufficient in addressing these serious issues. Expertise in selecting and delivering treatment options tailored to address all domains of quality of life is essential. To remain intact and whole while relieving intense pain and suffering, nurses must reflect on their own practice as they continue this meaningful work.

References

1. Al Kalaldeh M, Shosha GA, Saiah N, Salameh O. Dimensions of phenomenology in exploring patient's suffering in long-life illnesses: qualitative evidence synthesis. *J Patient Exp.* 2018;5(1):43–49.

2. Amonoo HL, Harris JH, Murphy WS, Abrahm JL, Peteet JR. The physician's role in responding to existential suffering: what does it mean to comfort always? *J Palliat Care.* 2020;35(1):8–12.

3. An E, Lo C, Hales S, Zimmermann C, Rodin G. Demoralization and death anxiety in advanced cancer. *Psychooncology.* 2018;27(11):2566–2572.

4. Beng TS, Ann YH, Guan NC, et al. The suffering pictogram: measuring suffering in palliative care. *J Palliat Med.* 2017;20(8):869–874.

5. Tan SB, Loh EC, Lam CL, Ng CG, Lim EJ, Boey CCM. Psychological processes of suffering of palliative care patients in Malaysia: a thematic analysis. *BMJ Support Palliat Care.* 2019;9(1):e19.

6. Chung BPM, Olofsson J, Wong FKY, Ramgard M. Overcoming existential loneliness: a cross-cultural study. *BMC Geriatr.* 2020;20(1):347.

7. De Laurentis M, Rossana B, Andrea B, Riccardo T, Valentina I. The impact of social-emotional context in chronic cancer pain: patient-caregiver reverberations: social-emotional context in chronic cancer pain. *Support Care Cancer.* 2019;27(2):705–713.

8. Zelaya CE, Dahlhamer JM, Lucas JW, Connor EM. Chronic pain and high-impact chronic pain among U.S. adults, 2019. NCHS Data Brief. 2020 Nov;(390):1–8. PMID: 33151145. https://www.ncbi.nlm.nih.gov/pubmed/33151145

9. Iskandar AC, Rochmawati E, Wiechula R. Patient's experiences of suffering across the cancer trajectory: a qualitative systematic review protocol. *J Adv Nurs.* 2021;77(2):1037–1042.

10. Devik SA, Hellzen O, Enmarker I. Bereaved family members' perspectives on suffering among older rural cancer patients in palliative home nursing care: a qualitative study. *Eur J Cancer Care.* 2017;26(e12609):1–9.

11. Gillsjo C, Nassen K, Berglund M. Suffering in silence: a qualitative study of older adults' experiences of living with long-term musculoskeletal pain at home. *Eur J Ageing.* 2021;18(1):55–63. https://doi.org/10.1007/s10433-020-00566-7

12. Davis MP, Rybicki LA, Samala RV, Patel C, Parala-Metz A, Lagman R. Pain or fatigue: which correlates more with suffering in hospitalized cancer patients? *Support Care Cancer.* 2021;29(8):4535–4542.

13. Siler S, Borneman T, Ferrell B. Pain and suffering. *Semin Oncol Nurs.* 2019;35(3):310–314.

14. Suso-Ribera C, Yakobov E, Carriere JS, Garcia-Palacios A. The impact of chronic pain on patients and spouses: consequences on occupational status, distribution of household chores and care-giving burden. *Eur J Pain (London, England).* 2020;24(9):1730–1740. https://doi.org/10.1002/ejp.1616

15. Bernhofer EI, Sorrell JM. Nurses managing patients' pain may experience moral distress. *Clin Nurs Res.* 2015;24(4):401–414.

16. Marterre B, Clayville K. Navigating the murky waters of hope, fear, and spiritual suffering: an expert co-captain's guide. *Surg Clin North Am.* 2019;99(5):991–1018.

17. Renz M, Reichmuth O, Bueche D, et al. Fear, pain, denial, and spiritual experiences in dying processes. *Am J Hosp Palliat Care.* 2018;35(3):478–491.

18. Glei DA, Weinstein M. Disadvantaged Americans are suffering the brunt of rising pain and physical limitations. *PloS One.* 2021;16(12):e0261375. https://doi.org/10.1371/journal.pone.0261375

19. Fagerlund P, Salmela J, Pietilainen O, Salonsalmi A, Rahkonen O, Lallukka T. Life-course socioeconomic circumstances in acute, chronic and disabling pain among young

employees: a double suffering. *Scand J Public Health*. 2023;51(1):257–267. https://doi.org/10.1177/14034948211062314

20. Paice JA. Risk assessment and monitoring of patients with cancer receiving opioid therapy. *Oncologist*. 2019;24(10):1294–1298. https://doi.org/10.1634/theoncologist.2019-0301

21. Paice JA. Pain in cancer survivors: how to manage. *Curr Treat Options Oncol*. 2019;20(6):48. https://doi.org/10.1007/s11864-019-0647-0

22. Centers for Disease Control and Prevention. Drug overdose deaths in the U.S. top 100,000 annually. Published November 17, 2021. Accessed March 15, 2022. https://www.cdc.gov/nchs/pressroom/nchs_press_releases/2021/20211117.htm

23. Enzinger AC, Ghosh K, Keating NL, Cutler DM, Landrum MB, Wright AA. US trends in opioid access among patients with poor prognosis cancer near the end-of-life. *J Clin Oncol*. 2021;39(26):2948–2958.

24. Treede RD, Rief W, Barke A, et al. Chronic pain as a symptom or a disease: the IASP Classification of Chronic Pain for the International Classification of Diseases (ICD-11). *Pain*. 2019;160(1):19–27.

25. D'Aiuto C, Gamm S, Grenier S, Vasiliadis HM. The association between chronic pain conditions and subclinical and clinical anxiety among community-dwelling older adults consulting in primary care. *Pain Med*. 2021;23(6):1118–1126. https://doi.org/10.1093/pm/pnab213

26. Burke AL, Mathias JL, Denson LA. Psychological functioning of people living with chronic pain: a meta-analytic review. *Br J Clin Psychol*. 2015;54(3):345–360.

27. Heathcote LC, Eccleston C. Pain and cancer survival: a cognitive-affective model of symptom appraisal and the uncertain threat of disease recurrence. *Pain*. 2017;158(7):1187–1191. https://doi.org/10.1097/j.pain.0000000000000872

28. Petrini L, Arendt-Nielsen L. Understanding pain catastrophizing: putting pieces together. *Front Psychol*. 2020;11:603420. https://doi.org/10.3389/fpsyg.2020.603420

29. Loffler M, Kamping S, Brunner M, et al. Impact of controllability on pain and suffering. *Pain Rep*. 2018;3(6):e694. https://doi.org/10.1097/PR9.0000000000000694

30. Bustan S, Gonzalez-Roldan AM, Schommer C, et al. Psychological, cognitive factors and contextual influences in pain and pain-related suffering as revealed by a combined qualitative and quantitative assessment approach. *PloS One*. 2018;13(7):e0199814. https://doi.org/10.1371/journal.pone.0199814

31. Bovero A, Sedghi NA, Opezzo M, et al. Dignity-related existential distress in end-of-life cancer patients: prevalence, underlying factors, and associated coping strategies. *Psychooncology*. 2018;27(11):2631–2637.

32. Bueno-Gomez N. Conceptualizing suffering and pain. *Philos Ethics Humanit Med*. 2017;12(1):7.

33. Gillsjo C, Nassen K, Berglund M. Suffering in silence: a qualitative study of older adults' experiences of living with long-term musculoskeletal pain at home. *Eur J Ageing*. 2021;18(1):55–63.

34. Granek L, Nakash O, Ariad S, et al. From will to live to will to die: oncologists, nurses, and social workers identification of suicidality in cancer patients. *Support Care Cancer*. 2017;25(12):3691–3702.

35. Grech A, Marks A. Existential suffering part 2: clinical response and management #320. *J Palliat Med*. 2017;20(1):95–96.

36. Hall M, Shannonhouse L, Aten J, McMartin J, Silverman E. Religion-specific resources for meaning-making from suffering: defining the territory. *Ment Health Relig Cult*. 2018;21(1):77–92.

37. World Health Organization. Palliative care. Published August 5, 2020. Accessed March 15, 2022. https://www.who.int/news-room/fact-sheets/detail/palliative-care

38. Cassell EJ. *The Nature of Suffering and the Goals of Medicine*. 2nd ed. New York, NY: Oxford University Press, Incorporated; 1994.
39. Stilwell P, Hudon A, Meldrum K, Page MG, Wideman TH. What is pain-related suffering? conceptual critiques, key attributes, and outstanding questions. *J Pain*. 2021;23(5):729–738. https://doi.org/10.1016/j.jpain.2021.11.005

5

Suffering of Infants, Parents, and Families

Elena Abascal and Frances T. McCarthy

Although the world is full of suffering, it is full also of the overcoming of it.
—Helen Keller

The Changing Landscape of Suffering for Infants, Parents, and Families

There was a time, not long ago, when the idea of a baby dying or being born ill, far from being shocking, was a part of everyday life. At the turn of the 20th century, nearly 30% of all deaths occurred in children under 5.[1] Suffering the loss of a baby was a tragic but not uncommon part of daily life. This commonality made public displays of suffering an acceptable and even encouraged part of mourning a child. Bereaved parents and families would wear black for months after the death of a baby, and they often commissioned artwork, jewelry, and later photography in remembrance of their child.[1] In one of the most recognizable portraits to arise from the 18th century, Marie Antoinette is seated with her three living children standing around her. Next to her, a large and opulent bassinet belonging to her infant daughter, who had died weeks earlier, lays empty.

Today, such profound suffering during this stage of life can seem almost inconceivable—in some ways, for good reason. Thanks to public health advances and social reforms, many pregnancy losses and infant deaths and illnesses can now be treated or prevented.[2] Advances in the fields of genetics and ultrasonography have made prenatal testing possible, providing individuals with insight into their baby's health long before birth. And thanks to advances in the fields of neonatology and pediatrics, today, many infants who historically would certainly have died can be saved.

However, despite these leaps forward, suffering during pregnancy and infancy is far from eliminated. The infant mortality rate in the United States remains higher than most other high-income nations, and disparities by race and ethnicity further complicate what is undoubtedly a health crisis.[3] Furthermore, the treatments currently available for medically complex babies can be painful and highly distressing for both the child and their parents, and an infant's inability to communicate their level of suffering can make caring for these patients enormously challenging. The nature of suffering during pregnancy and infancy has certainly evolved in response to medical and social advances, but its impact on patients has been anything but lessened.

Elena Abascal and Frances T. McCarthy, *Suffering of Infants, Parents, and Families* In: *The Nature of Suffering and the Goals of Nursing*. Second Edition. Edited by: William E. Rosa and Betty R. Ferrell, Oxford University Press. © Oxford University Press 2023. DOI: 10.1093/oso/9780197667934.003.0005

The Nature of Perinatal Suffering

For many families, pregnancy is one of life's most joyful periods. It can be a time of wondrous anticipation and hopeful preparation. But when circumstances change and a pregnancy ends in heartbreak, the physical, psychological, and social suffering can be devastating. Every issue that impacts those who are pregnant and their families deserves recognition and analysis from the nursing perspective. However, this section will focus on just two very specific causes of suffering during the perinatal period: perinatal loss (e.g., miscarriages and stillbirths) and loss of the "perfect" pregnancy due to prenatal diagnoses of life-limiting or life-threatening conditions.

When a pregnancy ends in loss, families grieve more than just the *idea* of their baby. These families grieve the hopes, dreams, and plans they had for their child. They grieve the excitement of imagining their new baby—what they will look like, which parent they will take after, and what their personality will be like. They grieve about the future they had planned together: family vacations, holidays, school graduations, weddings, and maybe even the birth of a grandchild many years down the road. There can also be the loss of social support and of important relationships, with many families feeling as though they have "disappointed" their loved ones by not achieving the perfect healthy pregnancy. It's impact on couples is especially visible, with as many as 22% of couples separating after a miscarriage and nearly 40% after a stillbirth.[4] There can be a loss of faith and of one's trust in a higher power or the natural order of life, or whatever one believes in. When a pregnancy is perfect, individuals and communities alike have a chance at renewed hope, unconditional love, and the opportunity to achieve more than they can alone. When pregnancies lose their ability to instill hope and joy, there can be enormous suffering for all of those who were invested in welcoming this new child.

Suffering, in whatever context it occurs, is never unidimensional. Even physical injuries, such as a burn, beget a range of experiences: pain alone does not explain the injured person's suffering. A burn is more than just a wound; it's an experience made up of sensations and emotions, such as the shock of touching a burning surface, the fear of wondering if the body has been irreparably damaged, and regret over the events that led up to the injury. Life-limiting or life-threatening prenatal conditions as well as perinatal losses are similarly multidimensional. There are physical, psychological, and social consequences of losing a pregnancy, facing the possibility of a baby's short life, or preparing for the birth of a child with medical needs. To understand the nature of perinatal suffering, nurses must look at the collective impact of these experiences.

Physical Suffering During Miscarriages and Stillbirths

Physical pain has a purpose. It alerts us when something is wrong, when we are injured, or when we are ill. It is an evolutionary trait that has helped humans survive by discouraging us from doing things that may cause us harm, for example, touching an open flame, and encouraging us to do things that will protect us from pain, such as wearing warm clothing in the winter. Pain can be tolerated when it has meaning and purpose. Medical procedures, treatments, or medications may cause great pain and discomfort, but patients endure them if they feel they have something to gain by doing so. Pregnancy and childbirth are undoubtedly physically uncomfortable and painful experiences. Regardless of how seamlessly a pregnancy progresses, there are still moments of great physical unpleasantness: nausea, swelling, and muscular pain, to name just a few. And no matter the method of childbirth, vaginal or cesarean, with or without anesthesia, there is always some amount of pain before, during, or after delivery. Yet, despite the known physical suffering of pregnancy and labor, it's estimated that 140 million babies were born in 2021.[5] What makes this pain tolerable for so many is the knowledge that their pain will soon be replaced by the joy of meeting their child. For those experiencing a perinatal loss, pain is endured without any such promise of reward.

Consider the experience of miscarrying. When an individual suffers a miscarriage, there can be physical pain coupled with immense anxiety and even fear. In the United States, miscarriages are managed either surgically (commonly dilation and curettage), medically (using pharmacological agents such as misoprostol), or expectantly (when patients are discharged from the hospital and miscarry at home).[6] Regardless of the method or management, women who have experienced a miscarriage often describe feeling ill-prepared by their clinicians for what it will physically be like to miscarry. They were not told how painful the experience can be, how long it can take, or what is physically taking place inside their body. Many have felt frightened by the amount of blood they lost, particularly because they did not feel prepared to recognize at what point emergency care should be sought out. Even after the miscarriage has occurred, women may continue to experience physical pain while also managing the aftermath of their loss, such as self-monitoring for signs of infection after surgical management or disposing of fetal remains at home. This unpreparedness for an experience as physically arduous as a miscarriage can cause enormous shame for those experiencing the loss.

For families who learn through prenatal testing that their child has a life-limiting or life-threatening condition, there can be enormous anxiety about the physical suffering of their unborn baby. Words such as "condition" or "syndrome" can have strong associations with pain and suffering, and so for some parents, prenatal diagnoses can conjure up images of a baby in agony. They may research the diagnosis online and find anecdotes from others whose children share the same diagnosis or images of older children with the condition. These may include detailed descriptions of invasive surgeries and procedures, stories about medical trauma, and imagery that can be shocking to those who are just learning about this condition for the first time. Families may not understand that although this information can provide some idea of what life *may* be like for their child in the future, they do not accurately reflect how their baby experiences the condition currently in the womb. The capacity to interpret pain and differentiate it from other sensations does not develop until the latter portion of the third trimester.[7] Moreover, even after a baby is born, there are many conditions that are associated with physical alterations but are not "painful." For example, Trisomy 21, the most common chromosomal alteration in humans, is not an inherently "painful" condition; in fact, research has found that people with Trisomy 21 experience acute and chronic pain with the same frequency as the general population.[8] To address suffering, nurses should be prepared to help parents distinguish between their own suffering and the suffering of their baby.

Psychological and Social Suffering in the Perinatal Population

Although suffering is a personal experience, it rarely happens in isolation from others. Friends and family members have the power to shape one's experience of suffering through their action or inaction. If others feel that one's suffering is justified, they will acknowledge, validate, and hopefully attempt to eliminate it. But when others do not empathize with one's suffering or if they perceive one's suffering as being disproportionate to the causative event, then they will likely disapprove of the kinds of behaviors that are associated with suffering (e.g., crying, grieving). For example, many perinatally bereaved families have faced criticism or a lack of understanding from well-intentioned relatives when they announce that they will be holding a memorial service for a baby who died in pregnancy. These responses can be incredibly isolating.

When others perceive that an individual's response to a loss is outside the bounds of what is socially acceptable, it is referred to as a "disenfranchised loss." This term broadly includes experiences of grief and suffering that others feel are abnormal, unreasonable, or aberrant (e.g., grieving a relative who died while driving under the influence of a substance). Because perinatal losses tend to occur outside of public view, those who have not directly experienced or witnessed a perinatal loss themselves may find it difficult to empathize with those who have. They may feel as though the perinatally bereaved never really "knew" their child, and they may struggle to comprehend how someone can mourn a person who existed so impalpably.

Additionally, many of the rituals and behaviors used to engage with those who are grieving are not socially acceptable in cases of perinatal loss, reinforcing the sense of "otherness" the perinatally bereaved often feel. For example, perinatally bereaved women have described the process of returning to work after a loss to be particularly isolating. Many of the behaviors colleagues may have engaged in for other forms of loss, such as signing a card or offering words of condolence in the hallway, are replaced with hushed tones and averted eyes. Women have described feeling ostracized in their workplaces, avoided by the same colleagues who just a few weeks prior had planned their baby shower or who had gladly covered their shifts during prenatal appointments. Even language limits our ability to engage with the perinatally bereaved: there is no equivalent of "widow" or "orphan" for parents who outlive their children, leaving the perinatally bereaved to wonder, *am I a parent or something else?*

Nurses can advocate for the perinatally bereaved by affirming their "right" to grieve and by using the best available evidence to support the legitimacy of their suffering. A prospective cohort study comparing 492 individuals experiencing a pregnancy loss and 87 individuals whose pregnancies progressed to term found that after 1 month, women in the pregnancy loss cohort were significantly more likely to be diagnosed with posttraumatic stress disorder, anxiety, or depression.[9] The authors noted that despite a decline in distress, it remained significantly elevated even 9 months later.[9] In addition to grief, the perinatally bereaved may experience a sense of powerlessness, fear about the future, or regret about the past.[9]

For families whose pregnancies continue in light of a prenatal diagnosis, there can be profound anxiety about the future. Typically, expectant families feel joy and wonder when they imagine their baby: *Will it be a boy or a girl? Will they have blonde, brown, or red hair? What color will their eyes be?* They imagine a life for their baby full of wondrous milestones—first steps, first words, learning to read or ride a bike—and these are just the early years. When a prenatal diagnosis is discovered, much of that excitement is replaced with fear and anxiety. Despite advances in the field of genetics, prenatal diagnoses are often unable to provide a clear picture of what a child's life will look like after birth. Families may be haunted by questions to which there often are no clear answers: *How long will they live? Will they be able to walk/talk/play? Will they be in pain?* It can be challenging to confront the feeling of futility that arises when a patient's suffering is so deeply rooted in questions we cannot answer and fears we cannot assuage.

Suffering in Newborns and Infants

Suffering is a human condition—from life in the womb to death at any age. But the suffering of babies and infants seems somehow unnatural. It creates tremendous grief for their parents and families that can be profoundly felt and influence their world-view for the rest of their lives. In perinatal palliative care (PPC), suffering of the un-born baby is, thankfully, almost never the case. Very few, if any, prenatally diagnosed life-limiting conditions are actually painful. Prenatally, babies remain blissfully una-ware of the suffering of their parents and families. This fact can be reassuring to the parents, but parental suffering is still very real.[10]

Unfortunately, postnatal suffering of the baby can and does occur. In the neo-natal intensive care unit (NICU), families that choose intensive care must accept that it comes with invasive procedures, tests, potential surgeries, and an interruption in parent-child bonding. Of course, this choice is made in service of the hope that the life of the baby will be spared or, at the very least, improved, and allow for some enjoy-ment and interaction between the baby and their parents, family, and environment. For infants in the pediatric intensive care unit (PICU), with genetic disorders, various syndromes, recovering from surgeries, or who have experienced accidents or injuries, physical suffering can be acute, can be lifelong, or may come and go with exacerbation or remission of underlying conditions. The suffering of infants cannot only be defined by physical pain. In fact, suffering may not involve pain at all, as is discussed in the perinatal section of this chapter. It is a state of being that encompasses emotional, psy-chological, and spiritual experiences, as well as possible physical pain.

Causes of Suffering in Newborns and Infants

What can cause suffering of newborns and infants? Approximately 3% of the more than 3.5 million babies born in the United States will have a congenital birth defect.[11]

This accounts for over 100,000 births per year.[11] Additionally, preterm births account for about 10% of all births in the United States every year.[11] In 2018, the infant mortality rate in the United States was 5.6 deaths per 1,000 live births.[11] More than 21,000 infants died that year.[11] The five leading causes of death in infants are birth defects, preterm birth and low birth weight, injuries, sudden infant death syndrome, and maternal pregnancy complications.[11] Whether born with congenital conditions, prematurity, genetic disorders, accidents, or injuries, newborns and infants can experience suffering long before the moment they may actually die.

The concept of suffering relates not only to physical pain but also to emotional, psychological, moral, and spiritual distress. Patients, parents, and staff alike may experience it. For bedside nurses caring for critically ill infants, suffering comes with the territory. One must expect that in caring for the most fragile and vulnerable population, that of critically ill newborns and infants, exposure to the pain and distress of their patients and of the parents and families of these babies can take a toll over time. Often, nurses spend more time with their tiny charges than parents can. Nurses certainly spend more time in hands-on care than any other member of the health care team and so they directly witness their patient's response to procedures, treatments, medications, and interventions. Some babies and infants are stable enough to tolerate vitals being taken, being suctioned, and being repositioned. In other babies their heart rates, oxygen saturation, or blood pressure drops when care is done. It can be daunting for the bedside nurse to do basic care for fear of the pain and suffering inflicted in keeping these babies alive. In addition, nurses must also care for the parents and families. While this care is not physical in nature, it requires nurses to be emotionally available, compassionate, and empathetic while providing excellent care to their actual patients, the babies.

It is the perception of suffering that can be problematic for both families and the health care workers who care for them and their babies. Who defines suffering: parents or staff? What does the family perceive as suffering? What happens when parents and caregivers don't agree? Almost all parents say that they don't want their babies to suffer, but what do they see as suffering? How can the health care team elicit an understanding of what suffering means to the parents? How much is too much suffering? These questions must be evaluated on an individual basis with parents and caregivers exchanging information, as well as their concerns and hopes for the baby's life.

Indeed, suffering is subjective to some extent and may be considered to be worth enduring, particularly if the end result will be improvement in quality of life, ultimate relief of suffering, or part of the process of healing from a surgery, injury, or illness. Effective communication between parents and caregivers helps to delineate what suffering means to the family. Having them describe how they perceive their baby's situation can give insight into their view of their baby's condition and response to treatment and their personal values and concerns. Asking the question "Do you think your baby is comfortable?" can provide a wealth of information to the health care team. Comfort of the baby is a priority for parents. In a study that examined providing the basic care elements of bonding, maintenance of body temperature, relief of hunger or thirst, and alleviation of discomfort in infants with life-limiting conditions, parents described comfort as more than the absence of pain.[12] They felt that these elements created a caring and supportive experience for their babies and that this was a source of comfort and satisfaction for the parents.[12] Similarly, other research has shown that grief scores were much higher in parents who perceived that their child suffered at the end of life.[13] This demonstrates the importance of utilizing appropriate medication at the EoL to relieve suffering in both the baby and family.

Liminality

Arnold van Gennep, French ethnographer and folklorist, first described liminality, from the Latin *limen*, meaning "threshold," in his seminal work *Les Rites de Passage* in 1909.[15] Liminality is the experience of being betwixt and between, and van Gennep used this term to describe the rites of passage, moving from one state to the next, which is identified by certain roles, rights, and obligations.[14] For families of acutely or chronically ill children or those with life-limiting conditions or injuries, they also inhabit the realm of liminality. They are wondering if, or how, their child will live. They are faced with uncertainty about their baby's prognosis, function, future medical needs, and possible outcomes. What will the future hold for their children and for their families? Are there supports that exist within the community that would allow the infant to return home? Is this a chronic or progressive condition? What impact does their child's condition have on other members of the family? In addition, family resources and socioeconomic status will impact many families' opportunities and decisions.

For families facing EoL decisions, liminality is also part of the process. EoL decision-making in the NICU or PICU is a complicated journey for parents and clinicians alike. How parents and clinicians navigate this journey can have profound effects on all of them. Shared decision-making is associated with lower grief scores in parents.[13] Grief scores have been shown to be higher in the cases of informed decision-making solely by physicians based on medical data. Intermediate grief scores were associated with paternalistic decision-making and no decision-making.[13]

The EoL decision-making process is a complicated one due to parental fear and reluctance of parents to make decisions that affect their child's fate while still wishing to be involved in these discussions and decisions. However, being involved in making these decisions may also help parents feel empowered and may ultimately lead to a sense of peace when the support of nurses and physicians occurs in the process. In practice, families should be given the opportunity to choose the type of decision-making that makes them most comfortable and allows them to make peace with whatever path they choose.

Suffering of Parents and Families

Parents of NICU babies face an environment that is foreign to them. Additionally, they may feel emotionally disconnected from a baby that is too small or ill to be touched or held. Parents can feel increased stress due to the inability to protect their child from pain as well as being unable to provide care for their infant. They perceive themselves as less competent and as having lost their parental role. The severity of their baby's condition also affects their levels of stress and anxiety.[15] Parents of infants in the PICU also face feelings of anxiety, sadness, and grief due to the circumstances of their child's hospitalization. Parents are often torn between care of their hospitalized child and other children at home. They have concerns about balancing the care of their child and maintaining a job, particularly if they are the main breadwinner. Lack of community-based support often leaves many families with few options for home care.

Siblings of hospitalized children also suffer. Young siblings who need care may have to be separated from their parents while they stay with a hospitalized sibling. The disruption of their usual routine, restriction from visiting their sibling, and concern for the well-being of their sibling can cause distress. Children can display a host of responses including somatic complaints, becoming withdrawn, displaying regressive behaviors, and acting out. But the experience is not unequivocally negative: children can also display altruistic behavior, display an increase in independent activities, and develop an understanding about the current situation.[16]

Both parents and families can experience posttraumatic growth. Trauma-informed care can help health care providers connect with families in a constructive and supportive alliance. Trauma-informed care views the traumatic life experiences of parents as having great influence on their interactions with the health care team. In the NICU and PICU, it is the parents' traumatic life experiences that must be understood. These past experiences can produce feelings of inadequacy, guilt, or distrust. These feelings can be exacerbated by the ICU experience and lack of understanding from health care providers. Families can be identified as difficult when in fact they are terrified or reliving past traumas.[17] Empowerment and engagement of families in the care of their babies helps to reinforce parent-child bonds that can help to mitigate this distress and enhance parental confidence.[17] Trauma-informed support is equally important for the well-being of nurses. Creating a supportive environment, reflecting on internal experiences, and debriefing and creating a work culture of awareness and acceptance are all ways to support staff in facing the challenging care of critically ill newborns and infants.[18]

Finally, the spiritual needs of families are an important aspect of care that is responsive to suffering. Spiritual beliefs can be a source of comfort and strength to families. Helping families express their spiritual needs and beliefs, particularly at the EoL, can help many parents find a sense of meaning and peace. Hospital chaplains are expert at supporting spiritual needs in both families and staff, and nurses should feel empowered to advocate for their presence.[19]

Case Exemplar 5.1

A full-term baby is born with a prenatal diagnosis of dysplastic cerebellum and other severe brain anomalies. The mother changed a prenatal plan for comfort care (bonding, maintenance of temperature, feeding/hydration, and medications as needed)[20] at her delivery and asked that the baby be resuscitated. The baby was born limp, with no respiratory effort, and was intubated and placed on a ventilator. No reflexes could be elicited; she had no purposeful movement and could not breathe independently. She was admitted to the NICU for care. In the first week of life, after evaluations by neonatologists and neurologists, a family meeting was held. The prognosis was grim. In addition to the minimally functioning cerebellum, the baby had hydrocephalus, absent corpus callosum, lissencephaly, and minimal cortical tissue. The family was heartbroken but insisted on continuing treatment. The grandparents were very vocal in their insistence that care be continued and their belief that "God would ultimately decide" the baby's fate. The medical and nursing staff voiced concern to each other and also to the family about the baby's future, her dependence on a ventilator, her increasing head size, and the potential for harm to the baby from continuous ventilation, lack of mobility, and difficulty moving and positioning her. This caused the family distress and they began to distrust the health care team. Many nurses felt uncomfortable caring for this baby and interacting with the family. Soon after, the grandmother pointed out that in 30 night shifts, the baby had been taken care of by 30 different nurses.

Eventually, the nurse manager asked an experienced nurse if she would work with this baby and family consistently. The nurse agreed and began to care for the baby whenever she was on duty.

Over time, general care caused the baby to tremor her oxygen saturations and heart rate to drop. In conversations with the mother, the mother expressed sadness and concern about the baby's condition but said, "I don't think I can take her off the breathing machine. I would feel like I killed her. God will decide what to do."

One evening, the grandfather came to visit and gently touched the baby's foot. She immediately began to have tremors that did not stop. Her oxygen saturation decreased and her heart rate slowed. The attending physician was called to the bedside and began to bag the baby with 100% oxygen. The nurse asked the grandfather to call the mother and tell her to come quickly.

When the mother and grandmother arrived, the baby's heart rate was hovering at about 99 bpm and her oxygen saturation was in the 50s. When the mother saw the monitor, she began to cry and asked to hold the baby. After the baby was placed in her arms, the attending physician asked if she would like to have the tube removed and see her baby's face. The mother immediately agreed. The tube was removed and the baby died quickly and peacefully in her mother's arms.

Case Exemplar 5.1 illustrates the need for effective communication in understanding the family's desires and goals of care, the importance of consistent caregivers, the discomfort that can be experienced by bedside nurses and the medical team, the persistent hope families have for a cure or "miracle," and the need for a multidisciplinary care team to create a safe-space environment for families and staff alike. It is not unusual for families to cling to a hope that their baby will get better, a belief that caregivers may deem unrealistic or even impossible. Perceived dismissal of the family's hopes and dreams can create conflict and distrust of the health care team. This results in increased anxiety in the family and staff alike.[21] A trauma-informed approach in this case could have gone a long way for the family and health care providers in establishing a trusting relationship. Debriefing after this case allowed bedside providers to understand the need for this family to be able to know they had done all they could for their daughter despite the outcome.

Responses to Suffering

For many families, pregnancy through infancy is a time of immeasurable joy. But when circumstances change, nurses should be prepared to journey alongside families as they chart a new course. Perinatal and infant suffering can feel senseless—and it very often is. It can be challenging for nurses to find a way to feel comfortable in situations where a positive pregnancy and neonatal period is not possible—as though supporting families faced by these issues implies that nurses have simply accepted this suffering as unavoidable. But responding to suffering through prevention and response is key for ensuring short- and long-term mitigation of suffering for this population.

Although suffering is painful, challenging, and disruptive, it is not universally negative. Posttraumatic growth is possible. The disruption of a person's worldview, whether in parents or caregivers, can be traumatic, but it can lead to personal growth through a reimagining of that worldview or the creation or adoption of a new worldview.[22] In one study, burnout of hospital health care providers was associated with units that had higher admission rates, number of beds, electronic health record (EHR) use, average lengths of stay, and regional level of the institution. It is possible that in larger, busier intensive care units in particular, nurses may feel decreased involvement in the management of patients, underappreciated workload in relation to admissions, and limited interpersonal interaction or time in direct patient care due to EHR use.[23]

Self-care is an integral part of resilience, along with other team and institutional interventions. Self-care requires that one make an effort to do something that benefits oneself. Physical activity, personal relationships, and mindfulness and spirituality practices can help nurses release the stress and anxiety that can build up when caring for newborns and infants in the ICU and reset emotionally, psychologically, and spiritually.[23–25] Engaging with leadership to provide support to staff is a good way to start. Official and unofficial debriefing should be done regularly, especially after an unexpected or prolonged loss. Fostering open communication and interaction with the entire health care team fosters camaraderie, cohesiveness, and trust among providers. This can be especially important when working with families facing difficult diagnoses and prognoses. Bearing witness to suffering, standing in the discomfort of EoL situations, and remaining available to patients and their families is a gift to them and to staff alike. Providing excellent care to patients, even when it can feel as though it's too much, is the bar that one must strive for. Suffering cannot be eliminated, but there is much that a nurse can do for patients and families that helps to shoulder the load. It is not in the province of the nurse to convince parents about what course they should take but rather to meet them where they are, share their thoughts transparently, and find ways to journey with patients and families while offering support, respect, and compassion at every step.

The intersection of perinatal loss with emotionally weighty subjects including abortion, parental rights, and child welfare can make it challenging for nurses to approach these families from a place of neutrality. And despite the hope nurses have that they will treat every patient the same way, it is easier said than done. How can nurses respond to the suffering of these patients without imposing additional distress?

This work is about "being with" families. This is not a passive process; it is not sufficient for the nurse to simply tolerate these patients or to approach them from a place of detachment. At the same time, being with a patient is not the same as seeing eye to eye with them under any circumstance. Nurses are not required to agree with every decision their patients make, nor do nurses need to suppress their beliefs and personal morals for the sake of others. Instead, when responding to the suffering of these families, nurses should remember that being with families is a process of actively engaging with those who view the world through a different lens than we do, of seeking common ground in light of varying perspectives. Being with patients who are suffering requires that nurses practice from a place of humility and curiosity. Beginning discussions with a question (e.g., can you tell me about your pregnancy/baby?) allows families to make sense of their situation in light of their personal beliefs and values, and to give language to their own experience of suffering. Additionally, nurses can invite families to explore who or what helps guide them when making difficult decisions, rather than implying that there is a "right" and "wrong" way to make this choice.

Historically, nurses have always been at the forefront of shouldering the pain of their patients. On the battlefield, in hospitals, or in the home, nurses have held the hands of so many in their darkest moments. Suffering is an ineliminable part of the human experience: to be alive is to be exposed to the possibility of suffering. Therefore, to be a nurse is to bear witness to it. Attending to the suffering of perinatal and neonatal patients can be incredibly challenging—it can force nurses to confront the limits of science, the unpredictability of life, and the bounds of their own abilities. However, there is also something incomparably rewarding about bearing witness to these journeys. Responding to suffering in the perinatal and neonatal period challenges the nurse to see beyond just a single patient and to think about how suffering affects not just the person right in front of them but also their family and their community. These patients allow the nurse to offer their attention and their presence to those whose suffering might otherwise go unnoticed. Experience and exposure to the many types of suffering and patients who suffer can help nurses develop a practice that meets the needs of their patients and themselves. It is essential for each nurse to find the balance between care and compassion for patients and their families and their own personal growth.

Conclusion

When suffering and joy coincide, as they sometimes do during the perinatal and neonatal period, it is both a professional duty and a profound privilege for nurses to be present for both. Suffering and hope are not incompatible—it is the ability to hold space for the full spectrum of human experiences that defines the very nature of nursing. This work is challenging, necessary, admirable, and rewarding. It is also worthy of respect and continued research as to the best approaches to relieve suffering in patients, families, and those who care for them. May all nurses who have held a dying infant, comforted a devastated parent, or reframed hope for a family in despair know that they have done sacred work. May all patients and their families be fortunate enough to be cared for by that nurse.

References

1. Kelly CE. Mourning becomes them: the death of children in nineteenth-century American art. *Antiques*. Published July 2016. Accessed March 14, 2023. https://www.themagazinea ntiques.com/article/mourning-becomes-them-the-death-of-children-in-nineteenth-cent ury-american-art/

2. Schanzenbach DW, Nunn R, Bauer L. The changing landscape of American life expectancy. The Hamilton Project. Published June 2016. Accessed 2022. https://www.hamiltonproject. org/assets/files/changing_landscape_american_life_expectancy.pdf

3. Healthy People 2030. US Department of Health and Human Services, Office of Disease Prevention and Health Promotion. Accessed February 2, 2022. https://health.gov/health ypeople/objectives-and-data/browse-objectives/infants

4. Gold KJ, Sen A, Hayward RA. Marriage and cohabitation outcomes after pregnancy loss. *Pediatrics*. 2010;125(5):e1202–e1207. doi:10.1542/peds.2009-3081

5. New Year's babies. UNICEF. Published December 2020. Accessed 2022. https://www.uni cef.org/press-releases/new-years-babies-over-370000-children-will-be-born-worldwide-new-years-day-unicef

6. Prager S, Micks E, Dalton VK. Pregnancy loss (miscarriage): management techniques. In: Post TW, ed. *UpToDate*; 2021. Accessed March 14, 2023. https://www.uptodate.com/ contents/pregnancy-loss-miscarriage-description-of-management-techniques?search= Pregnancy%20loss%20(miscarriage)&source=search_result&selectedTitle=6~150&usa ge_type=default&display_rank=6

7. Lee SJ, Ralston HJ, Drey EA, Patridge JC, Rosen MA. Fetal pain: a systematic multidisciplinary review of the evidence. *JAMA*. 2005;294(8):947–954.

8. McGuire BE, Defrin R. Pain perception in people with Down syndrome: a synthesis of clinical and experimental research [published online ahead of print, Jul 30, 2015]. *Front Behav Neurosci*. 2015;9:194. doi:10.3389/fnbeh.2015.00194

9. Farren J, Jalmbrant M, Falconieri N, et al. Posttraumatic stress, anxiety and depression following miscarriage and ectopic pregnancy: a multicenter, prospective, cohort study. *Am J Obstet Gynecol*. 2020;222(4):367.e1–367.e22. doi:10.1016/j.ajog.2019.10.102

10. Wool C. Systematic review of the literature: parental outcomes after diagnosis of fetal anomaly. *Adv Neonatal Care*. 2011;11(3):182–192. doi:10.1097/ANC.obo13e31821bd92d

11. National Vital Statistics Reports, Vol. 70, no. 17, February 7, 2022. CDC. http://www.cdc. gov/nchs/data/nvsr/nvsr69/NNVSR-69-7-508.pdf

12. Parravicini E, Daho M, Foe G, Steinwurtzel R, Byrne M. Parental assessment of comfort in newborns affected by life-limiting conditions treated by a standardized neonatal comfort care program. *J Perinatol*. 2018;38(2):142–147. doi:10.1037/jp.2017.160

13. Caeymaex L, Jousselme C, Vasilescu C, et al. Perceived role in end-of-life decision making in the NICU affects long term parental grief response. *Arch Dis Child Fetal Neonatal Ed*. 2013;98:F26–F31.

14. Carter BS. Liminality in pediatric palliative care. *Am J Hosp Palliat Care*. 2017; 34(4):297–300.

15. Harris R, Gibbs D, Mangin-Heimos K, Pineda R. Maternal mental health during the neonatal period: relationships to the occupation of parenting. *Early Hum Dev.* 2018;120:31–39. doi:10.1016/jearlhumdev.2018.03.009

16. Niinomi K, Fukui M. Children's psychosocial and behavioural consequences during their siblings' hospitalization: a qualitative content analysis from caregivers' perspectives. [published online ahead of print, Sep 14, 2021]. *J Clin Nurs.* 2022;31:2219–2226. doi:10.1111/jocn.16040

17. Hubbard DK, Davis P, Willis T, Raza F, Carter BS, Lantos JD. Trauma-informed care and ethics consultation in the NICU [published online ahead of print, Nov 9, 2021]. *Semin Perinatol.* 2021;151527. doi:10.1016/j.semperi.2021.151527

18. Sanders MR, Hall SL. Trauma-informed care in the newborn intensive care unit: promoting safety, security and connectedness. *J Perinatol.* 2018;38(1):3–10. doi:10.1038/jp.2017.124

19. Suttle ML, Jenkins TL, Tamburro RF. End-of-life and bereavement care in pediatric intensive care units. *Pediatr Clin North Am.* 2017;64(5):1167–1183. doi:10.1016/j.pcl.2017.06.012

20. Parravicini E, McCarthy FT. Patient care. Neonatal Comfort Care Program. Accessed February 15, 2022. http://www.neonatalcomfortcare.com/patient-care

21. Mills M, Cortezzo DE. Moral distress in the neonatal intensive care unit: what is it, why it happens and how we can address it [published online ahead of print, Sep 10, 2020]. *Front Pediatr.* 2020;8:581. doi:10.3389/fped.2020.00581

22. Picoraro JA, Womer JW, Kazak AE, Feudtner C. Posttraumatic growth in parents and pediatric patients. *J Palliat Med.* 2014;17920:209–218. doi:10.1018/jpm.2013.0280

23. Tawfik D, Phibbs S, Sexton JB, et al. Factors associated with provider burnout in the NICU. *Pediatrics.* 2017;139(5):e20164134. doi:10.1542/peds.2016-4134

24. Wei H, Roberts P, Strickler J, Corbett RW. Nurse leaders' strategies to foster nurse resilience. *J Nurs Manag.* 2019;27(4):681–687. doi:10.1111/jonm.12736

25. Grauerholz KR, Fredenburg M, Jones PT, Jenkins KN. Fostering vicarious resilience for perinatal palliative care professionals [published online ahead of print, Oct 8, 2020]. *Front Pediatr.* 2020;8:572933. doi:10.3389/fped.2020.572933

6

Suffering in Serious Pediatric Illness

*Kim Mooney-Doyle**

Introduction

Reflecting on child or adolescent suffering is unfathomable to many people. To imagine the scope, quantity, and nature of child or adolescent suffering is to ask for a heavy heart and perplexed mind. Yet, this is a stark reality for children and adolescents around the world, their families, and those who provide health and social care to them. Nurses, in particular, bear witness to suffering, walk with those affected, and take seriously the call to "cure sometimes, relieve often, comfort always."

This chapter provides a theoretical and linguistic overview of suffering in children, adolescents, and their families to consider how it is defined and conceptualized. A social ecological model of child and family suffering provides a contextualized depiction that is helpful in understanding antecedents to and consequences of suffering and determinants of comfort because it acknowledges that children and their families are nested within environments (e.g., extended family, health care providers, health care system, school, and sociopolitical-cultural context). The social ecological model also recognizes the bidirectional relationship between children/adolescents and their surrounding environments. The focus then narrows to children and adolescents living with serious illness and their families to provide an overview of evidence to date that describes their suffering and how nurses can respond effectively and empathically.

Defining Child, Adolescent, and Family Suffering

"Childhood suffering is one of life's disturbing realities ... and is uniquely tragic."[1(p137)] Yet, the field of pediatric health care and ethics does not have a definition of pediatric suffering. Suffering may be considered a state in which the child or adolescent is bearing a level of pain or distress beyond what might be expected from daily life. Examples of pain in daily life include pain at an immunization site, distress about not getting invited to the party peers are posting about on Instagram, or discomfort related to the common cold or influenza. Suffering is a subjective, complex phenomenon that inhabits the deepest, essential layers of a person's lived experience and can take different forms: physical, psychological, social, spiritual, and existential.

There is agreement among parents, professionals, and philosophers that children and adolescents of all ages and developmental abilities can suffer.[2] There are several challenges that arise in pediatrics. One challenge is the variation in development.

Kim Mooney-Doyle, *Suffering in Serious Pediatric Illness* In: *The Nature of Suffering and the Goals of Nursing*. Second Edition. Edited by: William E. Rosa and Betty R. Ferrell, Oxford University Press. © Oxford University Press 2023. DOI: 10.1093/oso/9780197667934.003.0006

Variations in development impact how a child or adolescent might define their suffering and their ability to engage in discussion about it. For example, the subjective experience of school-aged children or adolescents who can participate in conversation can be accessed, but we do not have the same ability when considering the suffering of young children and nonverbal children. In these cases, their behavioral cues are assessed and evaluated by parents or professionals. Of note, we may have some insights into what school-aged children and adolescents would consider suffering if they had shared these perspectives with us before becoming nonverbal (e.g., child with cancer who is engaged in discussions earlier in the trajectory who cannot speak for themselves once critically ill, intubated, and sedated), if such conversations are initiated. Another challenge in defining pediatric suffering is the question of who decides if a child or adolescent is suffering if they cannot provide such an answer themselves. Across these groups, parent or health care provider assessment of suffering is used as a proxy for the child or adolescent voice.

Salter describes child and adolescent suffering as "a negative, subjective experience that goes beyond the experience of pain."[3(p18)] Negative experiences encompass physical, psychological, emotional, social, spiritual, and existential suffering. This can be assessed by directly asking the child or adolescent who is capable of answering whether they are suffering (in a developmentally appropriate way and in child/adolescent-friendly language) or in an objective manner, as is often done by parents and health care providers, by observation of signs, symptoms, cues, and behaviors. This description is helpful because it both privileges the individual's lived experience and acknowledges the suffering of those children and adolescents who may not be able to communicate about their suffering but have others who report for them.[3]

Tate describes child and adolescent suffering as "a set of absences—absences of conditions that would otherwise constitute child flourishing."[1(p4)] For healthy children, without illnesses or disabilities, suffering may be understood as "the lack of conditions under which they can grow and develop normally into healthy youngsters, adolescents, and adults."[4(p155)] This understanding draws our attention to their vulnerability and reliance on adults in their families and communities. In addition, Tate's conceptualization of pediatric suffering draws in the relational and social dimensions of suffering because it acknowledges that "children are not responsible for their own suffering, nor can they allay it. Rather, children rely wholly on others to resist suffering, grow, and flourish."[1] The flourishing of children is interrelated with and bound to those around them.

Considering how child, adolescent, and family are inextricably linked, we must also consider family suffering. When we reflect on the suffering of families of children and adolescents with serious illness, Chesla reminds us that families living with serious illness "vacillate between hope and despair, suffering and possibility."[5(p371)] They live with a tension of encountering and confronting loss and leaning toward hope and possibility. Suffering for such families may exist in both "big moments," such as receipt of a life-threatening diagnosis or making a decision to withdraw life-sustaining therapies, and "small moments" of suffering, such as deciding whether to leave the bedside of a hospitalized child to attend the sports event of a healthy sibling of that child. These small moments of suffering illustrate the daily management and working-out of tensions that arise from the illness.

A Social Ecological Model of Child, Adolescent, and Family Suffering

Conceptualizing child, adolescent, and family suffering within a social ecological model acknowledges the "complex social, spiritual, historical, theological, psychological, physical, biological, and linguistic realities that bind children to their parents, parents to their children, and place both in the dynamic relationship of patient, doctor [nurse, *author addition*], and parent." [2] This theory-based framework describes how different layers of social systems or environments affect the daily lives of children, adolescents, and their families and has been used extensively in pediatric cancer and serious illness. It posits that the development of every child is influenced by personal characteristics and contexts, or social systems, in which they are nested as they develop over their lifespan. These social systems are referred to as the macrosystem, exosystem, mesosystems, and microsystems. [6] Figure 6.1 depicts a social ecological model of child, adolescent, and family suffering.

Professionals can most readily comprehend the impact of social determinants of health and the structural barriers (e.g., health policy, racism, health inequities) on child and family health outcomes using a social ecological lens. This understanding is incredibly important because it forces us to interrogate and articulate how forces that seem abstract affect the daily lives of children, adolescents, and their families. [7,8]

The macrosystem is the broadest context and is defined by the society and culture in which the child lives. Examples of macrosystem influences include cultural and ideological values and forces (e.g., individualism, systemic racism), the economy, health and social policy (e.g., provision for concurrent pediatric hospice care), and government regulations and law (e.g., nursing scope of practice regulations). The exosystem, more proximal to the child or adolescent, is composed of social systems that have an indirect yet significant impact on the child's or adolescent's life, such as parental workplace (e.g., benefits, leave policies) and local resources (e.g., community pharmacies that stock opioids for pain management). Microsystems are the most proximal social systems to children (i.e., the ones in which children are embedded and interact with consistently) and include family, school, and peer group. There is a bidirectional relationship between microsystems and individuals within them influence the child or adolescent at the center. When a child has a serious illness, the hospital or health care team becomes a microsystem within which the child develops. [9,10] Mesosystems may be understood as connections between microsystems. Examples of mesosystems include the connection between the health care team and family and the degree to which they work together to meet the needs of the ill child. These connections between microsystems are important in the coordination of efforts to diminish suffering and enhance child and family outcomes.

Responses to Suffering

The next section provides an overview of the literature and is organized by the domains of quality of life in palliative care as experienced by children, adolescents, and families to describe physical, psychological, social, and spiritual/existential suffering; consider

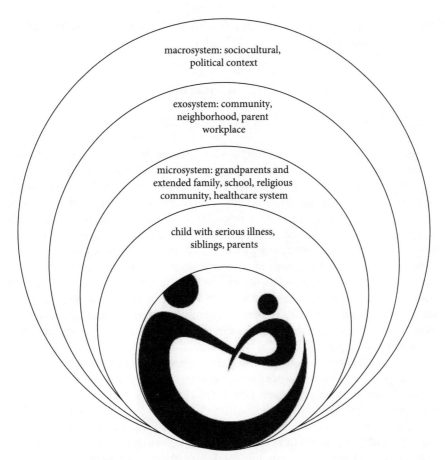

Figure 6.1 Social ecological model of child, adolescent, and family suffering.
Source: Adapted from Mooney-Doyle et al. (2022).

the consequences of unmitigated suffering; and reflect on how the experience of suffering changes the human experience.[11,12]

Broadly speaking, the evidence base that describes suffering in children, adolescents, and their families focuses predominantly on the experiences of physical suffering, manifested as pain and other symptoms that impact quality of life. There is less, but growing, attention paid to psychological symptoms that could contribute to suffering in serious illness. Experiences of psychological suffering in parents are more often explored in the literature than such experiences in seriously ill children and adolescents. Social, spiritual, and existential suffering are explored even less. Much of the literature focuses on children and adolescents with cancer and their families, but there is a growing presence of literature focused on the broader population of seriously ill children. Finally, the perspectives most often offered are those of parents, older children, and adolescents. The perspectives of young children or nonverbal children are absent, exemplifying Salter's point that we have little access to the perspectives of suffering in these two groups.[3]

Physical Suffering

Child and Adolescent

The preponderance of research on child and adolescent suffering centers on the assessment, identification, treatment, and experience of physical suffering. This emphasis on physical suffering in the form of pain and symptom management is unsurprising for a few reasons. First, bereaved parents and parents of seriously ill children have requested that more research be done that addresses child and adolescent symptoms so suffering can be minimized.[13] Second, nurses and other health care professionals have a robust history of investigating child and adolescent experiences of symptoms, symptom clusters, and methods of measurement.[14–16] Third, there is recognition that parents experience greater distress in bereavement when they perceive that their child's symptoms were not managed well.[17,18] Fourth, children experience multiple, simultaneous symptoms that can have a synergistic and aggravating effect on each other.[19] Thus, attending to the physical suffering of children and adolescents may be a way to bring some peace to patients, families, and clinicians.

Children and adolescents living with serious illnesses often experience polysymptomatology.[19] They can experience a variety of symptoms concurrently, which can impede and complicate management. Parent and child comfort and quality of life are diminished when symptoms are uncontrolled. Feudtner and colleagues found that, according to parent report, children and adolescents receiving pediatric palliative care experience a range of 6 to 12 symptoms on any given day.[19] The most commonly experienced symptoms were pain, low energy, irritability, drowsiness, and shortness of breath. Of note, nearly 75% of the sample in this study experienced at least five co-occurring symptoms. While there was some variation in symptom profiles, the authors found that symptoms for a variety of advanced serious illnesses may share common presentation. Children and adolescents who were technology dependent, those with metabolic conditions, and adolescents experienced the most symptoms. Thus, systematic assessment of symptoms for all seriously ill children and consideration of how treatment for one symptom can impact the experience of another symptom is needed.

Considering children and adolescents with cancer, fatigue, pain, and anxiety are among the most frequently experienced symptoms. Nearly 90% of children and adolescents with cancer experience fatigue,[14] but very few receive any treatment for it, and far less achieve successful treatment.[20] Pain is highly prevalent, secondary to underlying cancer, procedures, and anticancer treatment. Anxiety is recognized as having a substantial impact on the lives of children and adolescents living with cancer. Weaver makes an excellent point that the sheer ubiquity of these disquieting and unpleasant symptoms risk their "normalization as part of pediatric cancer,"[21] risks their underreporting, and can increase suffering. This would be a disservice since children and adolescents experience functional limitations, diminished quality of life, and relational strain because of uncontrolled symptoms.

Weaver and team found that the presence of fatigue, pain, and anxiety predicted moderate to high suffering for the child or adolescent. The high prevalence of these symptoms in children and adolescents with cancer is supported in a review by Eche and colleagues.[20] Through assessing child and adolescent reported outcomes, they found that fatigue most readily predicted membership in the medium-suffering group and anxiety substantially increased the likelihood of membership in the high-suffering group.

Family Suffering

Parents undertake complex mental and physical work when caring for their seriously ill child or adolescent. A recent systematic review by Hartley and team describes how parent physical health was negatively affected, most often by pain and sleep disturbances.[22] Over 80% of the studies they reviewed reported negative health effects for parents and caregivers, and this was directly related to caregiving duties. For example, parents describe back pain secondary to caregiving. Negative physical effects are influenced by support from spouse/partner, access to quality respite care, and health care professional support for their needs. [22]

Siblings can also experience physical suffering, but this has received less attention in the literature. Their physical suffering may be secondary to psychological distress or suffering. For example, abdominal pain can be a somatic manifestation of their psychological distress. Similarly, bereaved siblings who report being excluded from discussions and caring for the child with serious illness at end of life participated in more substance use or risk taking; these actions, while a result of psychological distress, can lead to physical suffering.[23-25]

Nurses caring for a seriously ill child and their family can be overwhelmed by encountering and addressing these symptoms. Yet, there are evidence-based steps they can take to mitigate suffering. According to the Children's Oncology Group, evidence-based approaches to addressing fatigue exist that can be readily implemented by nurses or taught to children and their families by nurses and may be transferable across disease states. These interventions include physical activity that includes resistance exercises, aerobic exercise, or neuromotor activities, like yoga or tai chi.[26] In addition, relaxation and mindfulness techniques can ameliorate fatigue and include activities like acupuncture, yogic breathing, and massage. Children whose fatigue does not improve with the introduction of physical activity, relaxation, or mindfulness may benefit from cognitive behavioral therapy.[26] Considering pain, skilled and thorough assessment are vital to minimizing suffering (COG). This assessment is the foundation for offering pain management that is child and family centered and tailored to the child's needs. Nurses can take a similar approach to mitigating the suffering that accompanies anxiety. Youth and family should routinely receive screening for psychosocial distress. Such screening can elucidate sources of risk and resilience, which can help mitigate the suffering from anxiety.[27]

The experience of fatigue, pain, and anxiety can be burdensome and decrease quality of life. Without mitigation of these frequently occurring symptoms, suffering from physical symptoms is amplified. Piette and team, in a systematic review of interventions to address quality of life at end of life in serious illness, found that electronic symptom monitoring, patient-controlled interventions, multidisciplinary palliative care, and provision of instrumental/logistic support to families enhanced child and adolescent quality of life, while moderate- and high-intensity chemotherapy and stem cell transplant near end of life led to a poor quality of life.[28]

Psychological Suffering

Child and Adolescent

The experience of life-limiting illness is stressful for children and adolescents. They report "feeling different" or fear stigma because of illness-related physical changes.[29(p20)] According to Weaver and team, anxiety has been described as "one of the most severe and long-lasting symptoms for children with cancer."[14] Child and adolescent social lives are often disrupted because of prolonged absence from school, extracurricular activities, and spending time with friends; they report feeling isolated.[29] This is particularly painful for adolescents who may feel more tethered to parents at a time when they simultaneously want more independence. Phenwan describes how this sense of isolation can amplify the adolescent experience of total pain and suffering.[30]

Like adults, children and adolescents worry about their relationships and loved ones. Adolescents with cancer have described "trying to be good patients" so they do not cause greater pain to their families.[31] Children and adolescents describe feeling worried about family members' fear, hopelessness, depression, and anxiety; they do not want to be a burden.[29] An important though understudied aspect of psychological distress includes concerns about romantic relationships and sexuality, the ability to have intimate relationships, and concerns about future fertility or prospects of having one's own family. These descriptions of psychological distress or suffering emphasize the need for age- and developmentally appropriate communication with children and adolescents to mitigate their suffering. Nurses can be a safe space for such conversations or can coach parents in how to use open-ended questions, active listening, and presence to help ameliorate their child's psychological suffering.

Psychological symptoms are prevalent but less likely to be treated in serious illness compared to physical symptoms that cause suffering. Addressing and attempting to diminish distress and suffering among children and adolescents is important because symptom-related distress is related to poor quality of life. This has downstream effects because parents' perceptions of poor child or adolescent quality of life or ineffective symptom management at end of life is associated with parent depression and grief.[20] Nurses can mitigate suffering in children and families through screening for psychosocial distress, providing a safe space that acknowledges the psychosocial impact of serious illness, and offering opportunities to enhance family cohesion and connection.

Family

"Cancer is a family disease. She has it. I feel like I have it. We wear it."[32]

Suffering of the family unit during serious illness has not received a great deal of attention. Yet, suffering is done within a social context and each individual has their internal experience with suffering.[5] This notion comes into stark relief when we explore parent suffering in serious pediatric and adolescent illness. Witnessing or perceiving one's child suffering instigates parental suffering. In the face of their child's suffering, parents experience uncertainty and powerlessness,[18] and their role as protector is challenged.[17] Parents also describe suffering, separate from the seriously ill child, when they consider the disruption to the family unit caused by the serious illness and caregiving demands.[18] Parents may feel they have to trade off one child's needs to meet those of another (most often putting siblings' needs on the backburner to attend to the needs of the seriously ill child or adolescent), and this can perpetuate distress.[32]

Just as suffering is relational and done in a social context, parents derive comfort and alleviation of their suffering when they are physically and emotionally close—in communion—with their child.[33] This sentiment is captured by a parent's quote: "If she's [patient] ok, then I'm ok."[34] Parents also experience comfort in receiving empathic care and support from nurses, witnessing expert symptom management from nurses for their child, connecting with other parents, returning to routines of home and "normal" life, and receiving instrumental help. By providing a consoling or comforting presence, nurses diminish parent and family suffering. This, in turn, enhances care and mollifies suffering of the child or adolescent.

Chesla describes "small suffering" as the everyday events and decision points of chronic illness management that bring about distress for patients and their family members.[5] This concept of "small suffering" is a helpful way to understand the suffering brought about by logistic challenges, bureaucratic hurdles, and time tax that families of seriously ill children and adolescents face. For example, parents of seriously ill children describe needing instrumental support for parking, food, and childcare for the healthy sibling.[35] These logistic challenges (e.g., pediatric home hospice being able to deliver needed equipment) or bureaucratic hurdles (e.g., insurance approval for medication) can impact parents' ability to manage the illness or symptoms, which can instigate parental psychological or existential suffering.[36,37] Parents report that skilled palliative care at home that can provide organized, individualized relational and instrumental support is helpful because it allows them to attend to the needs of the seriously ill child or adolescent and healthy siblings and regain a sense of normalcy.[36]

Siblings also experience psychological suffering. They have been described as "being on the outside looking in."[38] Their suffering is multipronged: they suffer negative emotions due to concern about the child with serious illness, they are concerned about parents they perceive to be distressed or overburdened, and they recognize the impact on their own lives from loss of routines or access to parent support or sibling confidante. In Case Exemplar 6.2, a bereaved sibling reflects on her experience from her current perspective as an adult who recently completed graduate study in child development to become a child life specialist.

Case Exemplar 6.1

Adolescent Survivor/Patient Case

When I consider suffering as a teenager with cancer, the first thing that comes to mind is the social impact and isolation from friends and school. Receiving a cancer diagnosis during high school, just at a time when you're trying to fit in and grow up, when friendships and building bonds outside home are so important, was painful. At a time when you're trying to grow up and get out, you're locked in at the hospital for treatment or at home because of neutropenia. This worsened during transplant, when I had to transfer to another center in another city. I was super-removed from life as I had come to know it.

The physical impact and suffering from cancer had downstream impacts on my social and psychological experience. Before diagnosis, I was tired and winded and knew something was not right. To have one's body not act as expected as a teenager is jarring. To not be listened to by health care providers added to the feelings of confusion and upset. I experienced both frequently and less frequently seen symptoms associated with treatment. In each case, nurses ameliorated my suffering through expert symptom management delivered with compassion and patience. Patience was key as we worked through different assessment, management, and evaluation modalities. For example, we used different communication strategies to communicate during my mucositis, a specialized wound care nurse cared for my radiation-associated burns, and the apheresis nurses had a steady rotation of warm blankets as my stem cells were collected for transplant.

As an adolescent with hopes and dreams, receiving a cancer diagnosis instigated emotional suffering that lasts through survivorship. The suffering can be long term because of the trauma of diagnosis and treatment. I struggled emotionally with the prospect of diminished fertility; it was so hard to imagine a future in which I was not a mother. My nurses, through these phases, helped me to stay focused on the present moment by reminding me that they would accompany me across the bridge to what was on the other side. These reminders kept me grounded in the moment and reminded me I was not alone.

Suffering also extended to my family. The nurses recognized this and scooped us up as soon as I was diagnosed with cancer. They welcomed my family and supported my family in caring for me. Since cancer can be difficult to talk about, the nurses helped my family and me discuss cancer and gave us the information about the disease and what to expect. This helped us share our cancer journey, which opened up a whole loving community to us.

The nurses were a lifeline through their ministry of presence. When an adolescent or young adult has cancer, nurses' showing up is monumental for healing. They sat with me and spent time with me, acknowledging the difficulty of the situation and meeting me where I was. They connected with me and my family and taught us what to expect, each step of the way. The nurses supported me in their individual interactions, helping to keep our hope grounded and afloat, and as members of the interdisciplinary team, they helped my family and me navigate the terrain of cancer.

Case Exemplar 6.2

Sibling's Voice: A Bereaved Sibling's Perspective

At the age of 7, I experienced the death of my little sister due to a stillbirth. My parents explained what happened, but I could not comprehend what everything meant. If I'm being honest, I did not fully understand that my little sister had died until the funeral occurred. Even though I was still slightly confused, the burial made everything click, which was when I began to cry. Throughout my grieving process, there was open communication with my parents, and we knew that we could talk about our feelings or ask questions. However, I remember worrying about talking about my sister because I didn't want to make anyone sad. I believe that this thought impacted my grieving process as time moved forward. At one point, my parents reached out to the community resources to help process and understand our grief, which was an impactful part of my grieving process. Even though my grief was complicated initially, the familial and community support I received helped me understand my reactions and control and cope with my emotions in different settings and around other people.

A few years later, my little brother was born, which brought me so much joy. I genuinely believe that my little sister gave us the gift of having my little brother and a second chance for me to be an older sibling. I do remember being nervous about my brother's birth and fearing that he would leave or that something could happen. After his birth, I was so excited to have a younger sibling and wanted to be an important part of his life. As I grew older, I noticed a few characteristics that I have portrayed that could be connected to experiencing my sister's death. First, I have found that I am very overprotective about my little brother and have felt anxious when he would be out or worried if he was feeling down because I felt the need to know he was okay. Our family has continued to have open communication and make it known that we can talk to each other about anything when we're ready, which I believe is important and was strengthened when coping with my sister's death.

Another aspect I noticed included experiencing waves of grief at unexpected times. For example, I have a friend who has the same birthday as my sister, and when that day occurred, I did not process or understand why I felt extremely sad and lonely. However, once I realized it was my sister's birthday, I felt a wave of grief wash over me that brought all the emotions back to the surface. This was a difficult realization that affected me for days where I felt that I was processing my grief again but as an adult. In addition, experiencing this grief at an older age was challenging and made me feel guilty about not realizing the event sooner. Even though the experience of my sister's death impacted me greatly, I believe that the strong support system and learned coping strategies that were developed and utilized after her death aided me in managing my grief more healthily and appropriately as an adult.

Spiritual and Existential Suffering

Child and Adolescent

For children and adolescents with serious illness, spiritual and existential suffering may be experienced as existential loss, worry about dying, not being at peace, uncertainty about the future, a desire to be remembered, and finding meaning, especially when children and adolescents feel their dreams and hopes for the future have been thwarted.[29] Children and adolescents may question God about their illness yet also report that faith or connection to the transcendent fosters resilience, maturity, and appreciation.[39] Interestingly, school-aged children and adolescents described existential loss, self-image, and the need for access to information as particular concerns.[29]

Family

For parents, spiritual and existential suffering can begin during the illness and follow them through bereavement.[40] This aspect of suffering is often neglected in the busy, daily world of illness management when the needs of the seriously ill child are paramount. Parents experiencing existential suffering may describe feeling "dread, powerlessness, solitude, and loss of control ... and extreme hopelessness ... and estrangement."[40] Nurses and other professionals can ameliorate these feelings in parents by maintaining a meaningful relationship and connection to the professionals in the child's care settings.

Despite the deep impact of existential and spiritual concerns, the evidence indicates that nurses and other health care providers may be uncomfortable having conversations with children about these topics and possess limited skills in doing so.[36,39,41] Not attending to child or adolescent existential or spiritual suffering can amplify their psychological and physical suffering. We can practice both attentive and preventive palliative care by encouraging and modeling family-based pediatric advanced care planning conversations and eliciting perspectives from children and adolescents in a developmentally appropriate yet meaningful manner.[29,42]

Social Suffering

Child and Adolescent

Suffering and comfort in serious illness can be socially determined. This means there are factors within the environments in which seriously ill children and their families live, work, and play that impact child and family suffering and comfort. A new term, the social determinants of comfort, articulates this intersection of the social determinants of health and pediatric palliative care, and can help nurses and other professionals understand factors that can ameliorate or exacerbate suffering for children and adolescents and their families.[43,44]

These social determinants of comfort can influence a person or family's ability to access resources, thereby exacerbating disparities or enhancing equity. Approaching child and family health from an ecological, public health lens, even in the midst of serious illness, provides a foundation for addressing factors that ameliorate or exacerbate suffering, improving outcomes, and achieving health equity. Social determinants of comfort are important for professionals to consider because they propel thoughts about factors beyond the clinical encounter that increase or decrease suffering or impede access to comfort. For example, nurses using this lens in discharge planning would consider how geography (e.g., rurality) impacts the availability of pediatric hospice or how family leave policy impacts parent employment and family financial stability. Thus, professionals are able to learn about the stressors families face other than the illness that are not usually part of the clinical encounter.

Namisango and team call for a person-centered framework for assessing and addressing child and adolescent symptoms because it acknowledges the child or adolescent in the context of their development and dynamic environments.[29] This begs the questions "Where is the family?" and "Who is assessing and addressing parent and family suffering?" Perhaps a person-centered framework can stimulate rethinking of a family-centered framework, so that parent and family suffering can be acknowledged and addressed. Without assessing and addressing family suffering, we may perpetuate trauma or distress that parents are experiencing in other spheres of their lives.[45,46]

Family

There has been limited exploration of parent health across social and economic contexts; such social determinants may impact parent health and physical suffering in the context of serious pediatric and adolescent illness. These findings are even more alarming when we consider the growing numbers of seriously ill children and adolescents, who are living longer, but with more complexity and increased needs,[47-49] as well as sources of health inequity that could preclude access to good-quality respite care.[22]

Conclusion

The US poet laureate Joy Harjo reminds us that "we are stewards of stories." One of the most meaningful and healing things we could ask of another person is to hear their story. We can ask children of varying ages and developmental abilities, and their parents, to share stories through a variety of media (e.g., drawings, photos, poems, voice recording). Once we hear these stories, about how parents "try to be good parents" to their seriously ill children and adolescents, our gaze may shift, our breath may be released, and we may be able to journey with, be present to, support, and provide comfort to a family as they navigate troubled waters and tough terrain.

Note

* With acknowledgments to Allison Fuson, MeD, and Jessica Thompkins, BSN, RN, CPN.

References

1. Tate T. Philosophical investigations into the essence of pediatric suffering. *Theor Med Bioeth*. 2020;41(4):137–142.
2. Tate T. Pediatric suffering and the burden of proof. *Pediatrics*. 2020;146(Suppl_1):S70–S74.
3. Salter EK. The new futility? The rhetoric and role of "suffering" in pediatric decision-making. *Nurs Ethics*. 2020;27(1):16–27.
4. Tate T. What we talk about when we talk about pediatric suffering. *Theor Med Bioeth*. 2020;41(4):143–163.
5. Chesla CA. Nursing science and chronic illness: articulating suffering and possibility in family life. *J Fam Nurs*. 2005;11(4):371–387.
6. Bronfenbrenner U. *The Ecology of Human Development: Experiments by Nature and Design*. Harvard University Press; 2009.
7. US Department of Health and Human Services Office of Disease Prevention and Health Promotion. Healthy People 2030. Published 2022. Accessed June 1, 2022. https://health.gov/healthypeople/objectives-and-data/social-determinants-health.
8. Mooney-Doyle K, Keim-Malpass J, Lindley LC. The ethics of concurrent care for children: a social justice perspective. *Nurs Ethics*. 2019;26(5):1518–1527.
9. Eriksson M, Ghazinour M, Hammarström A. Different uses of Bronfenbrenner's ecological theory in public mental health research: what is their value for guiding public mental health policy and practice? *Soc Theory Heal*. 2018;16(4):414–433.
10. Kazak AE. Families of chronically ill children: a systems and social-ecological model of adaptation and challenge. *J Consult Clin Psychol*. 1989;57(1):25.
11. Ferrell B, Paice J. *Oxford Textbook of Palliative Nursing*. 5th ed. Oxford University Press; 2019.
12. Khadra C, Le May S, Tremblay I, et al. Development of the adolescent cancer suffering scale. *Pain Res Manag*. 2015;20(4):213–219.
13. Lord B. Parent perspective and response to challenges and priorities for pediatric palliative care research. *J Pain Symptom Manage*. 2019;58(5):e9–e10.
14. Weaver MS, Wang J, Greenzang KA, McFatrich M, Hinds PS. The predictive trifecta? Fatigue, pain, and anxiety severity forecast the suffering profile of children with cancer. *Support Care Cancer*. 2022;30(3):2081–2089.
15. Mack JW, McFatrich M, Withycombe JS, et al. Agreement between child self-report and caregiver-proxy report for symptoms and functioning of children undergoing cancer treatment. *JAMA Pediatr*. 2020;174(11):e202861–e202861.
16. Reeve BB, Edwards LJ, Jaeger BC, et al. Assessing responsiveness over time of the PROMIS® pediatric symptom and function measures in cancer, nephrotic syndrome, and sickle cell disease. *Qual Life Res*. 2018;27(1):249–257.
17. Montoya-Juárez R, García-Caro MP, Schmidt-Rio-Valle J, et al. Suffering indicators in terminally ill children from the parental perspective. *Eur J Oncol Nurs*. 2013;17(6):720–725.
18. de Weerd W, van Tol D, Albers M, Sauer P, Verkerk M. Suffering in children: opinions from parents and health-care professionals. *Eur J Pediatr*. 2015;174(5):589–595.
19. Feudtner C, Nye R, Hill DL, et al. Polysymptomatology in pediatric patients receiving palliative care based on parent-reported data. *JAMA Netw Open*. 2021;4(8):e2119730–e2119730.

20. Eche IJ, Eche IM, Aronowitz T. An integrative review of factors associated with symptom burden at the end of life in children with cancer. *J Pediatr Oncol Nurs.* 2020;37(4):284–295.
21. Weaver M, Wichman C, Darnall C, Bace S, Vail C, MacFadyen A. Proxy-reported quality of life and family impact for children followed longitudinally by a pediatric palliative care team. *J Palliat Med.* 2018;21(2):241–244. doi:10.1089/jpm.2017.0092
22. Hartley J, Bluebond-Langner M, Candy B, Downie J, Henderson EM. The physical health of caregivers of children with life-limiting conditions: a systematic review. *Pediatrics.* 2021;148(2):e2020014423.
23. Lövgren M, Sveen J, Nyberg T, et al. Care at end of life influences grief: a nationwide long-term follow-up among young adults who lost a brother or sister to childhood cancer. *J Palliat Med.* 2018;21(2):156–162. doi:10.1089/jpm.2017.0029
24. Rosenberg AR, Postier A, Osenga K, et al. Long-term psychosocial outcomes among bereaved siblings of children with cancer. *J Pain Symptom Manage.* 2015;49(1):55–65.
25. Long KA, Lehmann V, Gerhardt CA, Carpenter AL, Marsland AL, Alderfer MA. Psychosocial functioning and risk factors among siblings of children with cancer: an updated systematic review. *Psychooncology.* 2018;27(6):1467–1479.
26. Robinson PD, Oberoi S, Tomlinson D, et al. Management of fatigue in children and adolescents with cancer and in paediatric recipients of haemopoietic stem-cell transplants: a clinical practice guideline. *Lancet Child Adolesc Heal.* 2018;2(5):371–378.
27. Kazak AE, Abrams AN, Banks J, et al. Psychosocial assessment as a standard of care in pediatric cancer. *Pediatr Blood Cancer.* 2015;62(S5):S426–S459.
28. Piette V, Beernaert K, Cohen J, et al. Healthcare interventions improving and reducing quality of life in children at the end of life: a systematic review. *Pediatr Res.* 2021;89(5):1065–1077.
29. Namisango E, Bristowe K, Allsop MJ, et al. Symptoms and concerns among children and young people with life-limiting and life-threatening conditions: a systematic review highlighting meaningful health outcomes. *Patient.* 2019;12(1):15–55. doi:10.1007/s40271-018-0333-5
30. Phenwan T. Relieving total pain in an adolescent: a case report. *BMC Res Notes.* 2018;11(1):1–4.
31. Weaver MS, Baker JN, Gattuso JS, Gibson DV, Hinds PS. "Being a good patient" during times of illness as defined by adolescent patients with cancer. *Cancer.* 2016;122(14):2224–2233.
32. Mooney-Doyle K, Deatrick JA, Ulrich CM, Meghani SH, Feudtner C. Parenting in childhood life-threatening illness: a mixed-methods study. *J Palliat Med.* 2018;21(2):119–273. doi:10.1089/jpm.2017.0054
33. Ångström-Brännström C, Norberg A, Strandberg G, Söderberg A, Dahlqvist V. Parents' experiences of what comforts them when their child is suffering from cancer. *J Pediatr Oncol Nurs.* 2010;27(5):266–275.
34. Mooney-Doyle K, Deatrick JA. Parenting in the face of childhood life-threatening conditions: the ordinary in the context of the extraordinary. *Palliat Support Care.* 2016;14(3):187–198. doi:10.1017/S1478951515000905
35. Mooney-Doyle K, dos Santos MR, Szylit R, Deatrick JA. Parental expectations of support from healthcare providers during pediatric life-threatening illness: a secondary, qualitative analysis. *J Pediatr Nurs.* 2017;36:163–172. doi:10.1016/j.pedn.2017.05.008
36. Greenfield K, Holley S, Schoth DE, et al. A mixed-methods systematic review and meta-analysis of barriers and facilitators to paediatric symptom management at end of life. *Palliat Med.* 2020;34(6):689–707.
37. Winger A, Kvarme LG, Løyland B, Kristiansen C, Helseth S, Ravn IH. Family experiences with palliative care for children at home: a systematic literature review. *BMC Palliat Care.* 2020;19(1):1–19.

38. Long K. On the outside looking in: a nationwide examination of barriers to and facilitators of implementing the standard of psychosocial care for siblings of children with cancer. *Psychooncology.* 2019;28:35. doi:10.1002/pon.4986 LK.

39. Ferrell B. Exploring the spiritual needs of families with seriously ill children. *Int J Palliat Nurs.* 2016;22(8):388–394. https://www.magonlinelibrary.com/doi/full/10.12968/ijpn.2016.22.8.388

40. October TW. Is all suffering equal or is it time to address existential suffering? *Pediatr Crit Care Med.* 2018;19(3):275–276.

41. Ferrell B, Wittenberg E, Battista V, Walker G. Nurses' experiences of spiritual communication with seriously iii children. *J Palliat Med.* 2016;19(11):1166–1170.

42. Friebert S, Grossoehme DH, Baker JN, et al. Congruence gaps between adolescents with cancer and their families regarding values, goals, and beliefs about end-of-life care. *JAMA Netw Open.* 2020;3(5):e205424–e205424.

43. Deatrick JA. Where is "family" in the social determinants of health? Implications for family nursing practice, research, education, and policy. *J Fam Nurs.* 2017;23(4):423–433.

44. Mendola A, Naumann WC, Mooney-Doyle K, Lindley LC. Social determinants of comfort: a new term for end-of-life care. *J Palliat Med.* 2021;24(8):1130–1131.

45. Mooney-Doyle K, Ulrich CM. Parent moral distress in serious pediatric illness: a dimensional analysis. *Nurs Ethics.* 2020;27(3):821–837.

46. Bloom SL. *Creating Sanctuary: Toward the Evolution of Sane Societies.* 2nd ed. Routledge; 2013.

47. Feudtner C, Zhong W, Faerber J, Dai D FJ. Appendix F: pediatric end-of-life and palliative care: epidemiology and health service use. *Dying Am Improv Qual Honor Individ Prefer Near End Life.* 2015:533–572.

48. Lindley LC. Multiple complex chronic conditions and pediatric hospice utilization among California Medicaid beneficiaries, 2007–2010. *J Palliat Med.* 2017;20(3):241–246.

49. Lindley LC, Cozad MJ, Svynarenko R, Keim-Malpass J, Mack JW. A national profile of children receiving pediatric concurrent hospice care, 2011 to 2013. *J Hosp Palliat Nursing.* 2021;23(3):214.

7

Suffering of Older People

Terry Fulmer, Amy Berman, Rebecca Slossberg, Teffin Benedict, and
Rumaysa Sharif

The concept of suffering is deeply personal, and by the time any of us reach what we call old age, there are often patterns and subjective feelings that have been established through the life course. It is not unusual to hear someone say, "Don't tell mom because she couldn't bear the news." In fact, there may be truth in the statement because family members have become accustomed to the reactions and patterns of intimate members in their family. However, usurping the older person's authority over information may cause even greater misery than the truth. In this chapter on suffering and older people, we discuss issues that provide the context for suffering in this age group and offer ideas for what needs to change in our aging society.

As a college professor, I (TF) was concerned that students might not have the opportunity to study the way that suffering is unique to older people. I created a course entitled "Comfort and Suffering" and taught it each fall semester to a first-year honors seminar in the College of Arts and Sciences and each spring to senior nursing students in the College of Nursing in their final semester. This seminar was meant to challenge how students think critically about what our society considers fair and just care and required full and active participation. We examined related readings through the lens of the health care system paradigm, and I used case studies to explore the wellness-illness continuum of human experiences. Students became familiar with conceptual frameworks used by nurses, physicians, and social workers as these professionals assist patients through the illness experience, which is continually balanced between comfort and suffering. Our discussions on the nature of comfort and suffering focused on writings from a variety of sources, including ancient works such as the Bible and the Quran, which were contrasted with contemporary editorials and publications, in order to examine historical changes in the way individuals think about these important dimensions of the human experience. We explored the scientific advances that have created heretofore unimaginable opportunities, choices, and suffering, and the psychological consequences that are inevitable when illness and care needs create complexity in our lives. We also debated the notion of "self-care," very popular in the health care literature, and contrasted it with the concept of "patient abandonment."

I personally wanted to learn from first-year students who were not in health sciences but rather in the liberal arts programs and then compare and contrast their views to those of senior nursing students who had observed suffering firsthand in the clinical setting over several semesters. The readings were the same and the syllabus for each course had similarities. However, the level of analysis and the examination expectations were radically different. With both student populations, I learned much

Terry Fulmer, Amy Berman, Rebecca Slossberg, Teffin Benedict, and Rumaysa Sharif, *Suffering of Older People* In: *The Nature of Suffering and the Goals of Nursing*. Second Edition. Edited by: William E. Rosa and Betty R. Ferrell, Oxford University Press.
© Oxford University Press 2023. DOI: 10.1093/oso/9780197667934.003.0007

about the way they think about older people and how the concept of suffering is so unique to each person. I learned a tremendous amount and was heartened by their compassion, sense of justice for all, and plans to make a difference in their future. Conversely, their eyes were opened to the prevalence of ageism in our country.

What Is Ageism and Why Is It So Important?

Robert Butler coined the term "ageism" in 1968 to describe discrimination against older people; the term was in keeping with other terms of prejudice such as sexism and racism. He defined "ageism" as prejudice by one age group toward other (older) age groups. He went on to say that ageism describes the subjective experience implied in the popular notion of *the generation gap* that reflects a deep-seated uneasiness on the part of the young and middle-aged, a personal revulsion to and a distaste for growing old, disease, disability, and fear of powerlessness, uselessness, and death.[1]

Prejudicial attitudes toward older people, old age, and the aging process include a number of discriminatory practices against older people such as job discrimination, infantilization, and institutional practices and policies that can also perpetuate stereotypes about older people and label them as "less than" younger people. Ageism allows younger people to see old people as "different."

The purpose of leading with a narrative about ageism is very intentional as an introduction to the unique aspects of suffering in older people. The added assault of ageism in the context of suffering can be unbearable. Nurses often make assumptions about what an older person would prefer in their clinical care and substitute their own choices for the older adult instead of asking them, which is often painful and insulting. Suffering is a subjective personal event, and that does not change with aging. What does change is the way society thinks about care for older people, especially those who need assistance with their activities of daily living (ADLs) including eating, feeding, bathing, grooming, and toileting. If the older person is living with dementia or even cognitive decline, there is even more substituted judgment for how the older person thinks and feels and what constitutes suffering for them.

We use terms with older people that are demeaning and infantilizing such as "honey, sweetie, young lady, or young man" and make reference to the appearance of an older adult as different from who they are. It is very common for people to say, "You don't look 90 years old" or "80 is the new 60," and while these are often meant to be complimentary, they may not be taken that way. What does 90 years old look like anyway? These types of comments tend to reflect nurses' concern about their own aging or are simply trite phrases that have been learned from others. Dr. Butler's book should be mandatory reading for every nurse in practice.

The Frameworks Institute is an exceptional organization in Washington, DC with international impact. That group has taken on the challenge of reframing aging, using a research-based approach to strategic communications. They do a deep dive into how people understand complex socio-political issues and then test ways to reframe them to drive social change.[2] In one of their powerful reports, "Finding the Frame: An Empirical Approach to Reframing Aging and Ageism," they discuss framing strategies to advance aging and address ageism as policy issues.[3] What this team has learned is that there are extraordinarily ingrained perceptions about aging in our country that need to be fundamentally changed. For example, the way that we use terms related to aging is very confusing. We refer to older people as "them" instead of "us," and that helps create the negative attitude of aging. Whenever we compartmentalize older people we marginalize them, and we dismiss them in ways that diminish our ability to understand their state of suffering. The Frameworks team also reminds us that our advertisements are full of content related to how to "fight aging." That phrase not only has a violent connotation but also rejects the very essence of older people in their experience.[3] We also use terms that are overwhelming such as "silver tsunami," and that term itself indicates that there is nothing we can do about our shifting demographics and likens this to a disaster.

Ken Dychtwald, the CEO of AgeWave (https://agewave.com/), has created an organization that promotes positivity and inclusiveness for older people and provides strategies and tactics to that end. The greatest success story of the 20th century is longevity, and nurses need to embrace the very special nature of this cohort and personalized care that ensures older people get the best care possible in the context of any suffering they are experiencing. Nurses have the ability to change the narrative from deterioration, loss of control, and dependency to staying active, using the accumulated wisdom of the years, and maintaining maximum mental and physical functioning in partnership with the health care team.

Racism

Another critical lens for examining suffering in older people is racism. Nurses and their patients exist in systems that reinforce racial discrimination, resulting in disparities in health outcomes well before their first clinical interaction with an older adult. Life expectancy for Black, Indigenous, and People of Color (BIPOC) is perpetually lower than for Caucasians in the United States.[4] There is no evidence to suggest that differences in mortality among people of color are genetic; rather, the underlying cause is structural racism. Structural racism leads to "differential access to the goods, services, and opportunities of society by race," determines societal values and power hierarchies, and underlies persistent health disparities in the United States."[5(p8)] Structural racism continues to create disparities in minority communities, leading to serious suffering.

Suffering in minoritized communities, particularly for older Black Americans, can often be attributed to a lifetime of structural racial discrimination. Nurses must be made aware of the accumulated suffering, also known to them as "weathering," that their older BIPOC patients have experienced. The American Psychological Association defines this accumulated suffering as race-related stress across the lifespan. "For [BIPOC] older people, these encounters are stored in memory and relived with each new racist and discriminatory experience."[6(p2)] Nurses spend far more time with patients, and in order to prevent any further race-related stress, providers must first understand the impact of racism on their patients.

One study including 619 Black older people residing in South Los Angeles found that economic strain was linked to five health outcomes. The most significant finding was that economic strain was associated with depressive symptoms, pain intensity, self-rated health, chronic diseases, and sick days. This pattern, alongside the higher rates of economic instability in Black communities in the United States than the general population, shows a disproportionate likelihood of suffering, especially in older people.[7]

In addition to the history of biomedical abuse, poor outcomes, and resulting distrust in health care experienced by the Black community, Black older people experience significant disparities in pain management. Up to 78% of Black older people experience chronic pain. However, often this pain is not adequately reported because minority groups can have different cultural beliefs when communicating their pain, which assessment tools don't capture and clinicians often misunderstand. When pain is measured accurately, Black older people are more likely to report higher levels of pain, suffering, and depressive symptoms than White people. Unfortunately, regardless of higher pain scores, Black patients are often given a lower dose of pain medications and experience longer wait times to receive those medications.[8]

To alleviate the suffering of vulnerable communities, nurses should mitigate racial bias in their institutions through evidence-informed advocacy and promoting cultural safety in practice. "Nurses must embrace a patient-centered approach responsive to the individual cultural needs and concerns of their patients and families."[9] A person-centered approach allows for the inclusion of cultural and socioeconomic needs in the care plan because the patient is willing to build further trust with the provider. Older people from vulnerable populations have endured weathering caused by structural racism, and the nursing field has a unique position to help address issues of racial equity. Unfortunately, social needs will continue to present themselves as a form of suffering in all clinical settings; it is our job to acknowledge the lived experiences of our patients and prevent any further harm.[10]

Responses to Suffering: Age-Friendly Health Systems

The Age-Friendly Health Systems movement mitigates suffering by directly addressing some of the underpinnings of structural racism such as health disparity. Older people suffer disproportionate harms and death because of suboptimal care, the lack of geriatric expertise in the health care workforce, and the provision of care that is not concordant with the older adult's goals and values. Age-Friendly Health Systems and its underlying 4Ms framework address these workforce disparities and the dearth of geriatric-expert clinicians by ensuring all clinicians providing care across the continuum are competently and reliably applying evidence-based assessments and actions that result in the avoidance of common harms and causes of suffering for older people.[11] Age-Friendly Health Systems is an initiative of the John A. Hartford Foundation and led by the Institute for Healthcare Improvement (IHI), in partnership with the American Hospital Association (AHA) and the Catholic Health Association of the United States (CHA).

Becoming recognized as Age-Friendly Health Systems entails reliably delivering the set of evidence-based elements of high-quality care, with corresponding assessments and actions, known as the 4Ms framework, as defined below:[12]

- *What Matters*—Know and align care with each older adult's specific health outcome goals and care preferences, including but not limited to end-of-life care.
- *Medication*—If medication is necessary, use Age-Friendly medication that does not interfere with What Matters to the older adult, Mobility, or Mentation across settings of care.
- *Mentation*—Prevent, identify, treat, and manage dementia, depression, and delirium across settings of care.
- *Mobility*—Ensure that older people move safely every day to maintain function and do What Matters.

Today more than 2,700 health systems and sites providing care to older people across the continuum, from hospitals and outpatient clinics to nursing homes and Program of All-inclusive Care for the Elderly (PACE) sites, have been recognized as Age-Friendly Health Systems by the IHI. The outcomes resulting from implementation of the 4Ms framework have been featured in a series of case studies produced by the AHA and featured in its Value Initiative. Sites recognized as Age-Friendly Health Systems reported reductions in length of stay, rehospitalization, delirium, falls, inappropriate medication use, and increased patient satisfaction.[13–15]

One of the greatest potential causes of harm in the seriously ill is the provision of care or treatment that conflicts with what matters to the older adult. The Age-Friendly Health Systems movement is predicated on What Matters as a critical element of the 4Ms framework. In eliciting what matters to the individual and integrating their goals and care preferences into treatment, the resulting aligned and age-friendly care reduces clinical harm and suffering caused by unwanted care and treatment. Further, in supporting what matters to the older adult, the movement supports autonomy and equity as it gives voice to the patient as a member of their own care team.

Why does What Matters matter and why does eliciting and acting on an older adult's goals and preferences reduce suffering? Eleven years ago, I (AB) was diagnosed with stage IV (incurable and widely disseminated) inflammatory breast cancer.[16] From the onset, I had the benefit of clinicians who asked what mattered to me. My prognosis was poor, with only an 11% to 20% chance of survival to 5 years. I told my oncologist that I did not want care and treatment that would strip me of my quality of life especially given that the treatment options would not cure me of cancer. I chose not to have my breast removed, which is almost a knee-jerk response to a breast cancer diagnosis. Why did I choose that? The cancer had already spread to my spine and coursed through every drop of my blood. Removing the breast would not remove the cancer and might lead to a new set of issues including lymphedema or surgical infection.

I asked my clinical team to focus on treatments that had fewer side effects. I asked for palliative care to address pain and symptoms related to the disease and treatment. And 11 years later I continue to work and live well in the face of life-limiting illness because what matters to me matters to my health care team. There is no better antidote to suffering in the seriously ill than attention to what matters to them.

Cultural Context for Suffering

Our lives are continuously influenced by culture. The Merriam Webster Dictionary defines "culture" as "the characteristic features of everyday existence (such as diversions or a way of life) shared by people in a place or time."

Culture is a way of life for a group of people, usually expressed in beliefs, values, and overall social constructs and norms in society. It is a backbone for everything we do and frames our perspective on life. The United States is often referred to as a melting pot of diverse cultures and backgrounds, depending on the region of the country. Urban areas where immigrants land or refugees come to live have a distinctly unique set of cultural elements that affect the expression of suffering. In other locations, there can be great homogeneity and therefore a greater capacity for nurses to anticipate what the belief systems might be. In the book *The Spirit Catches You and You Fall Down*,[17] the author portrays the heartbreaking story of a refugee family from Laos and the care of a child diagnosed with severe epilepsy. The interpretation of what the family believed and wanted was the antithesis of what the health care system understood as the goals of care or the expression of sadness and suffering. The author portrayed enormous suffering on the part of the family with little initial acknowledgment from the expert clinical team responsible. The American health care system has made little progress since this book was published.

When we discuss cultural competence, the meaning is often in the eye of the beholder. Cultural competence can be described using many different definitions, but they aim to address the idea that from both an individual and organizational perspective, we must be able to work with people of all different cultures and backgrounds.[18] This term sometimes is misunderstood to mean we all need to know everything about everyone's culture in order to properly care for patients and their families. However, cultural competence is about valuing the individuality of each person and recognizing the need for communication skills to effectively and respectfully care for each person based on what matters to them. It must be accompanied by cultural humility, cultural safety, cultural sensitivity, and respect. In nursing, it is impossible to be aware of the wide array of human conditions due to the many patients seen each day. However, it is hoped that each nurse knows how to effectively communicate to learn about the older person and their culture in order to respect what matters to them based on knowledge of and familiarity with the older person and their family's culture and background.

COVID-19

The COVID-19 pandemic brought into sharp focus the differences in access to care, vaccine availability, and culturally sensitive approaches to care for older people. This is very obviously entwined with the way a person experiences suffering.

The pandemic has also shed light on underlying ageism in both American society and globally, particularly in our health care system. The impact of the pandemic on older people was severe given the heightened risk for mortality if infected with the severe acute respiratory syndrome coronavirus 2 (SARS-CoV-2). This played a major role in health care decision-making, such as triage protocols, allocations of resources, and other emergency decisions that occurred during the height of the pandemic. Older people died at disproportional rates to younger Americans from COVID-19, which led to significant suffering experienced by older Americans and their families during this pandemic. Those disproportionate deaths also impacted health care professionals because of the overwhelming suffering they witnessed. Ageism became a default response to this virus due to the increased morbidity and mortality rates in this population. Health care systems resorted to using chronological age as a significant factor in medical decision-making because of the assumption that there is a correlation between chronological age and health outcomes.[19]

In addition to suffering caused by ageism, older Americans experienced mental suffering. For example, during the COVID-19 pandemic, older people in the United States were increasingly isolated and lonely due to increased restrictions in nursing homes and other home settings and from the deaths of friends and family members. Older people were isolated because community centers and places of social activity were closed. In this way, older people experienced suffering during the pandemic not just physically from those who were infected with the virus but also from loneliness and isolation while trying to avoid infection.[20]

Those older people who were hospitalized from COVID-19 may have experienced ageism in the form of discriminatory health care practices. Many hospitals had to create triage protocols that put older people at the bottom of the list for life-saving treatments, regardless of health status. Their suffering from these policies during the COVID-19 pandemic was a result of ageism. Unfortunately, societies have decided that when determining who should live and die, chronological age is a major factor, often favoring those who are younger.[20]

Dementia: The Experience of Caring, Comfort, and Suffering

There are over 6 million Americans living with Alzheimer's disease, and roughly one in three older people will die with Alzheimer's disease or another form of dementia.[21] Dementia is the loss of cognitive functioning, progressing from mild to severe stages, that often impacts a person's ADLs and instrumental activities of daily living (IADLs). People living with dementia often exhibit memory loss, confusion, wandering and getting lost, and acting impulsively, among other changes in cognition that affect one's ability to live. Given these large numbers of people living with cognitive impairment, this group of people accounts for a lot of the suffering that occurs in older people. Experiencing cognitive decline for the person themself can be scary and frustrating. Older people often report feeling vulnerable and frustrated by the inability to complete everyday tasks and express negative feelings toward becoming dependent and a burden on loved ones.[22] In addition to the personal suffering experienced by the one losing their cognition, the process also deeply impacts family, nurses, and caregivers.

People living with dementia often have a caregiver who spends a significant amount of time helping them with ADLs. Roughly 80% of caregivers are family members, with the other 20% being hired professionals. Given the complexity of caring for a person living with dementia, this can often have a negative impact on caregivers' own health. The World Health Organization has reported that over 264 million people globally suffer from major depressive disorder. However, the percentage of caregivers experiencing depression is much higher than that of the general population. Some of the effects of depression can include compromised physical health, reduced quality of life, and in some cases increased risk of caregiver suicide. This suffering by caregivers can not only be detrimental to their own health but also have negative impacts on their patient's health, including a more rapid cognitive decline. The shared experience of suffering from both the person with dementia and their caregiver shows just how impactful one's suffering is on the other.[23]

In acute care settings, nurses play a unique role in caring for patients with dementia. The nurses' experiences can be "characterized by frustration, overall job dissatisfaction, and feelings of powerlessness and guilt" given the complexity of caring for patients with cognitive impairment. [24] Patients admitted to the hospital with dementia often can show behavioral issues, leading nurses to employ physical and pharmaceutical strategies. However, in more recent years, there has been a shift to more person-centered approaches. Nurses are frequently very busy and have time constraints that make their jobs difficult. Especially when caring for a patient with dementia, nurses reported needing more time to carry out tasks, only adding to the stress of their workload. When patients with dementia exhibit aggressive behaviors or emotional challenges, this also impacts the experience of the nurse and can lead to suffering.[25]

End of Life and Medical Aid in Dying

The suffering experienced by an individual living with serious illness is often significant. For instance, older people with dementia may fear loss of control in decision-making, dependence on others for basic needs, and not being able to communicate their own suffering. Because of these fears, older people sometimes choose to formulate directives for medical assistance in dying, also referred to as assisted suicide. This is perceived as one way of avoiding the suffering they might experience if they were to progress into advanced stages of dementia. Further, older people often speak of "not becoming a burden to their loved ones." Clinical care is aimed at reducing the older person's suffering; however, what might decrease suffering for some can sometimes conflict with the religious, moral, or ethical beliefs of a clinician. For example, medical aid in dying (MAID) in a patient with dementia could reduce their suffering by shortening life in end stages of cognitive decline, but clinician reactions need to be considered and respected.

Globally, MAID is highly controversial, accepted by some and rejected by others. In the United States, Oregon was the first state to pass a death with dignity law in 1997, and in years after, states such as Montana, Vermont, California, Colorado, Hawaii, New Jersey, Maine, and the District of Columbia passed similar laws. In other states it has been ruled as illegal. Given this regional variation, there are limitations to this practice.[25]

The main arguments for MAID are respect for patient autonomy and relief of suffering, while others argue that this practice leads to what has been referred to as suicide contagion and overuse of the assistance. Older people living with dementia or other diseases from aging might request this practice to reduce suffering. However, this practice is contentious and political.[26]

Death and Dying: How Is It Different for Older People?

One aspect of suffering for older people that is more common is the experience of loss as they age. Watching dear friends or family members become seriously ill and die is a hallmark of aging. For many older people, losing a spouse can be a form of suffering that is particularly hard to emotionally overcome as the loss can pervade every aspect of life from an empty bed to challenges maintaining the home to social impacts as a single person. Some people describe the loss of their spouse as akin to losing a part of their own body. As emphasized throughout this volume, suffering is a highly individual experience. What one person experiences as suffering may not feel like suffering to another.

The experiences of structural discrimination may deepen the suffering of loss and bereavement in the face of structures that don't officially recognize some relationships and systematically disenfranchise some populations. The LGBTQ community has had to bear the brunt of this type of discrimination. The majority of studies that seek to describe the experience of end of life in older people has traditionally relied on nonrepresentative population samples (mainly Caucasian) that cannot be generalized to the rest of the public.

Another aspect of suffering related to serious illness, dying, and death is anticipatory grief related to fear of the loss of control or independence from illness. Older people recognize their mortality. Yet, this acceptance is ignored until one is diagnosed with a serious illness. The majority of deaths around the world are attributed to the older adult population, and as such, they experience disproportionate anticipatory grief beginning with a serious illness or poor-prognosis diagnosis, which can manifest depression, loss of physical and mental acuity, and conflict, in the same way people may experience grieving an actual death.[28]

Religion in the Context of Suffering for Older People

Spirituality is a belief in a transcendent power that controls at least some forces in individuals' lives. Religion consists of a group of people who have a shared system of beliefs, rituals, and practices, which strengthen their relationship with a sacred being. Even though religion and spirituality are different concepts, they do overlap in many ways. Many patients use religion and spiritualty as tools for their pain and suffering. In a recent study, 88% of patients with advanced cancer reported religion and spirituality to be personally important in adjusting to their illness. Religious coping can offer patients a sense of meaning, comfort, control, and personal growth while facing life-threatening illness. Research also indicates that religious factors affect medical decisions at a patient's end of life. In a survey of 1,006 members of the public, 68.3% of individuals stated that their religious beliefs would guide their medical decisions if critically injured, and 57.4% believed that God could heal a patient even if physicians had determined further medical efforts to be futile. Religious coping has been associated with increased preference for cardiopulmonary resuscitation, mechanical ventilation, hospitalization near death, and heroic end-of-life measures.[29] An interesting contrast is that even though most religious people choose life-prolonging interventions because they believe God can heal them even when doctors cannot, many patients from minoritized backgrounds do not believe in advance care planning because they believe only God controls their time of death.[30]

Researchers found that spiritual well-being significantly correlated with greater levels of physical, emotional, and functional well-being and a better quality of life. Greater spiritual well-being was associated with less decisional conflict, decreased uncertainty, a feeling of being more informed and supported, and greater satisfaction with one's decision. Most patients successfully implemented their decision and identified themselves as capable of early decision-making. Patients who were able to implement their decision presented lower decisional conflict and higher levels of spiritual well-being and quality of life.[31] It is very important for clinicians to have basic knowledge of patients' religious beliefs. By having this knowledge, it will allow clinicians to understand and respect patients' goals and behaviors and take them into consideration when making important end-of-life care decisions.[32]

Christianity, Islam, Judaism, Hinduism, and Sikhism are among the major religions in the world. These five religions strive for a peaceful end-of-life experience, discourage actions that can hasten death, and believe euthanasia to be morally and ethically wrong. However, it is important to note that these are not monolithic religions and patients may follow various interpretations based on their ethnicity and culture. While the modern approach to death is highly medicalized, it is important to remember that it is also a social experience defined by rituals, beliefs, and traditions. The involvement of family, community, and religious leaders is vital to some as it enables the provision of meaning, spiritual renewal, and comfort at the end of life.[32]

Conclusion

Our profession is keenly aware of the special needs of older people as they enter into a phase of their life where they have increasing disability, chronic disease, and in some cases social isolation and loneliness. Since the earliest days of visiting nurses, nurses were the leaders in the very special and intimate space that we think of as the alleviation of suffering for those who are at the end of life. The nursing profession should capitalize on our autonomy in this role and take back our practice. Nurses have been the leading generators of evidence for best practices in the care of older people and can unleash untold capacity and talent by ensuring nursing practice reflects our abilities and unique role in the care for older people, especially those who are suffering.

Case Exemplar 7.1

Mr. S, known to his friends as "Iron Mike," had been a rigorous athlete into his 80s despite a slowly progressing form of Parkinson's disease. His health took a dramatic turn over the past year when he experienced a series of vertebral fractures requiring extensive spinal surgery. In postsurgical rehabilitation, Mr. S did not have the strength to complete his physical therapy regimen. He suffered from several episodes of pneumonia over the year, caused in part by aspiration from the effects of Parkinson's and exacerbated by weakness and lack of physical activity. Each illness left Mr. S weaker than the time before.

It was difficult for him to speak beyond an occasional whisper. He spent much of the day sleeping. He was hospitalized for pneumonia yet again. The antibiotics caused severe intestinal discomfort and diarrhea. He had a loud rattle when breathing. The physician discussed hospice with his wife in his presence. Mr. S said he had "had enough" (treatment), which was the first time his wife ever heard him say that treatments were too much for him. His wife agreed to enroll him in hospice. His family had taken turns regularly visiting. His wife called the family and told them to immediately come see their father. The physician indicated that a hospice inpatient facility bed should be available in the next day or two.

Mr. and Mrs. S experienced a range of suffering with a number of mitigation strategies that provided support and comfort in his final days. Together, they experienced anticipatory grieving, loss of control and independence, fear, and loneliness from being disconnected from their circle of family and friends as they faced the end of life. Mr. S also faced physical suffering due to the labored breathing and effects of the antibiotic.

A nurse present for the physician's discussion with the husband and wife asked if the antibiotics could be discontinued and medication provided to ease his respiratory distress. The physician said that both steps would happen when he moved to hospice. The prescient nurse pushed the physician further.

"Are you saying that he should needlessly suffer until hospice has a bed?"

The young physician looked up and acknowledged the suffering, ordered the antibiotic to be discontinued, and added a medication to ease Mr. S's labored breathing. He seemed appreciative that the nurse reminded him of the goals of care and what he could do to ease the physical suffering.

Some members of the family arrived soon after. They helped Mr. S have video calls with the family who couldn't be there. Even though Mr. S could no longer speak, he smiled and his nonverbal responses showed the easing of his suffering. The nurse asked Mrs. S questions about Mr. S and the family; the use of reminiscence helped to ease Mrs. S's suffering by allowing her to share positive memories with Mr. S.

The family's rabbi visited that day to offer comfort and the support of their religious community and asked how best to offer spiritual support.

The next day, Mr. S died at home in hospice, although before he could be admitted to the inpatient setting. He was comfortable at home and had family with him. His wife said she was appreciative that the physician suggested hospice because during that conversation her husband said he was ready to stop treatment. It gave her comfort to know that "Iron Mike" was ready to die.

References

1. Butler RN. Age-ism: another form of bigotry. *The Gerontologist.* 1969;9(4 Part 1):243–246.
2. Frameworks Institute. Aging. Published 2022. Accessed March 15, 2022.
3. Sweetland J, Volmert A, O'Neil M. *Finding the Frame: An Empirical Approach to Reframing Aging and Ageism.* Frameworks Institute; February 2017.
4. Provisional life expectancy estimates for 2020. Washington DC: FrameWorks Institute; 2021.
5. Jones CP. Levels of racism: a theoretic framework and a gardener's tale. *Am J Public Health.* 2000;90(8):1212–1215.
6. Adomoko F. African American Older Adults and Race-Related Stress How Aging and Health-Care Providers Can Help [Fact Sheet]. Published December 1, 2018. https://www.apa.org/pi/aging/resources/african-american-stress.pdf
7. Assari S, Cobb S, Saqib M, Bazargan M. Economic strain deteriorates while education fails to protect black older adults against depressive symptoms, pain, self-rated health, chronic disease, and sick days. *J Ment Health Clin Psychol.* 2020;4(2):49–62.
8. Robinson-Lane SG, Booker SQ. Culturally responsive pain management for black older adults. *J Gerontol Nurs.* 2017;43(8):33–41.
9. ANA Ethics Advisory Board. ANA Position Statement: the nurse's role in addressing discrimination: protecting and promoting inclusive strategies in practice settings, policy, and advocacy. *Online J Issues Nurs.* 2019;24(3).
10. Cuevas AG, O'Brien K, Saha S. What is the key to culturally competent care: reducing bias or cultural tailoring? *Psychol Health.* 2017;32(4):493–507.
11. Fulmer T, Mate KS, Berman A. The Age-Friendly Health System imperative. *J Am Geriatr Soc.* 2018;66(1):22–24.
12. Terry Fulmer LP. *Age-Friendly Health Systems: A Guide to Using the 4Ms While Caring for Older Adults.* Institute for Healthcare Improvement; 2022.
13. Hochman R. Chair file: building Age-Friendly Health Systems to improve care for older adults. American Hospital Association. Published 2021. Updated June 14, 2021. Accessed March 15, 2022. https://www.aha.org/news/chairpersons-file/2021-06-14-chair-file-building-age-friendly-health-systems-improve-care
14. Age-Friendly Health Care improves value for older adults with fractures. AHA Members in Action Web site. Published 2021. Accessed March 15, 2022. https://www.aha.org/system/files/media/file/2021/02/value-initiative-member-in-action-case-study-cedars-sinai-medical-center-los-angeles-ca.pdf
15. Healthy Together care partnership embeds Age-Friendly framework into practice. Members in Action Web site. Published 2020. Updated December 2020. Accessed March 15, 2022. https://www.aha.org/system/files/media/file/2020/12/aha-cs-banner-health-1220.pdf
16. Living life in my own way—and dying that way as well. *Health Affairs.* 2012;31(4):871–874.
17. Fadiman A. *The Spirit Catches You and You Fall Down: A Hmong Child, Her American Doctors, and the Collision of Two Cultures.* Macmillan; 2012.
18. Shaya FT, Gbarayor CM. The case for cultural competence in health professions education. *Am J Pharm Educ.* 2006;70(6):Article 124. 10.5688/aj7006124
19. Kagan SH. Ageism, older people, and hospitalization: walking a path through the past, looking to lead in the future. *Geriatr Nurs.* 2020;41(5):654–656.
20. Monahan C, Macdonald J, Lytle A, Apriceno M, Levy SR. COVID-19 and ageism: how positive and negative responses impact older adults and society. *Am Psychol.* 2020;75(7):887–896.

21. Alzheimer's Association facts and figures. Published 2021. Accessed 2022. https://www.alz.org/alzheimers-dementia/facts-figures

22. Xanthopoulou P, McCabe R. Subjective experiences of cognitive decline and receiving a diagnosis of dementia: qualitative interviews with people recently diagnosed in memory clinics in the UK. *BMJ Open*. 2019;9(8):e026071–e026071.

23. Huang S-S. Depression among caregivers of patients with dementia: associative factors and management approaches. *World J Psychiatry*. 2022;12(1):59–76.

24. Pinkert C, Faul E, Saxer S, Burgstaller M, Kamleitner D, Mayer H. Experiences of nurses with the care of patients with dementia in acute hospitals: a secondary analysis. *J Clin Nurs*. 2018;27(1–2):162–172.

25. Dookhy J, Daly L. Nurses' experiences of caring for persons with dementia experiencing responsive behaviours in an acute hospital: a qualitative descriptive study. *Int J Older People Nurs*. 2021;16(4):e12379.

26. Cipriani G, Di Fiorino M. Euthanasia and other end of life in patients suffering from dementia. *Legal Med*. 2019;40:54–59.

27. Streeter JL. Gender differences in widowhood in the short-run and long-run: financial, emotional, and mental wellbeing. *J Econ Ageing*. 2020;17:100258.

28. Hottensen D. Anticipatory grief in patients with cancer. *Clin J Oncol Nurs*. 2010;14(1):106–107.

29. Phelps AC, Maciejewski PK, Nilsson M, et al. Religious coping and use of intensive life-prolonging care near death in patients with advanced cancer. *JAMA*. 2009;301(11):1140–1147.

30. Grace J, Kim LG. The effects of religion and spirituality on coping efficacy for death and dying. Published 2017. Updated November 9, 2017. Accessed March 17, 2022. https://www.practicalpainmanagement.com/resources/hospice/effects-religion-spirituality-coping-efficacy-death-dying

31. Rego F, Gonçalves F, Moutinho S, Castro L, Nunes R. The influence of spirituality on decision-making in palliative care outpatients: a cross-sectional study. *BMC Palliat Care*. 2020;19(1):22.

32. Choudry M, Latif A, Warburton KG. An overview of the spiritual importance of end-of-life care among the five major faiths of the United Kingdom. *Clin Med*. 2018;18(1):23.

8

Suffering Related to Mental Health Challenges and Traumatic Events

Barbara A. Harris

Introduction

In 2020, mental health challenges, in the form of mental illnesses and responses to trauma, affected as many as 52 million people in the United States.[1] The Substance Abuse and Mental Health Services Administration noted that in 2019, an additional 20.4 million Americans experienced or were diagnosed with a substance use disorder.[2] Hune and Kimball,[3] in their discussion of suffering and suicidality among persons with mental illness and substance use disorders, cite Cassell's[4] definition of suffering as the "state of severe distress associated with events that threaten the intactness of the person." Consider for a moment the phrase "the intactness of the person." To be intact is to be untouched, unharmed, undiminished. To feel harmed, damaged, less of a person, or less than whole is, as Hune and Kimball[3] assert, often central to the suffering of those with mental health challenges. The experiences and events that give rise to this suffering and the manifestations of suffering are the focus of this chapter. The central question that accompanies the discussion of these experiences is: how do we, as nurses, support persons suffering with mental health challenges to mend, or find a greater sense of wholeness, even in the face of illness, symptoms, or experiences that operate to take this away?

Mental health challenges in this chapter refer to the experience of symptoms of mental illness, substance use disorders, and psychological responses to trauma. While each of the three are distinct diagnostic categories and areas of human experience, people can be diagnosed in more than one category and suffer from the manifestations of more than one at a given time. In addition, having one may increase risk for another. For example, the connection between the experience of trauma and later substance use disorders is well documented.[5] Likewise, having a mental illness may predispose a person to substance use disorders because substances can sometimes be used as a way to manage symptoms or cope with psychological pain.[3,6] More importantly, there is overlap in the lived experiences of suffering within each category.

This chapter will describe and discuss the sources and nature of suffering for all three areas, with attention to the common dimensions of suffering across them. This chapter will also address how experiences of suffering among members of marginalized populations are shaped and often made worse by societal factors. It will conclude with a direct address of the question raised above: Given what we know about suffering with mental health challenges, how do we as nurses respond? How do we draw

Barbara A. Harris, *Suffering Related to Mental Health Challenges and Traumatic Events* In: *The Nature of Suffering and the Goals of Nursing*. Second Edition. Edited by: William E. Rosa and Betty R. Ferrell, Oxford University Press.
© Oxford University Press 2023. DOI: 10.1093/oso/9780197667934.003.0008

on both our humanity and knowledge of the person's suffering so that we are able to walk forward with them on their journey toward greater wholeness and less suffering?

The Suffering of Mental Illness

Mental illness includes several diagnoses that encompass a wide range of symptoms and experiences. Diagnoses can range from alterations of mood, such as depression and bipolar illness; to thought disorders, such as psychosis and schizophrenia; to disorders that stem from organic changes to the brain, such as dementia. Addiction and the psychological effects of trauma can also fall under the umbrella of mental illness but will be addressed separately in this chapter.

Much of the suffering related to mental illness can be exacerbated by the invisibility of its source, which can increase the burden of suffering. In addition, it is often harder for another person to understand suffering that does not have a visible source.[7] Further, as Verhofstadt et al.[8] note in their examination of euthanasia requests among persons with severe and persistent mental illness, not only is the source of suffering with mental illness often not visible to others, but also it may be hard to describe in ways to which others can relate. Almost everyone can relate to an experience of physical pain, but not all can relate to the psychic pain of despair, for example, or the unrelenting fear of a paranoid delusion. Hesitancy to share one's suffering out of fear of not being understood, or worse, being rejected can also occur, which, as discussed below, can lead to isolation, alienation, and disrupted relationships that can ultimately increase suffering.[8]

An experience of psychosis is a good example of an invisible source of suffering. Consider a person with an enduring delusion, or fixed, false belief, that they are being poisoned. They may not feel able to share this with others, or if they do, they may be told their fears are not real, though to them, the fears are very real. This person is experiencing the anguish of living with a very real fear that their body is being harmed inside and yet feels helpless to do anything about it. In addition, as Breggin and Stolzer[9] note, there is sometimes a propensity among clinicians to focus on the content of a delusion or its severity with the objective of resolving it or diminishing its severity to the exclusion of seeking to understand the distress it engenders for the person experiencing it. If the medical focus is solely on the delusion as an abnormality to be eliminated, it minimizes the human experience of suffering and can leave the person feeling defective.

A delusion or other symptoms of psychosis that alter a person's ability to perceive and interact with reality can significantly hinder their ability to function in the world. Preoccupation with a delusion can interfere with school, employment, and family, as can the emotions that frequently accompany these symptoms, such as fear and anxiety. The same can occur with the fatigue, apathy, and withdrawal that can accompany psychosis. If a person becomes severely psychotic, their behavior may cause harm to themselves or others. All these experiences can significantly interfere with a person's function in the world, leading to the distress of decreased self-esteem and diminished sense of efficacy and worthiness.[10] And all have the potential to contribute to a sense of brokenness and often helplessness.[9]

Persons with alterations of mood, such depression or bipolar illness, can experience unrelenting despair or hopelessness, even in the absence of real-world events that could cause this. Some feel defective or damaged or even guilty because they are aware they are not experiencing events that normally give rise to despair, yet they cannot simply "snap out of it" and feel better, as some family and friends may suggest.[8] There is, however, some evidence that persons with bipolar illness may experience the distress associated with adverse life events more keenly than those without mood disorders.[11] People around them who do not understand this may judge them as being overdramatic or unstable, increasing their despair and sense of themselves as damaged.

On the other end of the mood spectrum, persons who experience mania as part of their bipolar illness may find themselves acting in ways that, while part of the illness, wreak havoc with their lives and reputations. Hypersexuality and impaired judgement can place the person in unsafe and embarrassing or humiliating situations. Grandiosity (e.g., overestimation of worth and ability) can lead to overspending and result in financial damage. These are just a few examples of how bipolar mania can give rise to behaviors that, unlike some forms of mental illnesses, are visible to others, as are the consequences of the behaviors. The real-world consequences of the behaviors can be a significant source of suffering. Once the manic episode is resolved, a person can be left with criminal, legal, financial, and reputational problems that can be overwhelming. These life problems serve to intensify existing feelings of guilt, despair, and worthlessness.[12]

Isolation is not an uncommon response when people feel that what they are experiencing may be unacceptable, disgusting, or abhorrent to others. For example, a person who suffers with obsessive-compulsive disorder can experience repeated, intrusive, and obsessive thoughts of themselves being dismembered in accidents or through other violent methods. They may have no intention of acting on these thoughts and indeed spend tremendous energy suppressing these thoughts or performing compulsions, or repeated actions, to decrease the intensity of the thoughts and accompanying anxiety. Yet they can be very concerned about how the violence of their thoughts could alarm, disgust, or drive others away so they may choose to remain silent.[13] The same can occur with suicidal thoughts.[7] Isolation is further intensified when people around the suffering person sense something is wrong but the person does not reveal what that is. People around the suffering person may feel increasingly uncomfortable and helpless and eventually, either consciously or unconsciously, distance themselves from the person. This cycle of increasing isolation and alienation intensifies despair and helplessness. This can be seen in Case Exemplar 8.1. Peter struggles with fears that he will do something to disgust his coworkers. He certainly does not want to, but the anxiety and fear that he might is great. He attempts to manage the anxiety with repeated actions, or compulsions, yet these only serve to draw his coworkers' attention to him and eventually push them away. He does not explain his fear to them or the reason for the actions he takes. As a result, they withdraw from him. He can see no way to break this cycle and experiences isolation and alienation daily.

Case Exemplar 8.1

The Cycle of Isolation and Alienation

Pete is a 37-year-old clerical worker with a diagnosis of obsessive-compulsive disorder. He has recurrent, intrusive thoughts of a time when he vomited in the classroom during elementary school. These thoughts have generalized to fears he will lose control and do something "disgusting" that will repulse people. Pete understands his fear is not rational but cannot stop the thoughts. He attempts to decrease the anxiety of the thoughts with repeated actions, or compulsions, such as continually wiping his mouth. He avoids eating at work and when hungry will take tiny bites of food at his desk and chew each bite 30 times. His coworkers have noticed and occasionally make jokes at his expense. He feels alone and hopeless. Each day it is harder to sit at his desk alone and the intrusive thoughts become more intense. He wants to join in the regular workday socialization but knows his coworkers see him as "weird." He is wiping his mouth so much now that the skin is raw and red, and he knows his coworkers notice. He feels as though life is not worth living but cannot break free from his thoughts or compulsive behaviors. Pete visits his local community health clinic for his mouth, which appears infected. The nurse practitioner, Judy, carefully assesses his skin, talks to him about proper cleaning, prescribes him a topical ointment and analgesic cream—as the area has become very painful—and gently guides him in how he can care for the skin to avoid further irritation and infections. Judy sits with him to better understand what has led to the current condition. Pete begins to cry. He shares about his intrusive thoughts and compulsive actions, as well as his feelings of isolation and embarrassment. Judy sits and listens to Pete's story without interrupting. After acknowledging how hard it sounds like things have been for him, Judy normalizes his experience by sharing that several people struggle with similar challenges, and reminds him there is no reason to be ashamed—"You are safe here and you are not alone." She places her hand on his and asks if he would like to see the clinic case manager to arrange for some therapeutic support. Pete did not realize this was possible or that his insurance would cover these services. He tells Judy before he leaves that this is the first time—in a very, very long time—that he doesn't feel isolated or alienated. He feels seen.

Some people do choose to share their pain and the thoughts underlying the pain, only to find that those they share with are unable to, or appear to be unable to, handle the thoughts, feelings, or accompanying emotional intensity, leading them to greater isolation and increased sense of alienation.[7,8] Experiences like these may condition the person to expect only negative results from seeking help or sharing experiences. Isolation and alienation are potent sources of suffering for those with mental health challenges. Being unable to ease the burden of psychological pain through sharing as well as the fear that others will reject them if they do share reinforces a sense of brokenness and, for some, shame.[13]

There are other mental health challenges that hold the potential to contribute to isolation and alienation in different ways. At times, isolation is not a choice or self-protective action taken on the part of the person, but rather the result of other people's responses to them and their behaviors. Persons with obsessive-compulsive disorder may find themselves bullied in educational or employment settings because of what others perceive as odd behaviors. For example, a person with obsessive-compulsive disorder may get "stuck" performing a ritual that serves to decrease anxiety and the intensity of obsessive thoughts, which slows down their work performance, irritating their coworkers.[14] As a result of this or because their behaviors make others uncomfortable, they can become a target for bullying or harassment. Alternately, persons with obsessive-compulsive disorder may spend tremendous amounts of energy and endure severe psychological distress to resist acting on compulsions so as not to be targeted or labeled as different, resulting in stressful and draining workdays, or may believe that somehow their thoughts can be harmful to others and go to great lengths to avoid interpersonal engagement.[14] Some struggle to overcome the lack of interpersonal connection, often working hard to hide or mask psychological states that others might find off-putting. Isolation and alienation are problematic not only because of the suffering experienced as a result but also because lack of meaningful interaction and social support can intensify symptoms of mental illness and lead to poorer outcomes.[15] Social isolation and avoidance of help seeking can also be correlated with decreased quality of life.[16] As discussed above, Peter in Case Exemplar 8.1 cannot find a way to either explain his "weird" behaviors to his coworkers or stop them, leaving him without any way to connect with his coworkers. As a result, the suffering of his isolation grows and adds to the weight of hopelessness he feels.

Treatments for mental conditions can also be sources of suffering. Side effects of medications can cause physical discomfort, such as headaches or gastrointestinal disturbances. Other side effects, such as drowsiness, mental fogginess, or problems with vision and motor activity, including tremors and stiffness, can limit or decrease ability to function in the domains of work, family, school, and social life. For some, the side effects of medications are of a far greater magnitude than the actual effectiveness of the medication on target symptoms.[10] These side effects can clearly lead to distress, feelings of inadequacy, or feeling defective. Some medication side effects or long-term effects can cause visible disability. Tardive dyskinesia, for example, is a movement disorder characterized by involuntary movements that can result from the use of some antipsychotic medications. The visibility of tardive dyskinesia invites all of the same negative social reactions and associated suffering that persons with physical disability experience, including compromised physical function and being judged by others as less than capable, defective, or damaged. The experience of lack of control over side effects is also distressing, as is the awareness that stopping the medications to stop the side effects leads back to the distress of symptoms. Powerlessness and helplessness can be significant sources of suffering in these situations.

When perceptions of powerlessness and helplessness become unbearable, suicide can be perceived by a person as their only option for relief from the suffering of mental health challenges. In addition, when suicidality arises from largely invisible, psychological suffering, mental health providers may simply view it as a symptom of mental illness to be targeted with medication or somatic treatments, such as electroconvulsive therapy or transcranial magnetic stimulation.[9] As with the medicalization of delusions discussed above, medicalizing suicidal ideation as a symptom of illness divorces it from the human experience of suffering.[3] Over the past decade, however, there has been growing awareness that the suffering of mental illness is a type of existential crisis leading to suicidality in the same way that occurs with physical suffering. In their qualitative study of 26 people with mental health challenges and suicidality, Verhofstadt et al.[8] found that illness symptoms, medication effects, and isolation and disruptions of interpersonal relationships—and, significantly, feeling powerless to change these—were potent sources of the despair that gave rise to suicidality among their sample.

As demonstrated in the preceding paragraphs, there are many sources of powerlessness and helplessness that exist in the experiences of persons with mental health challenges. Isolation and alienation are also frequent sources of suffering among those with mental illness, which intensify or reinforce perceptions of powerlessness. The elusive and often invisible nature of suffering as well as the inherent difficulty of explaining it to others adds to the sense of powerlessness and can further fuel suicidality.[7]

The Suffering of Trauma Survivors

Trauma can be defined as an adverse experience that either harms or oppresses a person.[17] Events that cause trauma can vary in intensity and duration of time and can be either witnessed or personally experienced. These include a wide range of events such as natural disaster, war, torture, being a victim of a crime, violence of all kinds, and abuse, whether physical, psychological, or sexual. While the nature of harm or oppression stemming from the original traumatizing event may be either psychological or physical, or both, the focus in this chapter is on the psychological trauma that extends past the traumatizing event itself and continues to cause psychological symptoms and suffering for the person. Posttraumatic stress disorder (PTSD) is the commonly used psychiatric term for a lasting psychological response to a trauma. The nature, intensity, and length of the original trauma, as well as personal characteristics such as experience of previous traumas and possibly aspects of a person's personality, will all shape the person's response to trauma. Because of the multiplicity of factors that shape a person's response to trauma, it is essential to remember that a person's response may not be proportional to the original trauma; this should not overshadow attention to the unique, lived experience of suffering of trauma survivors.[18]

Trauma survivors' suffering is more likely than other mental health challenges to include physiological sources of suffering. Fibromyalgia and chronic pain disorders, for example, are not usually the direct physiological results of a trauma but occur at higher rates among trauma survivors than other groups and add to the burden of suffering.[19] Reynolds,[17] discussing the importance of understanding the lived experience of trauma for developing effective interventions, suggests that a major dimension of suffering among trauma survivors is a sense of brokenness, a belief that they were either too weak or too defective to prevent the trauma or to stop it. As can be seen in Case Exemplar 8.2, trauma survivors like Shanara may even feel that, in the case of abuse, they invited it. Living with this belief about oneself can cause pain, despair, and hopelessness. It can also lead to a sense of confusion as to what is right and wrong in morally ambiguous situations. Guilt can give rise to a view of self as morally broken or compromised. As Itzick et al.[6] remark about the experiences of trauma survivors struggling with addiction, one cannot underestimate the significance of suffering that arises from an inability to believe in oneself as a basically decent human being.

Case Exemplar 8.2

The Interrelated Nature of Mental Illness, Trauma, and Addiction, Compounded by the Effects of Marginalization

Shanara is a 23-year-old Black woman admitted to an in-patient psychiatric setting after overdosing on prescription medication. She reports a history of sexual abuse as a young teen, depression since she was 15, and suicide attempt and hospitalization when she was 17. She has a history of alcohol and drug abuse, job loss, and unstable interpersonal relationships. She is a lesbian and states she overdosed because her girlfriend of 6 months ended their relationship. Prior to the break-up, Shanara had started to see a psychiatrist and had begun taking an antidepressant. She had looked for an LGBT-friendly therapist but was unable to find one she could afford so began seeing a therapist at a local free clinic. She stopped going when the therapist asked her when she entered puberty, commenting that Black girls often develop early. She felt he was blaming her for the abuse and his attention to her body made her uncomfortable. She did not return. Now, as she sits with the nurse, relating these experiences, she questions again whether the abuse was her fault. She feels shame and believes this is why her girlfriend left her. She feels helpless to gain any control over her flashbacks and sees no way to get through the day besides drinking. She feels hopeless. The nurse's response is to listen calmly. She does not rush to try to make Shanara feel better; she lets her tell her story, listening without flinching when Shanara shares her experience of sexual abuse. When she finishes, the nurse validates her pain and shares how she sees Shanara as having been badly hurt, and not yet having had opportunity to find healthy ways to release her pain and begin to heal. She offers to start with Shanara wherever she is at, noting the journey will not be easy but offering hope by framing Shanara's honesty as evidence of her courage and desire to heal, strengths that will help her move forward.

Trauma survivors may also experience flashbacks to the original trauma experience, triggered by events or persons in their environments. Flashbacks can be terrifying, paralyzing, and, if witnessed by others, embarrassing, or lead to behaviors that impact function at work, school, or home. The unpredictability of flashbacks adds another dimension of suffering that can, as with the experience of mental illness, lead persons to isolate or withdraw from social situations. They may feel unable to trust themselves to stay in control or trust the responses of others around them should they have a flashback, or even trust that others will understand their need to withdraw to decrease distress.[17]

The Suffering of Addiction

Suffering in addiction, regardless of its original source, is often understood as a sense of something irreparably broken in a person's life, not unlike the sense of brokenness experienced by trauma survivors.[6,17] Both theoretical and empirical work on addiction suggest that trauma is often a contributor to addiction.[18,20] Shame is often central, with Ashcroft[7] suggesting that a sense of shame is both a potent contributor to suffering and a trigger for continued substance abuse.

It is important to note that the suffering experienced by persons with substance abuse can be both a result of substance abuse and a factor in its continuation. In other words, while suffering can arise directly from addictive behaviors and their consequences, suffering is also a trigger for the continuation of addictive behaviors. In addition, suffering from both mental illness and trauma have been identified as factors contributing to substance abuse.[5] In Case Exemplar 8.2, Shanara abuses alcohol to cope with memories of trauma and flashbacks. She relates, as is not uncommon with trauma survivors struggling with addiction, that she cannot find any other way to numb the pain or distance herself from traumatic memories enough to maintain a basic level of function or get through her day.[6,18] Thus, while the use of substances can numb a person temporarily to their suffering, whether the suffering arises from experience of mental illness, trauma, or addiction itself, the abuse of substances engenders helplessness and shame, which can perpetuate suffering, keeping the cycle of addiction going.[6]

While the ongoing nature of the cycle of addiction adds to the burden of shame that constitutes a significant portion of the addicted person's suffering, some theorize that suffering may be used as a doorway to change and sobriety.[6] It is often said that a person struggling with addiction must hit "rock bottom" to be motivated to make a change toward sobriety.[2] In other words, unbearable suffering may be what first opens the door to the possibility of change and release from addiction. Wiklund et al.[20] suggest that helping the addicted person see the craving for a substance not as a dead-ended urge leading to more substance use but as a yearning for relief can be a useful approach in substance recovery. Substance abuse treatment differs from treatment for mental health challenges in that the suffering of the former is embraced as a potential path toward healing, not just as the consequence of a symptom to be eradicated.

Marginalized Groups, Suffering, and Mental Health Challenges

A marginalized group is any group of people within society who are relegated away or kept from resources based on a common, usually readily identifiable, characteristic, such as skin color, race, sexual identity or preference, or disability status. This often includes persons with mental health challenges, particularly when their behaviors make the illness apparent, or when they share their experiences of illness with others. Thus, while marginalization contributes to the suffering of people with mental illness, trauma, and substance abuse, such suffering will be compounded for those who also identify with one or more other marginalized or minoritized groups.

Marginalized people are at risk to experience social stigma and internalized stigma. Stigma can be defined as social disapproval or discrimination against a person or group that possess a characteristic or identify in a way that makes them perceived as different from others in a negative way. Self-stigma refers to an internalized negative view of one's own identity. Self-stigma, also called internalized stigma, develops and takes root in people as a result of experiences of social stigma, becoming a significant source of suffering. The harsh, negative self-evaluation of internalized stigma causes suffering related to shame and guilt.[6] Intersectionality, in which multiple aspects of marginalized identity exist within a person, is responsible for an additive impact of both stigma and self-stigma.[22]

Beyond stigma, other effects of marginalization can occur in health care settings, potentially causing or intensifying the suffering of those seeking help. Cyrus[22] suggests that the oppression and discrimination experienced by members of marginalized groups can create stressful emotional experiences during health care encounters, which hold the potential to contribute to and worsen mental health challenges. Barriers to care as well as compromised quality of care can occur. For example, microaggressions, defined as intentional or unintentional insults or assaults on a person's identity, can create barriers to care in treatment settings when these invalidate identity, or make the person feel unsafe and unable to trust/engage further in treatment.[19] For example, in Case Exemplar 8.2, Shanara identifies as Black and lesbian, both identities that can be marginalized and stigmatized (e.g., intersectionality). She has difficulty finding a therapist who is LGBT friendly, and when she begins therapy, she experiences the therapist making inappropriate and unfounded comments about her racial identity that reignite her questions regarding her own guilt about her role in her sexual abuse. The experience is so negative that Shanara quits therapy, closing herself off from the only form of help and healing available to her at that time.

Quality of care can be compromised as well, as Doughty Shaine et al.[23] found in their study of transgender military veterans' attempts to seek mental health care. Several of those interviewed noted that when seeking help, they often needed to educate their providers on the nature of their lived experience, how it shaped their care needs, and what those needs were. When people seeking help need to take on the role of educator for mental health professionals, it can add to the burden they carry even as they seek help to lighten that burden. In addition, marginalized persons may be denied the authority to name and own their experiences of suffering by medical authorities.[23] This can both negate the human dimensions of suffering and hold potential for added harm to marginalized persons.

Anderson et al.[24] offer an example of how being denied the authority to name one's own suffering can lead to harm for marginalized persons. They outline how medicalizing addiction as a genetically mediated disorder for Black persons makes it easier for legal authorities to jump from a narrative of genetic propensity for addiction to one of propensity for repeated criminality. In other words, identifying addiction as a biomedical phenomenon makes it easier to link it with other biological characteristics, such as skin color or race, which can then feed or reinforce implicit racial bias of the law enforcement or judicial systems. This can also make people more hesitant to seek help for substance use disorders and can significantly interfere with treatment if the person does not feel they can trust professionals to act in their best interest. In a similar manner, the use of professional terminology around trauma, particularly for refugees who are survivors of war or war torture, can render the individual lived experience of the trauma, as well as cultural-specific meanings of experiences, invisible, adding to suffering by diminishing the person's worth and reinforcing a sense of helplessness and brokenness.[5] Having to overcome barriers to treatment, having to battle to name and own your experience of suffering, and being unable to trust providers all create significant additional suffering for persons who are members of marginalized groups seeking help for mental health challenges.

The overarching theme in this section is the way in which identifying or being identified as a member of one or more socially marginalized group can compound suffering for persons experiencing mental health challenges, trauma, or addiction. This can happen through stigma, through internalization of stigma, or more concretely through barriers to care or inequities in care encounters, all of which place an additional burden on those seeking care.

Responses to Suffering

Throughout this chapter, multiple forms of suffering have been described and discussed. Case Exemplar 8.2 shows how mental illness, trauma, and substance abuse can be interrelated. For Shanara, unresolved sexual trauma contributes to depression and substance abuse. Her identity as a Black woman who is a lesbian creates barriers that add to her suffering when she endeavors to seek help, leaving her isolated and hopeless. Case Exemplar 8.1 demonstrates how isolation can lead to hopelessness in a different way. The actions Peter takes to help cope with obsessive thoughts and related anxiety create a barrier between him and his coworkers that he finds impossible to breach despite his desire for interaction and connection. Both Shanara's and Peter's experiences are different, and unique to them, but both share a sense of being locked away, alone in their suffering. They are suffering alone in feeling broken and without hope that they can change things for themselves.

At the start of this chapter, the question was posed: Given what we know about suffering with mental health challenges, how do we as nurses respond? How do we draw on both our humanity and knowledge of the person's suffering so that we are able to walk forward with them on their journey toward greater wholeness and less suffering? Now that we have explored the nature of suffering experienced by persons with mental health challenges, trauma, and addiction, we know that while we may very much wish it to be, the answer does not lie in removing all sources of suffering for the person. While nurses may be able to alleviate some individual sources of suffering, for example, by helping a person find the most effective medication or dose for maximizing symptom control and minimizing side effects, the fullness of suffering related to mental health challenges, trauma, and addiction usually cannot be fully eliminated. The journey through suffering can be seen as a journey toward finding a new relationship with suffering and, most importantly, a way of being in the world that restores a sense of empowerment, or a way to move forward that removes barriers on a journey to greater wholeness. As Wiklund et al.[20] suggest, this journey can result in the restoration of dignity and wholeness with or despite suffering, while Itzick et al.[6] encourage those with substance use disorders to embrace suffering as an opportunity to begin their journey toward self-acceptance and self-care. The important point for nurses is that the suffering person cannot make this journey fully alone. Breaking the cycle of isolation and alienation is essential to moving forward. Interpersonal connection allows opportunity for both enhancement of individual agency or empowerment and making meaning of suffering and finding purpose within that.[3] Nurses can walk with the person on this journey by providing the interpersonal connection that creates opportunity for restoration of dignity, self-acceptance, and greater wholeness.

To walk with the suffering person in a helpful way, nurses must be prepared to be open to the suffering of others. Nurses can prepare themselves by addressing their own experiences of suffering as well as priming themselves to be open to difficult conversations.[3] Throughout this chapter, it has been noted that alienation is a significant source of suffering among those with mental health challenges. If nurses are not in touch with and comfortable with suffering, they may inadvertently shy away from the suffering of others. Withdrawing from a person or recoiling from the intensity of a person's suffering further increases alienation and sense of brokenness, ultimately increasing suffering.[21] Therefore, it is imperative that nurses are open to hearing anything and everything a person wants to tell them in an open and nonjudgmental manner and that they are prepared emotionally and spiritually to receive what the person brings. Unburdening to a nonjudgmental and accepting person is essential to regrowing a healthy sense of self-acceptance.[6] Talking through experiences gives rise to opportunities to make new meanings and restore mind-body-spirit connections.[3,10,21] And significantly, relating difficult life experiences and suffering honestly without experiencing rejection from the listener can dismantle the person's expectation of rejection and increase their future openness to sharing and connecting interpersonally.[8.] The nurse's response to Shanara in Case Exemplar 8.2 demonstrates all these actions. In addition, the nurse ends her interaction with Shanara with an offer to continue to move forward with her. She also offers realistic hope by acknowledging that while Shanara has a way to go on her healing journey, she has strengths that will help her to move toward health and wholeness.

It is also important that nurses transcend diagnostic and other terminology to truly witness people's suffering and establish trust.[17]

In other words, if the nurse can make an effort to think beyond what their patient's diagnosis entails to what their lived experience entails, the nurse is better positioned to respond from a place of human care. The person must feel safe and heard if they are to be able to engage in the process of making meaning from their suffering. It is important to note that this work can occur within the context of traditional psychiatric treatment. Psychiatric and substance use disorder treatment include diagnostic labels as well as labeling of behaviors for purposes of assessment. But a nurse willing to witness and walk with a person in their suffering will only use these as needed and put them aside while thinking about and responding to the person. Walking with and witnessing a person's suffering may not seem like significant actions in today's health care environments, where technology- and evidence-based intervention are given primacy, but it is one of the most elemental and human responses that can be offered to a suffering person.

Conclusion

Mental illness, trauma, and addiction are human challenges that each give rise to suffering in different ways. While the sources of suffering from each source may differ, the nature of suffering that results shares common dimensions. Common to all are isolation and alienation from others, emotional pain related to fear and helplessness, and guilt and a sense of being defective or broken. Suffering may also stem from a lack of meaning or purpose and a lack of vision to see a way forward. Suffering and hopelessness can be so all-encompassing as to lead to suicidal ideation. Persons suffering from mental illness, trauma, or addiction who also belong to marginalized groups can find their suffering compounded by social stigma, barriers to care, insensitivity, microaggressions, or even unsafe care. The ways in which these sources and forms of suffering intertwine produce a unique experience for each person. The nurse's response to suffering is rooted in acknowledgment of this uniqueness as well as the understanding that no one can fully relieve another's burden of suffering. By working to be in touch with their own experiences of suffering, nurses can meet the suffering person where they are with openness and steadfastness, as well as with a readiness to listen, witness, and walk with them on a path toward greater wholeness.

References

1. National Institutes of Health. Transforming the understanding and treatment of mental illnesses. Updated 2022. Accessed April 1, 2022. https://www.nimh.nih.gov/health/statistics/mental-illness
2. Substance Abuse and Mental Health Services Administration. Key substance use and mental health indicators in the United States: results from the 2019 National Survey on Drug Use and Health. Published 2020. Accessed April 1, 2022. https://www.samhsa.gov/data/sites/default/files/reports/rpt29393/2019NSDUHFFRPDFWHTML/2019NSDUHFFR090120.htm
3. Hune ND, Kimball TG. The role of suffering in relation to suicide in persons experiencing co-occurring substance use disorders and mental health conditions: a brief perspective. *Alcohol Treat Q.* 2022;40(1):93–99.
4. Cassell EJ. The nature of suffering and the goals of medicine. *NEJM.* 1982;306(11):639–645.
5. Kok T, De Haan HA, Sensky T, van der Meer M, De Jong, C. Using the Pictorial Representation of Illness and Self Measure (PRISM) to quantify and compare suffering from trauma and addiction. *J Dual Diagn.* 2017;13(2):101–108.
6. Itzick M, Segal JN, Possick C. Relationships in the lives of Israeli women coping with drug addiction: an ecosystemic perspective. *J Soc Pers Relationsh.* 2019;36(3):741–760.
7. Ashcroft R. Euthanasia and the nature of suffering in addiction. *Addiction.* 2018; 113:1181–1182.

8. Verhofstadt M, Thienpont L, Peters GY. When unbearable suffering incites psychiatric patients to request euthanasia: a qualitative study. *Br J Psychiatry*. 2017;211(4): 238–245.
9. Breggin PR, Stolzer J. Psychological helplessness and feeling undeserving of love: windows into suffering and healing. *Humanist Psychol*. 2020;48(2):113–132.
10. Le H, Awwad N, Vyas A. Shattered self: schizophrenia suffering, beyond logic and reason. *Psychiatr Times*. 2022;39(4):26–27.
11. Sato A, Hashimoto T, Kimura A, Niitsu T, Iyo M. Psychological distress symptoms associated with life events in patients with bipolar disorder: a cross-sectional study. *Front Psychiatry*. 2018;9:200. https://doi.org/10.3389/fpsy-2018.00200
12. MacKay K. The wounded healer: reflections on a personal journey. *Healthc Couns Psychother J*. 2019;19(4):11–17.
13. Mulhall K, O'Connor J, Timulakova K. Managing the monster in the mind: a psychoanalytically informed qualitative study exploring the experiences of people diagnosed with obsessive-compulsive disorder. *Psychoanal Psychother*. 2019;33(2):117–132.
14. Palombini E, Richardson J, McAllister E, Veale D, Thomson AB. When self-harm is about preventing harm: emergency management of obsessive–compulsive disorder and associated self-harm. *BJPsych Bull*. 2021;45:109–114. https://doi.org/10.1192/bjb.2020.70
15. Jordan AL, Marczak M, Knibbs J. "I felt like I was floating in space": autistic adults' experiences of low moods and depression. *J Autism Dev Disord*. 2021;51:1683–1694.
16. Thompson EM, Brierley ME, Destrée L, Albertella L, Fontenelle LF. Psychological flexibility and inflexibility in obsessive-compulsive symptom dimensions, disability, and quality of life: an online longitudinal study. *J Context Behav Sci*. 2022;23:38–47. doi:10.1016/j.jcbs.2021.11.004
17. Reynolds V. Trauma and resistance: "hang time" and other innovative responses to oppression, violence and suffering. *J Fam Ther*. 2020;42:347–364.
18. Proudfoot J. Traumatic landscapes: two geographies of addiction. *Social Sci Med*. 2019;228:194–201. https://doi.org/10.1016/j.socscimed.2019.03.020
19. Gilmoor A, Vallath S, Regeer B, Bunders J. "If somebody could just understand what I am going through, it would make all the difference": conceptualizations of trauma in homeless populations experiencing severe mental illness. *Transcult Psychiatry*. 2020;57(3):455–467.
20. Wiklund L, Lindstrom U, Lindholm L. Suffering in addiction—a struggle with life. *Theoria*. 2006:15(2):7–16.
21. Dawood R, Done J. An interpretative phenomenological analysis of service users' experiences in a psychosocial addictions intervention. *Psychol Psychother*. 2021;94:307–321.
22. Cyrus K. Multiple minorities as multiply marginalized: applying the minority stress theory to LGBTQ people of color. *J Gay Lesbian Ment Health*. 2017;21(3):194–202.
23. Doughty Shaine MJ, Cor DN, Campbell AJ, McAlister AL. Mental health care experiences of trans service members and veterans: a mixed-methods study. *J Counsel Dev*. 2021;99(3):273–288. doi:10.1002/jcad.12374
24. Anderson TL, Scott BL, Kavanaugh PR. Race, inequality and the medicalization of drug addiction: an analysis of documentary films. *J Subst Use*. 2015;20(5):319–332.

9

Suffering in Acute and Critical Care

Elizabeth G. Broden and Anessa Foxwell

Sources of Suffering in Acute and Critical Care

Admission to a hospital or other acute care setting suggests that a person is experiencing severe enough illness to require around-the-clock nursing and medical care. Whether the sick person is a child, adolescent, adult, or elder, their condition requires interventions only possible in a hospital setting. In addition to frequent assessment and treatment, a hospital admission also represents a vast shift from normalcy. This shift is characterized by diverse losses, such as separation from a person's home environment and social support, limitations on independence and functionality, and other changes. Even the language to describe a person shifts when they are admitted to a hospital. Language pivots from "person" to "patient," from "family" to "visitors," forcing explicit and implicit changes from agency to passivity upon them.

This chapter explores suffering in acute and critical care. These health care settings—characterized by sterile environments, strict policies, medications, constant monitoring, and invasive treatments—may themselves contribute to a person's experience of suffering, along with the aforementioned losses that accompany a hospital admission. The purpose of this chapter is to examine the multiple dimensions of suffering in acute and critical care settings, provide situation-specific considerations to help identify and alleviate suffering, and explore acute and critical care nurses' roles in attending to suffering. This chapter will describe suffering based on clinical and personal experiences, review the empirical and theoretical literature, and explore cases to illustrate the multidimensional elements of suffering.

Suffering is a profoundly personal experience defined by individually ascribed meanings. A closely related concept, "total pain,"[1] offers a framework to identify potential sources of suffering. Total pain includes physical, psychological/emotional, spiritual, and social domains. The sources and manifestations of suffering within each category are illustrated alongside an additional category, environmental, which encompasses the ways that the situational context of being admitted to the hospital impacts suffering. These domains likely overlap and amplify one another. Figure 9.1 represents this intersectional nature of suffering. Examples are provided under each domain of suffering. However, note that many potential sources of suffering are not finite; for instance, as previously suggested, total pain can contribute to physical, psychological, spiritual, and/or social suffering. The rest of the chapter will be grounded in this intersectional, multidimensional understanding of what it means to suffer in acute and critical care settings.

Elizabeth G. Broden and Anessa Foxwell, *Suffering in Acute and Critical Care* In: *The Nature of Suffering and the Goals of Nursing*. Second Edition. Edited by: William E. Rosa and Betty R. Ferrell, Oxford University Press. © Oxford University Press 2023. DOI: 10.1093/oso/9780197667934.003.0009

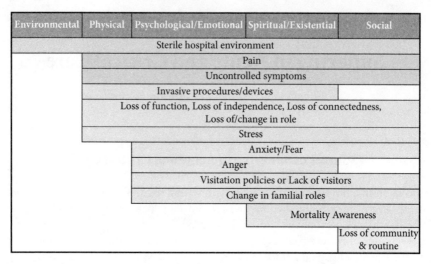

Environmental	Physical	Psychological/Emotional	Spiritual/Existential	Social
Sterile hospital environment				
	Pain			
	Uncontrolled symptoms			
	Invasive procedures/devices			
	Loss of function, Loss of independence, Loss of connectedness, Loss of/change in role			
	Stress			
		Anxiety/Fear		
		Anger		
		Visitation policies or Lack of visitors		
		Change in familial roles		
			Mortality Awareness	
				Loss of community & routine

Figure 9.1 The intersecting nature of suffering in acute and critical care.

In the model shown in Figure 9.1, the patient is at the center, with the dimensions of suffering depicted in overlapping circles. Under each domain, potential examples of suffering are in parentheses. First, the patient may experience physical suffering, for example, pain or uncontrolled symptoms. This physical suffering can also impact a person's experience of psychological/emotional, spiritual/existential, social, and environmental suffering. For each domain there is likely to be significant overlap; however, the experience of suffering is unique to each individual. The examples listed here are not exhaustive. See Case Exemplar 9.1 for further explanation.

Case Exemplar 9.1

A nonbinary person recently diagnosed with acute myeloid leukemia (AML) with FMS-like tyrosine kinase 3 (FTL3) is admitted to the inpatient oncology unit during the chemotherapy regimen for AML consisting of 7 days of cytarabine and 3 days of daunorubicin (7 + 3) via a peripherally inserted central catheter (PICC).

Scout is a 32-year-old nonbinary person who works in public relations. Until last week, their life centered around advancing their career, spending time with their friends, and staying healthy through regular spin classes and eating a primarily plant-based diet. Now, Scout is lying in a hospital bed, tethered to intravenous chemotherapy, uncomfortable, and lonely despite constantly being surrounded by people. They are learning a new language littered with acronyms for letters and numbers—AML, FTL3, 7 + 3, PICC.* They are trying to adapt to this new environment and be a "good patient" while also feeling a loss of self and silently suffering. They are struggling with constant nausea, pain from frequent phlebotomy, and questions about efficacy of treatment. This is the first time in Scout's life that they have been sick, but they are not just sick, they are very ill, and they wonder if they will make it out of the hospital. Scout has certainly faced adversity in their life, which has always been a source of strength and a badge of honor. Yet, this is the hardest thing Scout has ever experienced, and while the nurses and staff appear compassionate, Scout often feels like their concerns are minimized by everyone—family, friends, and health care workers. Scout wonders, "How is everyone so sure I'll get better, except me?"

Domains of Suffering

For the hospitalized patient, there are many sources of suffering—environmental, physical, psychological/emotional, spiritual/extensional, and social. Each person experiences and subjectively may define suffering differently. A recent systematic review identified more than 130 unique stressors experienced by critical care patients.[2] A key role in nursing is helping a patient to identify their sources of suffering and individualizing interventions to help alleviate associated distress.[3] In order for the nurse to care for a person experiencing suffering, they must first understand the potential domains of suffering.

First, the hospitalized patient is likely to experience environmental suffering as a function of being in an unfamiliar setting. Hospitals are typically sterile facilities that lack the comforts and familiarity of home. The environmental suffering that hospitalized patients experience may span all other domains of suffering. For many patients, the hospital environment is a constant reminder of illness and of disruption to normal life. The environment itself may also contribute to an individual's physical, psychological/emotional, spiritual/extensional, and social experience, as shown in Figure 9.1.

Second, physical distress that informs suffering could be caused by symptoms, including pain, nausea, constipation, diarrhea, fatigue, insomnia, and dyspnea, among others. Hospitalized patients, such as Scout, often experience additional sources of physical, as opposed to environmental, distress from "typical" hospital interventions. Scout is physically encumbered by the continuous intravenous chemotherapy infusing through a new central line. Hospitalized patients can feel "imprisoned"[4] by devices that limit their mobility, freedom, and privacy while under constant monitoring. Imagine patients in the intensive care unit (ICU) who typically are attached to, at times, dozens of devices: ventilator, multiple intravenous drips running through one or more central lines, an arterial line, a urinary catheter ... the list goes on. The ICU environment is a blur of lines connecting patients and machines, which frequently hinder, confine, and alarm. While each beep is an important warning for the ICU clinicians, the sounds and technology can be physically jarring for unfamiliar patients.

Third, patients in the acute care setting often experience psychological or emotional suffering. In fact, in the adult oncology population, one in two patients report experiencing psychological or emotional distress while coping with cancer.[5] Those with acute or chronic illnesses are susceptible to feeling psychologically distressed due to a loss of normalcy alone. Additionally, many patients experience fear, anxiety, feeling overwhelmed, uncertainty, and even anger. These emotions are normal responses to illness and hospitalization; however, unattended negative emotions can contribute to suffering. Research has shown that prolonged stress alone can lead to increased allostatic load—that is, the cumulative physiological changes that are caused by repeated stress and environmental factors—which contributes to poorer health outcomes.[6]

A fourth domain of suffering is existential suffering, which can be related to spiritual pain, demoralization, doubting one's previously held beliefs, or existential distress. In adults with cancer, the existential experience is fluid when considering one's mortality.[7] In the acute care context, spiritual pain can have similar sources to physical and psychological suffering that contribute to the loss of normalcy. Religion may be a source of comfort and ritual; without those traditions, people may feel lost. Moreover, when acutely ill, patients often ruminate on questions of "Why did this happen?" and "How did this happen?" For religious people, they may ask these questions of their God. In some traditions, such as Buddhism, illness is viewed in the context of karma (i.e., a cause or a punishment from one's actions in their previous life);[8] in others, suffering can be viewed as redemptive.[9] For all people, including those who are nonreligious (e.g., agnostic, atheist), questions of existential distress may center around a loss of meaning and purpose in life. For instance, in the case of Scout, if their work gave them meaning and purpose, being sick and unable to work could lead to a sense of purposelessness. Although hospitalizations are temporary, for many a diagnosis can be chronic and cause a shift in life goals and focus for years, and often for the rest of one's life. For those with serious, life-limiting illnesses, prognostic uncertainty and facing mortality is a common source of existential suffering.[7] People who believe in an afterlife (i.e., heaven) may find comfort in this belief, whereas others who may not have the same belief may struggle with the finality of death.

The fifth domain of suffering experienced by hospitalized patients is social suffering. Being hospitalized takes you away from your daily social interactions, causing change in familial, work, school, friend, and community relationships. The hospitalized person is seen as "sick" and a "patient" and therefore dependent on others for some degree of care. The hospitalized person's health is now managed by health care workers, which can cause suffering in a person's social sphere. For instance, in Scout's case they are no longer in a comfortable social situation of their choosing; further, they may fear being misgendered by health care team members who are guided by the biomedical model and outside their preferred—and safe—social circle. Visitor policies during the COVID-19 pandemic highlight another form of social suffering, where social networks were limited and minimized, contributing to hospitalized patients' isolation and therefore social suffering.

As previously noted, sources of suffering in acute care have much overlap. For example, when describing each domain, a common thread is the suffering due to "loss" or "change." It is important to note that loss of normalcy or change in role, for example, can cause suffering in one or more of the domains. In the case of Scout, they may identify physical suffering due to pain, psychological suffering due to diagnosis, existential suffering due to loss of meaning, and social suffering due to lack of social interaction with loved ones. As suffering is highly individualized, Case Exemplar 9.2, illustrating a case in pediatrics, in which similar domains of suffering are evident, shows how these domains manifest differently.

Case Exemplar 9.2

An emergent admission to pediatric intensive care unit (PICU) from the emergency department (ED) following febrile seizure.

This was Gabriela's second time ever in an emergency department. She held Luis, her 6-month-old, close. Luis was typically a happy, hungry, and active baby who hardly ever cried. She and her mother, her biggest helper in caring for Luis, often called him "gordo" or "gordito." So the last few days of alternating between barely keeping his eyes open, fussing constantly, and not keeping down any food was frustrating for him and Gabriela. Luis was awake now and had finally stopped crying after 2 hours in the ED waiting area. This morning, he had a fever of 104. He hadn't taken a full bottle in so many days now, despite Gabriela's best efforts. She'd always been able to make sure Luis had what he needed, but tonight, she felt at a loss. She brought him to the ED where she listed her concerns to an impatient triage nurse. It was a miracle that the nurse, "la enfermera," spoke Spanish; otherwise it would have been difficult to convey her fear and anxiety and how her baby was not acting like himself. But apparently Luis wasn't sick enough to see a doctor yet. So they waited. Suddenly, Luis began to jerk and shiver. Gabriela shouted for help. Two nurses rushed to her chair and grabbed Luis from her arms. She followed them to a room, where they quickly placed him on a bed and started attaching wires and monitors to him. He kept shaking. It felt like forever before he stopped. A bunch of people in white coats surrounded Luis's bed. Gabriela strained to see him. Without warning, they started wheeling his bed off. From what little she could hear, there were few words she could understand. "To the PICU," she overheard amid his cries. She didn't know what it meant. She couldn't get close enough to wipe his tears, let alone learn what was causing them. Two hallways, an elevator ride, and incessant beeps later, they were in another room, with another set of nurses and doctors, and Luis woke up screaming. She knew he must be so scared of all the people, the alarming monitors, the pokes from the needles. Before she could reach out to hold him, someone tried to secure a whooshing mask on his face. The crying and beeping continued . . . .

Situation-Specific Considerations

The sources of suffering in acute and critical care have common themes but require specialized consideration across different ages and settings. In Scout's case, the abrupt change to their daily routine and an unexpected confrontation with mortality precipitated psychological, existential, and social suffering. For Gabriela and her son Luis, their interaction with one another was drastically altered, leading to physical and psychological suffering for Luis and existential, social, and psychological suffering for his mom.[10] Depending on a patient's age and developmental level, environmental, physical, psychological/emotional, spiritual/extensional, and social sources and manifestations of suffering may differ. To provide a comprehensive examination of these important considerations, suffering is explored by population based on age/developmental level and then by setting and circumstance.

As explored more deeply in Chapter 6, identifying, assessing, and attending to suffering in children requires special attention to a family's lifecycle, including the developmental level of the child, parental roles, and the overall trajectory of the child and their family. In the hospital setting, many of the necessary interventions to diagnose, treat, and alleviate illness are painful, scary, uncomfortable, and completely unfamiliar to children, who may not yet understand various interventions (e.g., needlesticks, being NPO, etc.). Health care providers may take on primary caregiving roles, rather than parents or other loved ones. New parents working to establish their own roles are forced to continuously reevaluate how they fit into the team during seemingly never-ending invasive interventions.[11] Adolescents often find themselves straddling competing yet equally uncomfortable positions: dependence on (1) their parents, from whom they've worked hard to establish independence, or (2) nurses, who might be close to their own age, for intimate care tasks.

The ways in which the hospital environment forces a person to shift their way of being in the world can lead to multidimensional suffering. To adults who have established work and social routines, important cultural rituals, families or friends who depend on their presence at home, physical and mental health habits, and other such activities, a hospital admission for any length of time presents a thorough disruption to their everyday world. *Take Raquel, for example, who was recently admitted to the ICU for sepsis following an ambulatory surgical procedure. Raquel has struggled with anxiety and disordered eating since she was a teenager. She finds relief in regularity and routine. Cooking simple and small meals for herself has changed her relationship with food. She never misses salat and has a handwoven prayer rug for her grandmother that she typically kneels on, facing Mecca, for each of the five daily prayers. Being in the hospital has been harrowing on every level. Between the IVs, the blood draws what feels like every hour, and the debilitating fatigue, Raquel feels violated by the staff, who often enter her room without knocking, before she can put on her hijab. She is scared and anxious, finding no comfort in the hospital food. She's been unable to get into a position to pray because of constant pain and all the equipment on her and around her. Her suffering seems to go unseen by the nurses and doctors, who often talk at her as if she doesn't know English.*

Whether following an abrupt event or gradually worsening symptoms, the transition from being a "healthy person" to a "sick patient" is fraught with physical, emotional, and social changes and challenges that can cause immense suffering. Rather than family needs or work goals guiding a daily routine, in the acute or critical care unit of the hospital, a patient's activities are dictated by the biomedical model. Labs are drawn at 5 a.m., rounds are done at 10 a.m., and baths are given in the night shift. Medications are administered when ordered. Visitors are allowed only during strict hours, which has become even more limited in the wake of COVID-19. A person's life becomes completely consumed by their illness and its necessary treatment.

Gaining familiarity with the health care system through a hospital admission when you are sick is an unwelcome milestone that most people would elect not to experience. While the hospital unit constitutes a place of work for clinicians, the rooms, halls, and constant beeps become the entire life of a person admitted to it. In an acute care unit, characterized by stress and busyness, it may be hard for a person to get the necessary physical or emotional care and attention they need. Nurses may be on their feet for 12 hours straight while confronting short-staffing or other resource constraints, feeling like the to-do list is endless. For patients, these stretched-too-thin nurses might not be able to attend to their care needs, even those as basic and intimate as continence care. The nurses might seem too busy to ask for help. Environmentally, the hospital may be a complete departure from a person's typical life. They may be sharing a room, requiring help with intimate care, sleeping on a couch at their infant's bedside, or otherwise upended from well-established routines and coping mechanisms.

By design, patients admitted to a critical care unit find themselves strikingly close to the boundary of life and death. Patients may require invasive machines, high-risk medications, and constant monitoring to help keep them alive. Yet, all this technology may not help them heal. Nurses possess a uniquely holistic lens that grants them both clinical expertise and emotional intelligence. For example: *Zara was 13 when she was admitted to the ICU after her second bone marrow transplant with graft-versus-host disease. Her skin was completely covered in bandages that had to be changed every day. It was so deeply painful that she had to be sedated so that she wouldn't scream. As she'd fall asleep, she could hear her mother begging with her nurse, "Can we just leave it for today?" She wished her dad could be there too. Zara wished she could hold her mom's hand.* Bridging the gap between criticality and humanity for patients and their families by communicating, advocating, and liaising between multiple specialty and intensivist teams is among the most important but difficult of ICU nurses' tasks. Amid all these competing priorities, nurses can be present for families, offering emotional support in times of need. Achieving this quality of care is increasingly difficult in a fragmented health system that constantly operates with bare-minimum staffing.

Transitions in care across the wellness-illness continuum can heighten suffering and illuminate changes and loss. Whether experiencing an abrupt or gradual shift from very healthy to very sick, navigating a new diagnosis, dreading returning to the hospital again, adjusting to new equipment or medication, going home with a body or soul forever changed, or any other anticipated or unanticipated transition, such changes can precipitate suffering spanning from the physiologic to the existential. Perhaps one of the most profound transitions is the transition to and through the dying process.

Dying in the hospital medicalizes the experience in ways that can range from helpful (easy access to pain medication and symptom management experts) to awkward (transferring from the ICU to the floor for "comfort care only") to intrusive (dying in a shared patient room) to downright miserable (excruciating pain from traumatic injuries followed by failed cardiopulmonary resuscitation).[12] Parents whose child dies in the hospital are particularly at risk of adverse outcomes[13] and often perceive high levels of suffering.[14] Bearing witness to a loved one's death can be grueling. Being in the hospital during any part of the dying process can exacerbate suffering.[15] As the bedside providers with the most frequent interaction with dying patients and their families, nurses are well placed to help facilitate an end-of-life experience that is meaningful for families by anticipating and attending to symptoms and circumstances leading to different dimensions of suffering during the dying process.[16]

Clearly, assessing and attending to suffering is a complicated task for the bedside nurse. A general but adaptable framework of guiding questions based on self-reflection, intuition, and patient assessment can help nurses identify suffering and wholly attend to it by collaborating with interdisciplinary colleagues. To conclude this section, questions to guide a focused but comprehensive examination of suffering are offered (Box 9.1). These questions provide a quick and feasible way to approach suffering within each patient and family interaction and can be integrated throughout a nurse's shift.

Responses to Suffering

Hospital-based nurses juggle many responsibilities with a primary goal of caring for complicated patients. For the novice nurse, their focus is on completing tasks, and it may be daunting to imagine adding one more task, such as responding to suffering. Initially, interventions for suffering may be nebulous. However, there are a few communication principles that are key when responding to suffering: (1) therapeutic presence, (2) empathic communication, and (3) individualized care (Figure 9.2).

Therapeutic presence is a tenet of nursing care that is often underestimated when nurses are being pulled in many directions. Therapeutic presence can include active listening, nonverbal communication (i.e., sitting with the patient and having open body language), and being a source of support.[17] Empathic communication entails acknowledging and responding to emotion. While clinicians often worry that talking about emotions will be time-consuming, studies have shown that making space to respond to emotion adds only 21 seconds to a clinical encounter and increases trust in clinicians.[18,19] Box 9.1 provides examples of naming and responding to emotions in italics. Naming a patient's emotion (i.e., "I can see this is scary for you") tells the patient you are listening, builds trust, and allows them to explore their own feelings. Individualized care is at the heart of nursing and responding to suffering; Box 9.1 provides a roadmap to offer such patient- and family-centered care.

Nurses in acute and critical care settings are particularly well suited to help patients *feel like people* in an often-dehumanizing hospital unit. For children, adolescents, and their family members, it's important to explain procedures, include parents' and/ or adolescents' perceptions in their assessments, and ensure that parents are able to complete some of their child's basic caregiving activities (changing diapers, feeding, etc.) to the extent that brings each comfort. To help the child or adolescent experience less suffering, nurses can minimize painful procedures, cluster invasive or uncomfortable care, provide medication when possible, and incorporate developmentally appropriate play and/or social opportunities when possible. For adults, taking the time to learn about their story and how their illness fits into it can be a helpful way of acknowledging their personhood and their suffering. Partnering with families is critical to understanding and attending to the unique ways that suffering may impact an individual child, teenager, or adult. Many challenges can prevent a nurse from holistically attending to suffering—whether staffing issues, a language or cultural barrier, or a nurse's own moral distress. Advances in technology have made some issues easier to

---

Box 9.1 Assessment of Patients' Multidimensional Suffering*

Step 1. Prework

Outside of the patient room, ask yourself, *"What do you think is the primary source of the patient's suffering (past, present, and future)?"*

Step 2. Situational Awareness

Consider these questions about communication, timing, and environment:
- Communication: *What is the best way for the patient to communicate? What accommodations should you think about (i.e., ventilated, language barrier, cultural considerations, family dynamics)?*
- Timing: *Is this the best time to engage the patient? (Considerations: Did they recently receive sedating medications, do they need to use the bathroom, etc.?).*
- Situational awareness: *Who is in the room? And who does the patient want in the room (check in with patient)?*

Step 3. Talking with the Patient

When exploring sources of suffering, give the patient time and space to talk about sources of suffering while exploring values, preferences, and concerns. Communication examples:
- If patient names suffering, ask: *What is contributing to your suffering the most right now?*
- Adaptation: *What is bothering you the most? What concerns you when thinking about the future?*
- Acknowledge stress, suffering, or any emotion the patient is experiencing.
- Think back to "Step 1" for potential areas to focus on.

Step 4. Co-construct a Therapeutic Plan.
- Acknowledge emotion and praise patient for sharing with you.
- Consider offering interdisciplinary support tailored to primary source of suffering (i.e., chaplain for existential distress, psychology for emotional, child life specialist, etc.).
- Tips for ending conversation: repraise, reacknowledge emotions, and set a plan.
  "I'm grateful you've shared this with me."
  "I'm honored you've shared this with me."
  "I know this must have been hard to share."
  "It sounds like you are carrying a lot right now."
  "We've talked about some tough stuff; I'll be back soon and we can talk more if you want."
  "We've talked about some tough stuff; I'm going to go look into how and who can help and check back in soon."

Step 5. Implement Plan

Share results with team; check in with and reassess patient later.

*Example language in italics.

---

overcome, such as phone and electronic interpretation over videoconferencing software,[20] but some issues have become more pervasive with time, such as nurse staffing and burnout. Though these challenges are complex and difficult to overcome, the tenets underlying therapeutic presence, empathetic communication, and individualized care offer a method to acknowledge and alleviate suffering that transcends these barriers.

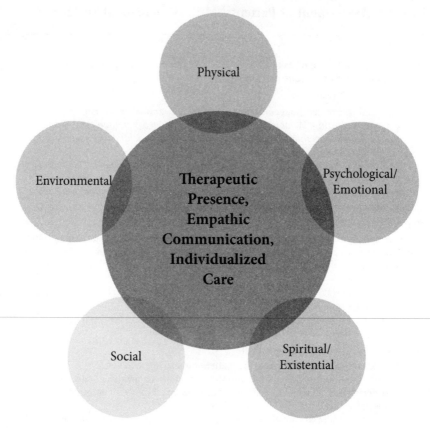

Figure 9.2 Responses to suffering.

Case Exemplar 9.1

Revisited

It's 7 a.m. Nurse Joyce is getting report from the night shift. She knows the first two patients from last week and previous admissions—an older man with multiple myeloma who is here for pain management and a middle-aged woman with CNS lymphoma getting her 10th round of methotrexate. But the third patient is new: Scout, a 32-year-old with new AML, struggling with chemo-induced nausea and diarrhea currently. Joyce blurts out, "I have a nonbinary sibling," shocking both herself and her colleague. She realizes she hasn't shared this with anyone at work. "OK," the night shift nurse continues with report, more shocked by the interruption than the confession. They finish up with report and check in on the patients. All three are still sleeping, but the hustle and bustle of the hospital will wake them soon enough. Joyce returns to the nurse's station to check orders and get prepared for the day. Scout rings their call bell. Joyce goes to the room and cheerily introduces herself. Scout says a groggy hello and asks for something for nausea. Joyce offers an as-needed antiemetic and leaves to prepare the medication. She returns to the room, making small talk while administering medications and doing the morning assessment. Scout engages with Joyce, but it's clear that they are uncomfortable beyond the outward physical sense. Later, Joyce is in the room for rounds. Scout sits up in bed, nods their head when cued, and at the end asks, "How much longer will I feel this bad?" The oncologist responds with, "Be strong. You'll get through this." The team leaves the room, but Joyce stays behind as she normally does with newly diagnosed patients because she knows that rounds can be intimidating and sometimes it's helpful to debrief. Joyce says, "Do you have any questions about what the team said?" Scout says, "I don't know" while hanging their head. Joyce takes a seat and leans in. She waits. Then Scout says, "I feel awful. I've never felt this bad. How is he so sure I'll get better when I don't feel it?" Joyce says, "This must be so hard for you. I'm sure everything changed in an instant. Have you had time to process all this?" Scout replies, "All I do is think. What else am I supposed to do?" Joyce says, "It must be overwhelming." Scout sighs, "It is."

The two sit in silence. Joyce isn't sure what Scout is thinking but thinks about her sibling, only a few years younger than Scout. What if they were in this bed and suffering as Scout is? Joyce's heart ached for Scout. After what felt like 5 minutes (but was probably 30 seconds), Joyce breaks the silence and says, "My sibling is nonbinary too." Scout raises their head and smiles, "Oh yeah?" They ask questions about Joyce's family and they talk for a while. Scout shares that they volunteer at the lesbian, gay, bisexual, trans, and queer/questioning (LGBTQ+) youth center. After a natural pause in conversation Joyce says, "I need to check on my other patients, but thank you for sharing a part of your story with me." Scout replies, "Thank you for making me feel like a person again . . . and not just a patient."

Case Exemplar 9.2

Revisited

Lin had just gotten back from an already late lunch break when she made eye contact with the charge nurse. He smirked. "Six-month-old coming up from the ED. Seems like he's in status; they've given him a couple of doses of Versed but haven't been able to break it. The mom's been difficult too. Only speaks Spanish. Sorry." Lin sighed and went to the break room to start gathering supplies. A flashlight, stethoscope, IV supplies. It was already 4:00. The end of this shift was going to be crazy. When they rolled up from the ED, Lin could see that the little boy was crying now. He looked scared; his mom did too. Lin followed the ED team and the stretcher into the room and started hooking the child up to the monitors while another nurse started looking for an IV. "It's OK, Luis," Lin whispered. "I've just got some special stickers to put on." He kept crying. Lin could see his oxygen saturation dropping and called for a respiratory therapist to start continuous positive airway pressure. This was always the worst part. "I've got a million things to do, for Luis and my other patient, and I wish I didn't have to make him cry. I wish I could explain to his mom how sorry I am," Lin thought to herself. "Those little things go by the wayside when there is a language barrier though. They shouldn't, but the reality is that they do. Once I get him settled I'll call an interpreter and give her a full update…."

Conclusion

Nursing responses to suffering within each domain of suffering can be woven together throughout a nurse's shift to attend to a person's suffering holistically and feasibly while they are admitted to an acute and/or critical care setting. Between the tasks that often dictate a nurse's shift, there are fleeting moments when these responses can be quickly and adeptly incorporated. While the blood pressure cuff is inflating, assessing respirations and perfusion, drawing labs, helping the patient ambulate, or transporting a patient to a procedure, or during the first 15 minutes of blood transfusion—these short, often unnoticed pauses in the endlessly busy shift are when the nurse can offer therapeutic presence or empathetic communication for the patient and their loved ones if present. Sometimes it can help to delegate tasks to another nurse, nursing assistant, or other interdisciplinary colleague so that the primary nurse can attend to a patient or family's psychosocial suffering. Rather than attempting to address the full spectrum of a patient's suffering in one fell swoop, it may be more feasible to conceptualize alleviating or minimizing suffering as a constant duty that nurses work to uphold throughout the entirety of their care.

References

1. Saunders C. Care of patients suffering from terminal illness at St. Joseph's Hospice, Hackney, London. *Nursing Mirror*. 1964;14(2). https://scholar.google.com/scholar?hl=en&as_sdt=0%2C5&q=Saunders+C.+Care+of+patients+suffering+from+terminal+illness.+Nursing+Mirror.+&btnG=

2. Krampe H, Denke C, Gülden J, et al. Perceived severity of stressors in the intensive care unit: a systematic review and semi-quantitative analysis of the literature on the perspectives of patients, health care providers and relatives. *J Clin Med*. 2021;10(17):3928. doi:10.3390/jcm10173928

3. Rosa WE, Buck HG, Squires AP, et al. American Academy of Nursing Expert Panel consensus statement on nursing's roles in ensuring universal palliative care access. *Nurs Outlook*. 2021;69(6):961–968. doi:10.1016/j.outlook.2021.06.011

4. Spichiger E. Being in the hospital: an interpretive phenomenological study of terminally ill cancer patients' experiences. *Eur J Oncol Nurs*. 2009;13(1):16–21. doi:10.1016/j.ejon.2008.10.001

5. Mehnert A, Hartung TJ, Friedrich M, et al. One in two cancer patients is significantly distressed: prevalence and indicators of distress. *Psychooncology*. 2018;27(1):75–82. doi:10.1002/pon.4464

6. Guidi J, Lucente M, Sonino N, Fava GA. Allostatic load and its impact on health: a systematic review. *PPS*. 2021;90(1):11–27. doi:10.1159/000510696

7. Tarbi EC, Meghani SH. Existential experience in adults with advanced cancer: a concept analysis. *Nurs Outlook*. 2019;67(5):540–557. doi:10.1016/j.outlook.2019.03.006

8. Xu J. The lived experience of Buddhist-oriented religious coping in late life: Buddhism as a cognitive schema. *J Health Psychol*. 2021;26(10):1549–1560. doi:10.1177/1359105319882741

9. Balboni MJ, Sullivan A, Enzinger AC, et al. U.S. clergy religious values and relationships to end-of-life discussions and care. *J Pain Symptom Manage*. 2017;53(6):999–1009. doi:10.1016/j.jpainsymman.2016.12.346

10. October TW. Is all suffering equal or is it time to address existential suffering? *Pediatr Crit Care Med*. 2018;19(3):275–276. doi:10.1097/PCC.0000000000001447

11. Weaver MS, October T, Feudtner C, Hinds PS. "Good-parent beliefs": research, concept, and clinical practice. *Pediatrics*. 2020;145(6):e20194018. doi:10.1542/peds.2019-4018

12. Lasater KB, Sloane DM, McHugh MD, Aiken LH. Quality of end-of-life care and its association with nurse practice environments in U.S. hospitals. *J Am Geriatr Soc*. 2019;67(2):302–308. doi:10.1111/jgs.15671

13. Snaman J, Morris SE, Rosenberg AR, Holder R, Baker J, Wolfe J. Reconsidering early parental grief following the death of a child from cancer: a new framework for future research and bereavement support. *Support Care Cancer*. 2020;28(9):4131–4139. doi:10.1007/s00520-019-05249-3

14. Clark OE, Fortney CA, Dunnells ZDO, Gerhardt CA, Baughcum AE. Parent perceptions of infant symptoms and suffering and associations with distress among bereaved parents in the NICU. *J Pain Symptom Manage*. 2021;62(3):e20–e27. doi:10.1016/j.jpainsymman.2021.02.015

15. Su A, Lief L, Berlin D, et al. Beyond pain: nurses' assessment of patient suffering, dignity, and dying in the intensive care unit. *J Pain Symptom Manage*. 2018;55(6):1591–1598.e1. doi:10.1016/j.jpainsymman.2018.02.005

16. Breen LJ, Szylit R, Gilbert KR, et al. Invitation to grief in the family context. *Death Studies*. 2019;43(3):173–182. doi:10.1080/07481187.2018.1442375

17. Ellison DL, Meyer CK. Presence and therapeutic listening. *Nurs Clin North Am*. 2020;55(4):457–465. doi:10.1016/j.cnur.2020.06.012

18. Kennifer SL, Alexander SC, Pollak KI, et al. Negative emotions in cancer care: do oncologists' responses depend on severity and type of emotion? *Patient Educ Couns*. 2009;76(1):51–56. doi:10.1016/j.pec.2008.10.003

19. Tulsky JA, Arnold RM, Alexander SC, et al. Enhancing communication between oncologists and patients with a computer-based training program: a randomized trial. *Ann Intern Med*. 2011;155(9):593–601. doi:10.7326/0003-4819-155-9-201111010-00007

20. Rajiv P, Riggs E, Brown S, Szwarc J, Yelland J. Communication interventions to support people with limited English proficiency in healthcare: a systematic review. *J Commun Healthc*. 2021;14(2):176–187. doi:10.1080/17538068.2021.1890518

10

Suffering in Chronic Illness

Avery C. Bechthold and J. Nicholas Dionne-Odom

Background

This chapter describes the concept and experience of suffering within the context of chronic illness and the role of nurses in addressing suffering. To do this, distinctions are first made among the nomenclature of "disease," "illness," and "sickness," reflecting professional, personal, and social perspectives on how we refer to an individual who is not "healthy."[1] These three states will be collectively referred to as "unhealth," a term coined by Dr. Marshall Marinker in 1975.[2] Since the 1950s, there have been discourses about these terms in medical sociology, medical anthropology, and the philosophy of medicine.[1] In this chapter, the authors integrate the nursing perspective to these multidisciplinary viewpoints. Hence, the goal of this chapter is to first illuminate distinctions among the terms "disease," "illness," and "sickness." Subsequently, the term "suffering" is defined and explored as it relates to the subjective experience of chronic illness. The chapter concludes with a discussion of how nurses in clinical, research, and education roles may effectively respond to the suffering of patients with chronic illness.

Disease, Illness, and Sickness

Defining disease, illness, and sickness has been argued to be a critical reflection in the health care field as it dictates the objectives and actions that clinicians take toward addressing them.[1] Further, it has been noted that distinguishing and defining disease, illness, and sickness is more difficult than might first appear. For example, it might be questioned whether heart failure describes a specific pathology or a syndrome of objective pathological processes in combination with presenting subjective symptoms. Consistent with other recent discussions on this topic and for the purposes of this chapter, "disease" is defined as a physical or mental health condition resulting from a combination of genetic, physiological, environmental, and behavioral factors that persists beyond 1 year and requires ongoing monitoring or treatment and/or limits activities of daily living.[3] Disease is frequently described in objective physical terms, such that it can be observed (i.e., seen, touched, measured, and smelled), mediated, and measured.[1,2] Its basic phenomena consist of physiological, biological, genetic, and mental entities.[1] Health care professionals aim to cure disease through classification, detection, control, and treatment, ultimately enhancing a person's survival.[1]

Avery C. Bechthold and J. Nicholas Dionne-Odom, *Suffering in Chronic Illness* In: *The Nature of Suffering and the Goals of Nursing*. Second Edition. Edited by: William E. Rosa and Betty R. Ferrell, Oxford University Press. © Oxford University Press 2023. DOI: 10.1093/oso/9780197667934.003.0010

Conversely, "illness" is defined as the subjective feeling or emotional experience of impaired or diminished physical, emotional, intellectual, social, developmental, or spiritual functioning.[1,2] Such subjective experiences are made apparent to others through communications and verbal reports based on introspection.[1,2] Health care professionals often seek to address a patient's illness experience by employing strategies to enhance coping, thereby optimizing a person's quality of life.[1] Although illness may exist in the absence of disease, it often exists alongside it.[2] Manifestations of illness include anxiety, fear, pain, *and suffering.*[1]

Finally, "sickness" is a social construct that is governed by the culture and laws established by social institutions and societal norms.[1,2] Such norms determine an individual's entitlement to treatment, economic rights, exemption from social responsibilities (e.g., sick leave), and legal accountability.[1,2] The basic phenomena of sickness include expectations, conventions, policies, and social norms and roles.[1] While disease and illness are confined to an individual, sickness is determined by relations with others and the society and culture in which one lives.[1,2] For example, diagnosis with a so-called self-inflicted disease, such as chronic obstructive pulmonary disease (COPD), can have a judgmental aspect where one treats the diagnosis as reflective of one's way of life.[4]

Nurses and other health care professionals play a key role in addressing the social determinants of health, defined as the conditions that people are born into and live under that affect their health (e.g., environment, socioeconomic status, access to health care).[5] At the patient level, nurses may identify patient needs (e.g., transportation, legal assistance) and partner with other health care professionals, such as social workers, to address such needs, which may help alleviate patient stress, foster patient- and family-centered care planning and delivery, and promote better outcomes.[6] At a system level, nurses may advocate for health equity through inclusive policy advancement, partner with national and international professional associations to raise awareness and improve education about the social determinants of health, and hold systems accountable for ensuring the workforce is supported, respected, and treated equitably.[6]

While disease, illness, and sickness each demand action, this chapter will focus on the individualized, subjective experiences of suffering in chronic illness.[1,2] This aligns most closely with the scope of suffering, which has also been described as an individualized experience.[7-9]

Suffering

Definition

Recognizing that suffering is an experience frequently encountered in clinical practice,[7] nurses across the world have sought to define the concept of suffering and identify its attributes.[7-9] Across the scientific literature, suffering has been consistently described as a negative, individualized (or subjective), and complex experience.[7-9] Synthesizing the previously discussed definitions of suffering, the remainder of this chapter will refer to suffering as an individualized experience of loss, damage, or pain that is dependent on inner factors, significant others, exterior circumstances, and stimuli, and one's meaning of life; consists of physical, psychological, social, and spiritual aspects and threatens an individual's self-integrity and induces withdrawal, feelings of helplessness, despair, and changes to one's value system and sense of reality.

Guided by this definition, the remainder of the chapter will focus on exploring the suffering of patients with chronic illness and clarifying the nurse's role in responding to patient suffering.

Suffering and Chronic Disease

Chronic diseases are ongoing or recurrent, are potentially characterized by periods of exacerbation and recovery, and typically persist for as long as a person lives.[10] While many chronic diseases may not be noticeable in the early stages, most can eventually be diagnosed using laboratory procedures.[10] As chronic diseases progress, their management often becomes complex and overwhelming.[10]

Five major concerns often accompany chronic diseases: (1) impaired cognitive functioning (i.e., attributable to either medications or the illness), (2) loss of independence and the perception of burdening others, (3) alterations in body image, (4) inability to maintain social roles (e.g., loss of employment, identity, family cohesiveness), and (5) uncertainty about the future (e.g., physical or mental limitations, financial demands).[10] Additionally, many patients perceive their illness and care needs as a burden to others and a cause of hardship, which may lead to frustration, worry, distress, feelings of responsibility, and a diminished sense of self.[11] As the number of family caregivers providing care to loved ones with chronic illness continues to increase, it is critical for nurses to consider self-perceived burden as a potential source of suffering.[11,12] Patients from diverse cultures have uttered the statement, "I do not want to be a burden."[12] Thus, self-perceived burden appears to be a universal form of suffering among patients with chronic illness that transcends cultural differences.[11]

The subsequent sections will detail patients' experiences with suffering in the context of five of the most prevalent chronic diseases worldwide: (1) heart disease, (2) stroke, (3) Alzheimer's disease, (4) chronic lung disease, and (5) chronic kidney disease.

Heart Disease

Heart disease, a broad term for conditions affecting the heart's structure and function, includes, among others, coronary heart disease (the most common type), arrhythmias, and valvular disease.[13] Approximately one in four deaths in the United States—that is, about 659,000 people each year—are due to heart disease.[13] Heart disease is among several conditions that may lead to heart failure, a condition that develops when the body receives insufficient blood, either due to inadequate filling or weak pumping.[13] Heart failure affects over 6 million adults in the United States.[13]

Suffering and Heart Failure

Patients with heart failure have identified the following as causing suffering: burdensome symptoms (e.g., fatigue [42%–82%], dyspnea [18%–88% prevalence], pain [14%–78%], delirium [15%–48%], depression [6%–59%], impaired sleep); anticipatory grief related to an uncertain clinical course, marked by acute exacerbations (i.e., hospitalization), progressive disability, and near-death experiences; feelings of loss (e.g., achieving life goals, previously enjoyed activities, roles, and employment), hopelessness (i.e., knowledge of having a progressive, life-limiting illness), and isolation; and depression and worry about increasing dependence and burden.[14,15]

Stroke

In the United States, strokes account for approximately 1 of every 19 deaths, with an estimated 7.6 million Americans self-reporting having had a stroke.[13] Each year, approximately 610,000 are first attacks and 185,000 are recurrent attacks.[13] Ischemic strokes are the most prevalent (87%), followed by intracerebral hemorrhagic (10%) and subarachnoid hemorrhagic strokes (3%).[13]

Suffering and Stroke

Stroke survivors experience numerous debilitations, including paralysis or reduced control of their movements, sensory disturbances (e.g., pain), problems speaking or understanding language or both (e.g., expressive, receptive, or global aphasia, respectively), difficulties with thinking and memory, and emotional disturbances.[16,17] Additionally, approximately one-third of all stroke survivors experience poststroke depression.[18] Patients have expressed distress over the suddenness of their stroke and a lack of forewarning; feelings of powerlessness (e.g., recurrence is beyond their control), reduced autonomy, and dependence; undesirable side effects from new medications (e.g., bleeding, gastric pain); frustration related to difficulties with communication; and fear of death or future occurrences and profound disability (e.g., physical or ability to communicate).[16,17] Feeling disempowered and at the mercy of others may also alter the patient's identity, including their occupational identity, and devalue their self-concept.[16] Patients may experience role reversal, intergenerational changes, or an altered position in the family and may no longer be able to participate in their valued occupation.[16]

Alzheimer's Disease

More than 6 million Americans are living with Alzheimer's disease, a progressive type of brain disease, and the most common cause of dementia (i.e., a particular group of symptoms, including difficulties with memory, language, and problem-solving).[19] Initially, patients are unaware of brain changes, which begin many years before symptom presentation.[19] However, after many years of neuron damage or destruction, patients begin to experience memory loss and language problems.[19] Gradually other parts of the brain are damaged or destroyed, and eventually, basic bodily functions (e.g., walking and swallowing) are affected.[19] As the disease progresses, family caregivers must increasingly advocate; provide hands-on assistance with care and mobility, social support, and medical care; and manage behavioral symptoms.[19]

Suffering and Alzheimer's Disease

Currently, Alzheimer's disease remains irreversible and incurable.[19] Patients in the early stages of Alzheimer's disease have described suffering in terms of inevitable, unwanted changes in personality, life, and behaviors, such as forgetfulness, not recognizing loved ones, loneliness, loss of dignity, and feeling "lost in one's own life and in the mazes of one's own mind."[20,21(p1464)] As Alzheimer's progresses, patients may become unable to communicate their suffering.[20] Thus, pain or other symptoms may manifest as agitation, aggression, wandering, sleep disturbances, withdrawal, resistance to care, hallucinations, or delusions.[20] Agitation or other restless behaviors should be considered as evidence of discomfort such as pain, urinary retention or incontinence, or constipation until proven otherwise.[20] Other sources of potential suffering include choking and swallowing problems (e.g., infection, aspiration), recurrent infections (in the terminal stages), urinary retention or incontinence (i.e., due to infections and cortical damage), and falls (i.e., related to pain, medications, environmental factors).[20]

Chronic Lung Disease

Chronic lung disease is a slow, progressive disease that affects the airways and other structures of the respiratory system.[22] COPD, asthma, occupational lung diseases, and pulmonary hypertension are among some of the most common types.[22] More than 16.4 million Americans have been diagnosed with COPD, a group of diseases that impact airflow and breathing (i.e., chronic bronchitis, emphysema).[22,23]

Suffering and Chronic Lung Disease

Common sources of suffering for patients with COPD include unpleasant and distressing symptoms (e.g., dyspnea [90%–95% prevalence], fatigue [68%–80%], depression [37%–71%], anorexia [35%–67%], pain [34%–77%], delirium [18%–33%]); feelings of powerlessness and guilt from dependence on others, loss of social roles, and the inability to conduct many day-to-day activities (e.g., shopping, walking); fear about the future with an incurable disease (i.e., deterioration and death); social isolation, including stigmatization within society and the health care system; and feelings of shame and guilt due to the perception of self-inflicted disease (i.e., due to smoking).[4,24] Patients have doubted their deservingness of receiving care and comfort from others due to what they perceive as a personal weakness or a "self-inflicted" disease.[4] Further, some patients reported not feeling welcomed or outwardly rejected and accused of bringing about their own situation by health care professionals or family.[4] A persistent cough and the use of supplemental oxygen are particularly "eye-catching" barriers to hiding their disease, although some have reported concealing their disease as a less stigmatized disease, such as asthma.[4]

Chronic Kidney Disease

Chronic kidney disease (CKD) involves slow, progressive loss of renal function, whereby the kidneys are damaged and unable to adequately filter blood.[25] Eventually this loss of function can lead to early cardiovascular disease and renal failure, which requires dialysis or a kidney transplant to manage the buildup of excess fluid, toxins, and waste products in the body, and ultimately, to sustain life.[25] In the United States, over 37 million individuals (one in seven American adults) are estimated to have CKD and millions of others are considered at risk.[25]

Suffering and Chronic Kidney Disease

Patients with CKD have reported demanding lifestyle changes, including managing symptoms (e.g., fatigue [73%–87% prevalence], pain [47%–50%], anorexia [25%–64%], dyspnea [11%–62%], depression [5%–60%]) and self-care in relation to diet, fluid, and physical well-being, and monitoring medication side effects.[24,26] Other identified sources of suffering include prognostic uncertainty; worry about catastrophic events, including death, as a result of surgery or missing treatments or immunosuppressive medications; anxiety due to altered social roles, burden (e.g., logistics of CKD and treatment, asking friends or family for a living kidney donation), and the inability to perform daily tasks; financial burden (e.g., lack of insurance to pay for dialysis or transplant surgery) and dependence due to loss of employment or reduced work hours; frustration at the receipt of fragmented and mechanistic care and feeling unheard or misunderstood; and concern about a lack of readily accessible and understandable CKD-related information.[26] Patients have also reported distress over the looming possibility of reaching kidney failure and being forced to choose between dialysis, transplant, or conservative care, which was described as "life or death."[26] Additionally, fear of social stigma and prejudice was another source of suffering.[26] Reasons for stigma included CKD being perceived as a self-induced disease and being labeled with the "patient stamp" (i.e., the stigma of being sick) and perceived as weak or inferior.[26] Patients reported worry of social exclusion due to physical and medical restrictions, and that others would not take them seriously or use their illness against them.[26]

Responses to Suffering

Nursing as a professional discipline has long regarded suffering and addressing those experiences as a central focus of its role.[7,27] According to the American Nurses

Association, the Nursing Scope and Standards of Practice consists of "the protection, promotion, and optimization of health and abilities; prevention of illness and injury; facilitation of healing; alleviation of suffering through the diagnosis and treatment of human response; and advocacy in the care of individuals, families, groups, communities, and populations."[27] Thus, in the scope and standards of nursing itself, registered nurses and advanced practice registered nurses are expected and deemed competent to attend to patient suffering.[27] But what exactly does alleviation of suffering entail?

Nurses spend a significant amount of time with chronically ill patients compared to other health professionals. Therefore, they are uniquely situated to respond to suffering deriving from chronic illness. Addressing suffering requires nurses to care for patients in a holistic fashion, beyond physical symptoms.[3] Instead of attempting to fix, change, or eliminate suffering, nurses should first empathize with patients to understand their experience of suffering and then assist with coping and reframing suffering in a way that is meaningful and promotes overall well-being. Although caring for a suffering person requires extensive effort on the nurse's part, the act of caring can serve as the fuel needed to provide compassionate care.[28] See Case Exemplars 10.1 and 10.2 for case studies demonstrating how to address suffering in heart failure and dementia, respectively.

Case Exemplar 10.1

Addressing Suffering in Heart Failure

Emily, a registered nurse in the cardiovascular stepdown unit, has been assigned to care for John, a 63-year-old Caucasian male with advanced heart failure, recently admitted from home due to worsening breathlessness, orthopnea, and lower extremity edema. Emily greets a disheartened-looking John and his wife. She asks John if there is anything that she can do to make him more comfortable. Emily listens attentively as John replies, "No. Well, I don't know. I'm just so frustrated that I keep ending up in the hospital. When my condition gets bad, I can't do the things I enjoy like tending to the garden. To top it off, my wife has to help me out even more. I just don't know what to do." Hearing that John is feeling a sense of loss and hopelessness, Emily responds, "John, that sounds frustrating. You can't do the things that you once enjoyed, and you don't want to burden your wife. Is there anyone else that you can reach out to for support? Family? Friends? Neighbors?" John pauses and replies, "Well, my church is a very tight-knit group. We always help each other out. I haven't been able to go lately but I'd really like to be able to go again. I used to go every week." Emily encourages John and his wife to reflect on some tasks they might be able to delegate. Later, they go over the ideas together. Emily informs John and his wife about some options while he is admitted: having their pastor or the hospital chaplain visit or tuning into their church's services online or by radio. John and his wife are thrilled to learn about these options. Toward the end of her shift, Emily informs John and his wife that she will be leaving shortly and handing his care over to the night shift nurse. They thank Emily profusely for being so kind and attentive.

Case Exemplar 10.2

Addressing Suffering in Dementia

Maria is a registered nurse who has worked on the dementia unit in a nursing home for several years. She is preparing to give medications to Frannie, a 68-year-old, ambulatory resident with early-stage Alzheimer's disease. As she enters the room, she finds Frannie frantically tearing through her closet. Maria greets Frannie, "Hello Frannie, what are you looking for?" Frannie turns to Maria looking visibly upset. She exclaims, "I've lost my purse! Oh, what am I going to do!" They search the room until they locate the purse under the bed. Frannie quickly pulls out a photograph and lets out a sigh of relief. Maria asks Frannie to sit with her and chat. After a few moments of silence, Frannie shares that she often worries about her worsening memory and fears the day she is unable to recognize her loved ones, which is why she keeps their photograph in her purse. Maria listens attentively as Frannie shares her fears about the progression of her Alzheimer's. She empathizes with Frannie's concerns and thanks Frannie for confiding in her. Maria asks if this can be an ongoing conversation between them. In the meantime, they agree that the purse should always be kept in the same place in Frannie's room. At the end of the conversation, Frannie thanks Maria for listening to her story.

Clinical Responses to Suffering

In the clinical setting, nurses can help patients find meaning in their suffering by (1) listening to and witnessing suffering, (2) connecting suffering and spirituality, (3) facilitating values elicitation, and (4) delivering primary palliative care.

Listening to and Witnessing Suffering

Unbearable suffering has been described as a type of suffering that is silent and hidden and experienced as a "single pole," for example, only death, dying, or darkness.[29] An experience may seem unbearable due to its duration (i.e., mismatch in the expected and actual duration of suffering) or intensity.[30] Suffering begins once a patient acknowledges their trying situation and continues until they engage in an existential caring encounter,[29] which is characterized by (1) presence and active listening, (2) recognizing the uniqueness of each patient and their needs, and (3) treating the patient as a fellow human rather than a patient.[31] For example, the nurse may sit and listen to the patient's story; engage in small talk or use humor; or use gentle touch, such as holding the patient's hand.[31] This encounter serves as a turning point toward what is known as "bearable suffering"—that is, the patient suffering becomes conscious and expressible, and they struggle between paradoxes such as hope and hopelessness, meaning and meaninglessness, and reconciliation and broken-heartedness.[28,29]

Many factors challenge a nurse's ability to be fully present with patients, including time constraints and distractions such as electronic health records, computers, cellular phones, and modern diagnostic technology.[32] However, when a patient is hospitalized, nurses are the only health care professionals in direct contact with patients 24/7, which places them in an ideal position to facilitate an existential caring encounter.[32]

Suffering does not resolve quickly; however, giving the space for patients to narrate their stories and voice their suffering provides relief from frustration, guilt, and shame; fosters peace and acceptance of the past; preserves dignity; minimizes feelings of loneliness and abandonment; increases a sense of human connection; and creates meaning and begets hope, which makes the patient's present and future bearable.[28,32-34] Nurses should listen empathetically to the patient's story and encourage the leveraging of any resources and abilities.[34] In this way, the patient can create meaning in their life situation, which includes their chronic illness.[34]

Connecting Suffering and Spirituality

Religion and spirituality have been suggested to affect a patient's beliefs about their suffering, influence their experience of suffering, and help them to endure suffering as well as find meaning in their journey.[28] Finding meaning in suffering offers patients a means of control, spiritual growth, and increased empathy for others.[28] Spiritual distress—that is, suffering due to unmet spiritual needs or an impaired ability to find meaning in life through connectedness with oneself, others, the world, or a Superior Being—has been found to contribute to worsening physical and emotional symptoms.[33] Thus, a patient's spiritual well-being should be treated as equivalent to their physical or emotional well-being.[33]

While chaplains are charged with in-depth exploration of a patient and caregiver's spiritual, religious, and existential suffering, nurses can conduct a spiritual screening (i.e., one to two questions at admission to determine the need for a referral to a spiritual care professional) or spiritual history (i.e., a clinical history to develop care or treatment plans), promote spiritual well-being (e.g., encourage connectedness), and initiate specialist referrals.[32,33] Providing attentive, spiritual care helps patients sort through their experiences and feelings related to their illness and to regain perspective.[28,32,33] Elements of spiritual care include active listening, compassionate presence, authenticity, kindness, respect, vulnerability, service, honesty, and empathy, which align closely with the nursing philosophy of care.[32,33]

Because spirituality and religion can vary considerably by culture, region, and individual, nurses should explore each patient's particular spiritual and religious background to gain insight into how the patient makes meaning of suffering.[28] Nurses should support patients who wish to engage in religious or spiritual rituals and consider leveraging spiritual care colleagues, such as chaplains, for more intensive support.[28,32,33] There may also be patients who are too ill to attend religious services, in which case the nurse might suggest a visit from the chaplain or religious leader, or listening to religious services on the television or radio or online.[32] Note that rituals may be nonreligious by nature, such as birthday cakes, bedtime stories, or coffee or tea while reading.[32] To promote spiritual well-being, nurses should find some private, uninterrupted time for the patient and family's unique needs and desires.[32]

Nonreligious patients can be assisted to find meaning in their suffering based on their past and present situation.[28] Relaxation responses, breath work, and meditation techniques are some body and mind health approaches that may help in finding peace, increasing one's understanding of self, and finding balance.[32] Integrative practitioners with experience in these modalities may be available for specialist consultation and support in some health settings.

Facilitating Values Elicitation

Often, patient values, defined as abstract and subjective core beliefs that function within a system and a priority that can be changed under certain circumstances,[35] are unknown to the health care team, which may result in uncertainty, unwanted care, increased costs of care, avoidable suffering, and futile treatments at the end of life.[36] However, nurses can engage in values elicitation and assist in incorporating patient values into care through the delivery of person-centered care, an approach to care guided by the patient's values and preferences.[37,38] In this approach, patient decision-making is informed by others, including people important to them and relevant providers, to the extent to which they desire.[37] Shared decision-making and advance care planning represent two person-centered decision-making programs that recognize the uniqueness of each patient and are driven by the patient's values, goals, and preferences.[39]

Given recent controversies surrounding advance care planning,[40] there has been renewed emphasis that advance care planning is not synonymous with the completion of advance directives, which are legal documents that may arise from advance care planning.[41,42] Advance care planning involves (1) understanding and sharing one's personal values, life goals, and preferences regarding future medical care and (2) aligning care with one's expressed wishes.[39] These conversations should focus on understanding what patients consider acceptable and unacceptable in life, rather than identifying in-the-moment treatment preferences or hypothetical situations.[43] This includes facilitating the elicitation of patient values, goals, wishes, surrogate(s), and prognosis prior to a medical crisis.[43] If the patient is unable to participate in active decision-making due to mental or physical incapacitation, the health care team should link the patient's values and life goals to the care plan and partner with the patient and surrogate(s) to ascertain the best course of action given these articulated wishes.[39,43] Care decisions made by the health care team and surrogate should be guided by the patient's expressed wishes.[43]

Research Implications

Despite a modest amount of scientific literature examining suffering among patients with chronic disease, few articles explicitly detail the nurse's role in responding to suffering.[30] Researchers should consider detailing the clinical implications of their findings, including common sources of suffering among patients with a particular disease and actionable items for nurses. Further, authors should avoid phrases such as "patients suffering from ...", "patients who suffer from ...", or "sufferers of ..." within their title or full text unless they intend to explore this concept. Suffering is an individualized, subjective experience; therefore, researchers should not overgeneralize and assume all patients with a particular diagnosis are suffering. Avoiding the use of such phrases will also assist other researchers when searching the literature.

Educational Implications

While it is essential for nursing students to develop skills related to the identification and planning of care for patients who are suffering, the complexity of the concept, as well as a scarcity of clinical sites and adequate exposure to patients during clinical rotations, necessitates imaginative and innovative learning activities.[44] For example, one assignment included William Utermohlen's nine self-portraits, which chronicle his deterioration from Alzheimer's disease, as a strategy to increase their awareness of the mental and physical impact of Alzheimer's disease.[44]

Conclusion

In this chapter, we defined the terms "disease," "illness," and "sickness"; explored suffering as it relates to the subjective experience of chronic illness; and discussed how nurses in clinical, research, and education roles may variously address the suffering of patients with chronic illness. Although patient suffering is a unique, individualized experience, nurses may apply similar approaches to address patient suffering, including listening to and witnessing suffering, connecting suffering and spirituality, facilitating values elicitation, and delivering primary palliative care. Further, nurses in research roles should detail the clinical implications of their findings and avoid referring to entire patient groups as suffering.

References

1. Bjørn H. Disease, illness, and sickness. In: Solomon M, Simon JR, Kincaid H, eds. *The Routledge Companion to Philosophy of Medicine*. Routledge; 2016:16–26. Accessed April 22, 2022. https://www.routledgehandbooks.com/doi/10.4324/9781315720739.ch2
2. Marinker M. Why make people patients? *J Med Ethics*. 1975;1(2):81–84. doi:10.1136/jme.1.2.81
3. World Health Organization. Noncommunicable diseases. Published April 13, 2021. Accessed March 26, 2022. https://www.who.int/news-room/fact-sheets/detail/noncommunicable-diseases
4. Jerpseth H, Knutsen IR, Jensen KT, Halvorsen K. Mirror of shame: patients experiences of late-stage COPD. A qualitative study. *J Clin Nurs*. 2021;30(19–20):2854–2862. doi:10.1111/jocn.15792
5. Schillinger D. The intersections between social determinants of health, health literacy, and health disparities. *Stud Health Technol Inform*. 2020;269:22–41. doi:10.3233/shti200020
6. Schneiderman JU, Olshansky EF. Nurses' perceptions: addressing social determinants of health to improve patient outcomes. *Nurs Forum*. 2021;56(2):313–321. doi:10.1111/nuf.12549

7. Rodgers BL, Cowles KV. A conceptual foundation for human suffering in nursing care and research. *J Adv Nurs.* 1997;25(5):1048–1053. doi:10.1046/j.1365-2648.1997.19970251048.x

8. Liu G, Hsieh H, Chin C. Concept analysis of suffering. *Hu Li Za Zhi.* 2007;54(3):92–97.

9. Ortega-Galán ÁM, Ruiz-Fernández MD, Roldán-Rodríguez L, et al. Unbearable suffering: a concept analysis [published online ahead of print, Feb 7, 2022]. *J Hosp Palliat Nurs.* 2022;24(3):159–166. doi:10.1097/NJH.0000000000000844

10. Weiss GL, Lonnquist LE. *The Sociology of Health, Healing, and Illness.* 8th ed. Pearson; 2017.

11. Rehmann-Sutter C. Self-perceived burden to others as a moral emotion in wishes to die. A conceptual analysis. *Bioethics.* 2019;33(4):439–447. doi:10.1111/bioe.12603

12. Bigger SE, Vo T. Self-perceived burden: a critical evolutionary concept analysis. *J Hosp Palliat Nurs.* 2022;24(1):40–49. doi:10.1097/njh.0000000000000805

13. Tsao CW, Aday AW, Almarzooq ZI, et al. Heart disease and stroke statistics-2022 update: a report from the American Heart Association. *Circulation.* 2022;145(8):e153–e639. doi:10.1161/cir.0000000000001052

14. Marks SM, Chambers B, Hunter B, et al. Relieving suffering in patients with heart failure. Published February 3, 2019. Accessed January 17, 2022. https://www.capc.org/training/relief-of-suffering-across-the-disease-trajectory/relieving-suffering-in-patients-with-heart-failure/launch/

15. Higashitsuji A, Matsudo M, Majima T. Suffering and attitudes toward death of patients with heart failure in Japan: a grounded theory approach. *J Hosp Palliat Nurs.* 2021;23(5):421–428. doi:10.1097/NJH.0000000000000783

16. Martin-Saez MM, James N. The experience of occupational identity disruption post stroke: a systematic review and meta-ethnography. *Disabil Rehabil.* 2021;43(8):1044–1055. doi:10.1080/09638288.2019.1645889

17. Manning M, MacFarlane A, Hickey A, Franklin S. Perspectives of people with aphasia post-stroke towards personal recovery and living successfully: a systematic review and thematic synthesis. *PLoS One.* 2019;14(3):e0214200. doi:10.1371/journal.pone.0214200

18. Woranush W, Moskopp ML, Sedghi A, et al. Preventive approaches for post-stroke depression: where do we stand? A systematic review. *Neuropsychiatr Dis Treat.* 2021;17:3359–3377. doi:10.2147/ndt.S337865

19. National Academies of Sciences, Engineering, and Medicine; Division of Behavioral and Social Sciences and Education; Board on Behavioral, Cognitive, and Sensory Sciences; et al. *Reducing the Impact of Dementia in America: A Decadal Survey of the Behavioral and Social Sciences.* National Academies Press; 2021. https://www-ncbi-nlm-nih-gov.ezproxy3.lhl.uab.edu/books/NBK574341/?report=reader

20. Marks SM, Chambers B, Hunter B, et al. Relieving suffering in patients with dementia, and their caregivers. Published January 29, 2019. Accessed January 17, 2022. https://www.capc.org/training/relief-of-suffering-across-the-disease-trajectory/relieving-suffering-in-patients-with-dementia-and-their-caregivers/launch/

21. de Beaufort ID, van de Vathorst S. Dementia and assisted suicide and euthanasia. *J Neurol.* 2016;263(7):1463–1467. doi:10.1007/s00415-016-8095-2

22. Centers for Disease Control and Prevention. Chronic obstructive pulmonary disease (COPD). Published April 28, 2020. Updated April 22, 2022. Accessed April 22, 2022. https://www.cdc.gov/tobacco/basic_information/health_effects/respiratory/index.htm

23. American Lung Association. Learn about COPD. Updated March 5, 2021. Accessed November 30, 2021. https://www.lung.org/lung-health-diseases/lung-disease-lookup/copd/learn-about-copd

24. Marks SM, Chambers B, Hunter B, Rosielle D, Melhado L, Higgins P. Relieving suffering in patients with chronic obstructive pulmonary disease (COPD). Published January 29, 2019. Accessed January 17, 2022. https://www.capc.org/training/relief-of-suffering-acr

oss-the-disease-trajectory/relieving-suffering-in-patients-with-chronic-obstructive-pulmonary-disease-copd/launch/

25. Centers for Disease Control and Prevention. Chronic kidney disease basics. Updated February 28, 2022. Accessed April 22, 2022. https://www.cdc.gov/kidneydisease/bas ics.html

26. de Jong Y, van der Willik EM, Milders J, et al. Person centred care provision and care planning in chronic kidney disease: which outcomes matter? A systematic review and thematic synthesis of qualitative studies: care planning in CKD: which outcomes matter? *BMC Nephrol.* 2021;22(1):309. doi:10.1186/s12882-021-02489-6

27. American Nurses Association. *Nursing: Scope and Standards of Practice.* 4th ed. American Nurses Association; 2021.

28. Deal B. Finding meaning in suffering. *Holist Nurs Pract.* 2011;25(4):205–210. doi:10.1097/HNP.0b013e31822271db

29. Rehnsfeldt A, Eriksson K. The progression of suffering implies alleviated suffering. *Scand J Caring Sci.* 2004;18(3):264–272. doi:10.1111/j.1471-6712.2004.00281.x

30. VanderWeele TJ. Suffering and response: directions in empirical research. *Soc Sci Med.* 2019;224:58–66. doi:10.1016/j.socscimed.2019.01.041

31. Holopainen G, Nyström L, Kasén A. The caring encounter in nursing. *Nurs Ethics.* 2019;26(1):7–16. doi:10.1177/0969733016687161

32. Gillilan R, Qawi S, Weymiller AJ, Puchalski C. Spiritual distress and spiritual care in advanced heart failure. *Heart Fail Rev.* 2017;22(5):581–591. doi:10.1007/s10741-017-9635-2

33. Clark CC, Hunter J. Spirituality, spiritual well-being, and spiritual coping in advanced heart failure: review of the literature. *J Holist Nurs.* 2019;37(1):56–73. doi:10.1177/0898010118761401

34. Lindqvist G, Hallberg LR. "Feelings of guilt due to self-inflicted disease": a grounded theory of suffering from chronic obstructive pulmonary disease (COPD). *J Health Psychol.* 2010;15(3):456–466. doi:10.1177/1359105309353646

35. Karimi-Dehkordi M, Spiers J, Clark AM. An evolutionary concept analysis of "patients' values." *Nurs Outlook.* 2019;67(5):523–539. doi:10.1016/j.outlook.2019.03.005

36. Sedini C, Biotto M, Crespi Bel'skij LM, Moroni Grandini RE, Cesari M. Advance care planning and advance directives: an overview of the main critical issues. *Aging Clin Exp Res.* 2021;34(2):325–330. doi:10.1007/s40520-021-02001-y

37. American Geriatrics Society Expert Panel. Person-centered care: a definition and essential elements. *J Am Geriatr Soc.* 2016;64(1):15–28. doi:10.1111/jgs.13866

38. Bechthold AC, Montgomery AP, Fazeli PL, Dionne-Odom JN. Values elicitation among adults making health-related decisions: a concept analysis [published online ahead of print, Apr 17, 2022]. *Nurs Forum.* 2022;57(5):885–892. doi:10.1111/nuf.12730

39. Sudore RL, Lum HD, You JJ, et al. Defining advance care planning for adults: a consensus definition from a multidisciplinary Delphi panel. *J Pain Symptom Manage.* 2017;53(5):821–832. doi:10.1016/j.jpainsymman.2016.12.331

40. Morrison RS, Meier DE, Arnold RM. What's wrong with advance care planning? *JAMA.* 2021;326(16):1575–1576. doi:10.1001/jama.2021.16430

41. House SA, Ogilvie WA. *Advance Directives.* StatPearls. StatPearls Publishing; 2021. https://www.ncbi.nlm.nih.gov/books/NBK459133/?report=reader

42. Dobbins EH. Advance directives: replacing myths with facts. *Nursing.* 2019;49(10):11–13. doi:10.1097/01.NURSE.0000558102.43538.8f

43. Morrison RS, Meier DE, Arnold RM. Controversies about advance care planning-reply. *JAMA.* 2022;327(7):686. doi:10.1001/jama.2021.24754

44. Harrison EM. Understanding suffering: utermohlen's self-portraits and Alzheimer's disease. *Nurse Educ.* 2013;38(1):20–25. doi:10.1097/NNE.0b013e318276dfa0

11

Suffering in the Context of Cancer

Renee Wisniewski and Blima Marcus

Background

Over the past several decades, progress in cancer detection and treatment has led to earlier diagnosis, decreased mortality rates, and longer survival. Despite this progress, cancer incidence remains high, with 442.4 per 100,000 men and women each year diagnosed in the United States alone.[1] Worldwide, cancer is among the leading causes of death with over 18.1 million new cases and 9.5 million cancer-related deaths.[1] This chapter presents an overview of the suffering caused by cancer and cancer treatments throughout the trajectory of a patient's journey from initial diagnosis through survivorship, while examining the unique experiences of "the sandwich generation"; adolescents and young adults (AYAs); Black, Indigenous, and People of Color (BIPOC); and lesbian, gay, bisexual, transgender, and queer/questioning (LGBTQ+) cancer survivors. As of January 2019, there were an estimated 16.9 million cancer survivors in the United States, with this number projected to increase to 22.2 million by 2030 and reach 26.1 million by 2040.[1]

A cancer diagnosis may immediately incite significant distress or suffering for the patient and their family. According to the National Comprehensive Cancer Network (NCCN), everyone with cancer has some level of distress, which is considered normal, common, and expected and can range from mild to extreme.[2] Symptoms of suffering commonly experienced by patients with cancer include physical discomfort and symptoms, emotional and psychological distress, and existential pain. Lesser-studied sources of distress include financial struggles, discrimination, and role changes for family members.

The role of the nurse in the cancer context is to provide holistic person- and family-centered care, nurture, assess and manage symptoms, educate, and alleviate suffering. Nurses can use the NCCN 2020 Guidelines for Patients Distress During Cancer Care to familiarize themselves with common symptoms of distress, the causes, risk factors, and triggers of distress; times when distress is more likely; and to learn to incorporate distress screening into their symptom assessment.[2] The NCCN recommends using a two-part patient-reported distress screening tool consisting of a Distress Thermometer and a Problem List.[2] The patient is able to rate their level of distress on the thermometer over the past week from 0 to 10; 0 equates to no distress and 10 correlates with extreme distress. Patients can self-select from a list of problems associated with distress that is stratified into five categories: practical problems, family problems, emotional problems, spiritual/religious concerns, and physical problems. Nurses are on the front line of cancer care and often the

Renee Wisniewski and Blima Marcus, *Suffering in the Context of Cancer* In: *The Nature of Suffering and the Goals of Nursing.* Second Edition. Edited by: William E. Rosa and Betty R. Ferrell, Oxford University Press. © Oxford University Press 2023. DOI: 10.1093/oso/9780197667934.003.0011 first to detect patient distress.[2] The goal of this tool is to identify and assess distress in patients, allowing nurses to intervene accordingly and help provide referrals to chaplains, social workers, psychologists, psychiatrists, physical therapists, occupational therapists, and other critical interdisciplinary team partners based on patient responses.[2]

Defining Suffering and Distress in Patients with Cancer

"Distress" and "suffering" are used interchangeably in this chapter with the purpose of describing the widest possible range of experiences. The National Cancer Institute (NCI) defines distress as emotional, social, existential, or physical pain or suffering that may cause a person to feel sad, afraid, depressed, anxious, or lonely.[1] People in distress may also feel that they are not able to manage or cope with changes caused by normal life activities or by having a disease, such as cancer.[1] According to the NCI, patients with cancer may have trouble coping with their diagnosis, physical symptoms, or treatment due to their distress or suffering.[1] People with uncontrolled symptoms from cancer, treatment, or a combination of both are more likely to be distressed.[2] This definition demonstrates how the expression of suffering is imbedded in the subjective experience of distress.

Physical suffering is common among patients throughout their cancer experience. Weakness, fatigue, pain, loss of appetite, insomnia, respiratory distress, invasive procedures, and gastrointestinal disturbances related to cancer or cancer treatment can reduce a patient's ability to perform activities of daily living (ADLs), socialize, and enjoy available pleasures, and may cause overall suffering. From antiemetics to analgesics to appropriate referrals, there are many useful pharmacological and nonpharmacological management options for these symptoms. For instance, nurses assess patients for symptoms of physical suffering during routine encounters, from which specialist referrals for nutrition or rehabilitation therapy are often initiated.

Emotional suffering that accompanies a cancer diagnosis may contribute to and exacerbate a patient's physical and existential distress. Anxiety is a common symptom experienced by patients at various times and in varying degrees throughout their cancer experience. For patients undergoing cancer treatment, anxiety can heighten the expectancy of pain and other symptoms of distress, increase sleep disturbances, and be a major factor in anticipatory nausea and vomiting.[3] Anxiety can manifest at various times during cancer screening, diagnosis, treatment, and recurrence.[3] The NCCN recommends screening for distress at every health care visit but especially at transition times when distress is likely.[2]

Emotional suffering is reported as a source of distress for most patients diagnosed with cancer, regardless of age, race, gender, or type of cancer. The risk of suicide among people with a cancer diagnosis is higher, transcending sociodemographic characteristics and clinical risk factors (e.g., depression, cancer site, and time since diagnosis).[4,5] Depression is one of the most common psychiatric complications among people with cancer and has been reported to increase risk of mortality.[6] Many academic cancer centers have psychiatrists, psychologists, and social workers to assist patients with their mental health, but in rural communities and resource-poor cancer clinics worldwide, there is a dearth of mental health support for these patients. The NCCN Problem List screening tool can be utilized by nurses to assess causes of psychological/social suffering during each care encounter. Oncology nurses are often enlisted to provide emotional support for patients with cancer and their families throughout the trajectory of their disease course.

Existential distress occurs frequently among patients with cancer, especially in advanced stages. In the face of a cancer diagnosis or progression of disease, various aspects of life may lose their former meaning, and one's sense of stability, familiarity, and safety may become questionable and precarious.[7] Basic assumptions of the world that once seemed controllable may now be shattered, former goals may no longer be achievable, and one's sense of meaning may unravel.[7] A cancer diagnosis, unlike other illness diagnoses, forces patients to confront their mortality, making the process of finding meaning more difficult and at the same time more urgent.[7] Various evidence-based interventions in the psycho-oncology field have sought to address and alleviate existential grief. Meaning-centered psychotherapy (MCP), inspired by the work of Viktor Frankl, is a structured intervention that organizes and distills existential concepts so that they are more accessible and relevant to patients' lives.[8,9] Concepts utilized to facilitate MCP include creating meaning, fostering the will to find meaning, having the freedom to choose how suffering is experienced, and exploring sources of meaning from the domains of everyday life.[8,9]

Cancer pain, which has the potential to become severe, excruciating, and unrelenting, comprises not only physical components but also psychological, social, emotional, and existential components as described by Cicely Saunders.[10,11] She coined the concept of "total cancer pain," which encompasses all of the above aspects of pain for an individual.[10,11] The contribution of each component varies with each individual and their circumstances.[10] Nurses are able to utilize their assessment skills and validated screening tools to understand their patient's subjective experience of suffering and distress and provide referrals to aid in alleviating these symptoms.

Systemic stressors and structural injustices—such as financial stress and racism at myriad levels—may lead to uniquely intense pain or distress for patients, and it behooves providers to be familiar with these issues while incorporating the social determinants of health into oncology care planning and delivery. Often, providers may be able to assist patients with additional resources and bear witness to their suffering while providing safe spaces for their narratives and personal experiences to be seen, heard, and acknowledged.

Financial distress is also common in oncology. Studies have shown that when compared to patients with other diagnoses, patients with cancer experience more significant financial burdens.[12] Overall cancer mortality in counties with persistent poverty was 7.4% higher than in counties experiencing current but not persistent poverty.[13] Financial stress can contribute to emotional distress and worse outcomes; bankruptcy is associated with a 79% increase in early mortality among people with cancer.[14] Studies on medication adherence related to finances found that 19% of oncology patients only partially filled prescriptions, 24% avoided filling prescriptions altogether, and 27% reported poor medication adherence.[15] Making financial concessions to cancer care may lead to an increase in physical suffering, as palliative chemotherapy or palliative radiation therapy visits may be canceled or prescriptions for pain or nausea unfilled.

Another poignant example is the discrimination, implicit bias, and racism (interpersonal, institutional, systemic, structural) that continues to impact care for Black, Indigenous, and People of Color (BIPOC). Even after controlling for health care barriers and socioeconomic status, BIPOC experience poorer outcomes and poorer experiences in the health care system. Minoritized people experience more employment discrimination, leading to more uninsured BIPOC, more Medicaid coverage, less access to care, more delayed diagnoses, and worse outcomes.[16] Decades of studies on pain management among Black people consistently found that racial bias impacted providers' opioid prescribing habits, with Black people consistently being undertreated for pain.[17] Experiencing microaggressions and disrespectful interpersonal treatment while navigating a cancer diagnosis will contribute to increased emotional suffering for the racialized patient dealing with cancer. Providers need to acknowledge the impact that racism and implicit bias have on health outcomes while advocating for needed changes to dismantle racist structures and promote inclusive, community-oriented, and people-centered cancer care. Remaining cognizant of these biases by engaging in self-reflection may enhance patient care, including management of side effects and treatment. Nurses in leadership must ensure that their institutions have diversity, equity, and inclusion training, with a particular focus on creating welcoming environments and developing empathic, culturally sensitive communication skills.

Suffering with an Initial Diagnosis of Cancer

Despite an overall decline in the cancer death rate, a diagnosis of cancer is often associated with increased distress. For many people, cancer is still viewed as "a death sentence." Distress can first manifest during routine preventive screenings or when getting tests for a symptom or lump.[2] The lag time between taking the test and receiving the results can be distressing for patients who are existing in a space of unknowing. Patients' responses to a cancer diagnosis include shock, worry, fear, and sadness.[2] Additional tests, surgery, or imaging may be needed to learn more about the cancer diagnosis, causing further distress.[2] Waiting for cancer treatment to start and receiving treatments can trigger distress due to complications or side effects.[2] Transitions in care or changes in treatment are sources of distress, for example, learning that a cancer treatment did not work, hospital admission or discharge, completing cancer treatment, and shifting from frequent treatment visits to less routine follow-up visits.[2] Nurses are present in the clinical setting, chemotherapy suites, and inpatient setting to assess symptoms of distress and utilize resources available to alleviate patient suffering. Nurses can help mitigate financial stress by having open conversations with the patient about their financial concerns, considering treatments with lower copays, utilizing social workers or case managers who may offer services, and seeking funding assistance for their patients.

Sandwich Generation

The sandwich generation has been defined as "the middle-aged generation who are responsible for caring for elderly parents and dependent children,"[18] "individuals aged 35-75 with adult children and living parents who may face competing demands on their time and finances from two generations of family,"[19] and "mid-life individuals [who] are sandwiched between multiple generations, providing care for multiple generations."[20] For this chapter, the sandwich generation is defined as individuals between the ages of 35 and 75 providing care (time and/or money) to multiple generations of family including grandchildren, children, and parents/in-laws.

Maria Rivera's parents (Case Exemplar 11.1) are part of the 33% of individuals who are providing care to multiple generations of family;[19] in this case they are caring for three generations of family members. Maria's mother was unable to engage in paid work due to the responsibilities of multigenerational caregiving and made the decision to quit her job to devote more time to caring for her daughter and grandson. The challenges of balancing competing demands of raising or supporting children while caring for aging parents/in-laws has led to negative effects on caregivers' overall well-being.[21] Caregiving responsibilities impact health-related outcomes including sleep disturbance, physical health, fatigue, and stress.[18,21]

Case Exemplar 11.1

Maria Rivera was a 32-year-old Latina diagnosed 2 years ago with metastatic colon cancer and hospitalized with a large bowel obstruction on fourth-line treatment. She was a single mother to a 7-year-old son. One month prior to her death, Maria and her son moved in with her mother, father, and grandmother because Maria was experiencing a decrease in functional status, impacting her ability to work and to care for her son, due to chemotherapy treatments. Three months prior to hospitalization, Maria's mother quit her job to stay home and care for Maria, Maria's son, and her mother, who was losing her vision due to diabetes.

Prior to Maria's hospitalization, her mother was providing physical and emotional care to Maria, Maria's son, and Maria's grandmother approximately 60 hours per week while Maria's father worked full time in maintenance facilities at a university. Maria was hospitalized in the fall of 2020 during the COVID-19 pandemic, impacting her ability to have her son and extended family at her bedside in the last days of her life. Fortunately, Maria's mother was able to be at her bedside during the final days of her life to provide emotional and physical support to her daughter.

During Maria's final days, she experienced severe physical and emotional suffering because of her widely metastatic disease and likely bowel perforation, which required high doses of multiple pain medications and sedatives to manage her symptoms. Her hospitalization and death were challenging for the oncology nurses and other clinicians caring for her due to her age, high symptom burden, and intense suffering requiring around-the-clock symptom management on a busy stepdown unit.

Sandwich generation members are less likely to check food labels, exercise, use seat belts, and choose food based on health value while experiencing increased job burnout, financial and emotional stress, and feeling overwhelmed.[18,19,21] Maria's mother had to make a choice between caring for her family or working, and for Maria's mother, family and her daughter were most important. Maria's father was struggling to balance his job and his desire to be with his daughter in the final months and days of her life. Often caregivers are forced to make difficult choices about how they spend their time if they continue to work and how to balance caring for themselves. Oncology patients require time for transportation, cancer treatment, multiple doctors' appointments, tests, and recovery from treatments. Family, friends, and paid help are often required to support a patient throughout their treatment.

Being a caregiver contributes to increased physical and psychological distress, which can result in feeling overwhelmed. The responsibilities and stress of the sandwich generation will likely continue to increase as the population ages and rates of new cancer cases increase worldwide, along with increased incidence of AYA cancers.[1] An increase in the incidence and prevalence of cancer worldwide and the large percentage of sandwich generation members already providing care for multigenerational family members cause concern about rising rates of financial, emotional, and physical suffering among this population.

Assessing the distress of the patient and their caretakers is a central role of nurses. Nurses can assist in alleviating distress associated with a wide range of problems, such as practical matters like needing a ride to appointments, lack of knowledge about cancer, physical symptoms and illnesses, complex health care systems, and mental health symptoms and disorders.[2] Nurses and other clinicians can collaborate in assessing the emotional and physical health of caregivers, familiarize themselves with support available to caregivers, and provide referrals to social work, chaplaincy, and case management when appropriate and available.

Cancer Suffering Among Adolescents and Young Adults

Maria accounted for one of the 9,270 cancer deaths during 2020 in the AYA population.[22] Cancer in AYA is defined as a cancer diagnosis in young people aged 15 to 39.[35,36] According to the NCI, 89,000 young people are diagnosed with cancer each year in the United States, accounting for 5% of all cancer diagnoses in the United States.[23] The AYA cancer population is expected to grow due to the significantly increased incidence of 6 of 12 obesity-related cancers (multiple myeloma and colorectal, uterine, gallbladder, kidney, and pancreatic cancers).[23,24] This population is at risk for emotional, physical, and financial distress due to age at diagnosis and the unique life transitions experienced during adolescence and young adulthood. A cancer diagnosis and oncology treatments can cause substantial disruptions in school and career as well as changes in functioning and appearance, making the transition after treatment a longer process.[22,23] Fertility issues, sexual dysfunction, and body image, particularly among women, are common among AYA cancer survivors.[22] Compared with both younger and older patient populations, AYA cancer survivors report worse overall psychosocial functioning, which may reflect difficulty in coping with cancer during early life transitions.[22] Psychological distress among the AYA population includes fear of recurrence or being different, feeling different, cancer-related disclosure, distress of diagnosis, and control of treatment.[25]

AYA patients with cancer generally experience more financial hardship, spending more on out-of-pocket medical costs due to higher rates of uninsured AYAs compared to other groups; this can contribute to significant delays in diagnosis and lead to poorer outcomes and more extensive treatment.[22] Compared with older survivors, young survivors have higher rates of bankruptcy and more frequently forgo needed medical care because of cost.[22] Paid work is associated with a higher quality of life, self-esteem, and social status, and is often experienced as a sign of recovery after a long period of treatment.[26]

Utilizing a multidisciplinary approach, using open communication, and involving family members are key elements in alleviating suffering in the AYA population. Primary palliative care (i.e., non-specialized palliative care) promotes stronger primary clinician/nurse-patient relationships and reduces fragmented care using four domains: assessing/treating physical symptoms; addressing psychological, social, cultural, and spiritual aspects of care; serious illness communication; and care coordination.[27] Health care providers participating in one qualitative study described the challenges of engaging AYAs/families in a palliative approach to care, an increased sense of tragedy treating this group of patients, and the emotional proximity experienced when caring for them.[28] Nurses caring for Maria (Case Exemplar 11.1) reported distress about the patient's young age, concern about the patient's son losing his mother at a young age, and distress about not being able to alleviate Maria's suffering.

Access to primary palliative care remains a barrier to improved quality of life for many patients with cancer throughout the trajectory of their treatment. Nurses can screen for distress using the NCCN Distress Thermometer to identify areas and levels of distress among their patients, caregivers, and families. Providing nurses with education about primary palliative care and involving palliative care specialists in AYA care as needed may improve quality of life and reduce distress for the patient, their family, and health care clinicians.

Suffering in Survivorship

A cancer diagnosis can ignite a sequelae of physical, emotional, and existential suffering persisting well into survivorship. Cancer survivorship focuses on the physical, mental, emotional, social, and financial effects of cancer that begin at diagnosis and continue through treatment and beyond with family, friends, and caregivers included in the survivorship experience.[29] Over the past several decades, prevention and improved cancer screening, detection, and treatments have contributed to an increase in the number of cancer survivors worldwide. Cancer is a highly heterogeneous condition, and recognition of the diversity of survivorship experiences is crucial to optimizing care.[30] The suffering and lived experience of cancer survivors are varied in relation to age, gender, cancer diagnosis, and occupation, yet some symptoms are shared among all populations. Survivors living with cancer were more likely to report lower levels of physical functioning, self-rated health, and quality of life and slightly higher psychological distress than those without cancer, with considerable variation across cancer types, time since diagnosis, treatments, and stages.[30]

Research over the last decade has, to a large extent, focused on treatment side effects such as physical and psychosocial damage, emotions, coping, quality of life, and how the workplace is experienced among cancer survivors.[31] Physical, emotional, and cognitive fatigue was found to be prevalent in many cancer diagnoses for at least 2 years after diagnosis and higher than in the general population.[32] The type of fatigue and level of fatigue varied depending on cancer diagnosis. Patients with stomach cancer have demonstrated higher levels of physical and emotional fatigue; patients with bladder cancer had the highest prevalence of emotional fatigue and among the lowest prevalence of physical fatigue; and physical fatigue levels were significantly higher among patients with stomach, lung, pancreas, and kidney cancers compared to breast cancer.[32]

Fear of recurrence is among the top reported causes of distress among cancer survivors. People want to return to the life they had before cancer, but many people find this experience difficult because they continue to experience side effects of cancer treatment and long-term effects of their therapy.[31] When cancer treatment ends, patients enter a period where they must adapt to their new life on their own with decreased support from health care clinicians.[31] Suffering patients sometimes feel they need to protect others from their suffering and therefore suppress it, which can lead to compounded suffering.[31] Cancer survivors are often perceived as "healthy" and their illness as "a thing of the past," causing a conspiracy of silence that breeds more suffering.[31] Based on the 2021 study by Ueland et al., survivors may try to accept the limitations and find their subjective meaning in the new delimited and narrowed life space; this population is an example where meaning-based interventions, such as MCP, may be utilized effectively by trained nurses to explore and create meaning amid the transition to survivorship.[31]

Age and gender are commonly studied in relation to the suffering experienced by cancer survivors. In a 2021 study of cancer survivors 65 years and older with two or more additional comorbid conditions, 45.7% of those studied reported worse pain and fatigue and greater physical function limitations compared to survivors reporting only one comorbidity and survivors without any additional comorbidities.[33] The AYA population also experiences suffering related to physical, psychological, and quality-of-life changes caused by cancer diagnosis and treatment. This population often has a longer survivorship trajectory due to their age at diagnosis and developmental stage, impacting their experience, level of suffering, and survivorship needs. According to the NCI, the transition after treatment for the AYA population took longer and was more challenging than they anticipated, with many young people reporting prolonged side effects from treatment, long-term side effects, and late effects.[23] A systematic review in 2016 reported that AYAs desired information concerning possible late and long-term side effects of treatment, their capacity to pursue family and work-related goals in the future, the transition to survivorship and what to expect, guidance on which health professionals to seek out for various issues, and access to supportive care to manage challenges in reintegrating to school and work roles.[25] Older AYAs were more likely to follow up with oncological care, females were generally more likely to comply with recommended oncological follow-up (but also experience greater cost barriers) compared to men, males were more likely to experience unmet service needs, and non-white AYA survivors were more likely to experience unmet service needs.[25]

Between 420,000 and 1,000,000 LGBTQ+ cancer survivors are estimated to live in the United States.[34] The LGBTQ+ community comprises a historically excluded and poorly researched population with cancer survivorship needs that are important to explore and recenter. Minority stress—defined as the chronic, underlying worry about discrimination and prejudice that an LGBTQ+ person may experience because of their stigmatized sexual or gender identities—is important to recognize when caring for these survivors.[34] Many cancer survivors experience continued anxiety, depression, psychological distress, and the stress of integrating a new identity postcancer; for LGBTQ+ cancer survivors, this distress may be magnified by underlying, chronic minority stress.[34] For instance, transgender survivors have experienced a lack of information regarding guidance about the continuation of hormone therapies and population-specific screening/monitoring guidelines. Both LGBTQ+ and AYA survivors report unmet information needs related to fertility, coordinating follow-up care, and dealing with late effects of treatment.[25,34] It is well documented that LGBTQ+ young people face increased risk of suicidality, mental ill-health, substance misuse, smoking, bullying, sexual abuse, disordered eating, and sexually transmitted diseases.[35] Screening LGBTQ+ patients with cancer, specifically young adults with cancer, to assess for distress may improve health outcomes throughout the trajectory of their treatment and survivorship. Transitioning from active treatment to survivorship presents unique challenges to all patients with cancer and is associated with ongoing management of physical, emotional, social, and psychological distress. Cancer survivors reflect the heterogeneity of the general population, highlighting the importance of understanding the unique suffering and concerns of specific people and populations. Nurses can assess the individual needs and suffering of patients by implementing a patient-centered approach to survivorship care. Patient-centered survivorship care may facilitate improved referral and access to interdisciplinary professionals who can best address the type of suffering being experienced. Training nurses in meaning-making techniques may be helpful in alleviating the distress survivors feel during the transition phase from active treatment to less frequent visits and support of the health care team.

Responses to Suffering

Suffering in its many forms is prevalent among all ages and at any stage of care (from diagnosis through survivorship) in the oncology population. Taking time to understand the unique challenges that contribute to the increase in suffering of each patient and the people who support and care for them will help nurses provide high-quality, patient-centered oncology care. Nurses should be familiar with the resources available to their patients and issue appropriate referrals as needed to help alleviate their suffering. Asking values questions, which are questions about patients' beliefs and principles that guide how they live their lives and make decisions, and receiving training to provide holistic, primary palliative care, which addresses physical, social, spiritual/

existential, emotional and psychological, cultural, and legal/ethical concerns, are tools to better understand the patient as a person with a cancer diagnosis.

Bearing Witness

The palliative care field has grown considerably in the last few decades, and there is more awareness of pain and symptom burden and its management. However, some symptoms and some forms of suffering cannot be helped with treatment, traditional symptom management, or further referrals or resources. This is where bearing witness can be a crucial way to be with the patient and be present, alleviating suffering by sharing in their experience. Bearing witness is defined as being present and attentive to the truth of another's experiences.[36] Many authors who have sustained trauma, from Elie Wiesel to Maya Angelou, have described bearing witness as necessary to their healing and survival. This is where the true calling of nursing and the art of nursing lies: in compassionate connection, therapeutic touch, being with, being present, reflective listening, and the art that is oncology nursing.[36] Nurses must practice this art, for when there is nothing left to "fix, cure, or mend," entering into another's suffering as sojourner and witness may provide the greatest comfort.

Compassionate Silence as Presence

"Compassion" literally means "to suffer with." "Compassionate silence" is the intentional approach of creating an empathic and quite space to acknowledge and honor another's suffering.[37] Compassionate silence can be used by providers to participate meaningfully and establish connection with another person during difficult conversations.[37] Long speaking pauses can convey bearing witness and tangible listening and absorb the suffering of others. It requires a shift from doing something for the patient to simply being with the patient. Nurses should accept the limits of the spoken word and acknowledge that at times, a therapeutic silence may provide the patient with more comfort than meaningless or empty words. Compassionate silence may be useful in conversations when patients ask rhetorical questions, such as, "Is this the end for me?" Knowing the answer, the patient and nurse can choose to sit together in meditative silence, avoiding unnecessary and inconvenient answers in order to process, to grieve, and "to suffer with."

Nurturing Resilience Among Oncology Nurses

Oncology nurses experience moderate to high levels of moral distress due to their frequent exposure to end of life, challenges with symptom management, and conflicts about goals of care.[38] Moral distress is defined as a complex issue in health care that occurs when an individual faces a moral event, such as moral uncertainty or conflict, and experiences psychological distress, putting the individual at risk for burnout and compassion fatigue.[38] More research is being conducted on moral distress among oncology nurses in an effort to identify strategies to mitigate negative effects: decreased job satisfaction, avoidance, compassion fatigue, and turnover. McCracken et al., in their study examining moral distress among oncology team members, found that improved team collaboration, early and ongoing palliative care, goal-of-care discussions, and accessible organizational and unit-based resources were important strategies in supporting oncology health care professionals' ability to find meaning in their work. Facilitating the meaning of work may be an important strategy to mitigate moral distress, burnout, and compassion fatigue for those in oncology practice.[38] But, ultimately, alleviating moral distress among nurses will require both individual nurses' commitment to their own mental and emotional health and system-level changes that invest in workforce wellbeing and sustainability.[39]

Conclusion

Suffering—physical, psychological, emotional, social, spiritual, and existential—is prevalent among all people with cancer across the lifespan and at any stage of disease. However, nurses can serve as a compassionate and consistent presence throughout the cancer trajectory. They are in the unique position to heal, nurture, and alleviate that suffering in the face of distressing symptoms, in the large and small transitions, and in the quiet moments. Taking time to understand and assess the unique challenges that contribute to the suffering of each patient, and the people who support and care for them, will help nurses provide high-quality, patient-centered oncology care. Nurses should be familiar with the resources available to their patients and issue appropriate referrals as needed to help anticipate and alleviate their suffering. Asking questions about a patient's values and providing holistic, primary palliative care (Case Exemplar 11.2) are some of the tools nurses can employ to better understand the patient as a person with a cancer diagnosis.

Case Exemplar 11.2

Kevin, a 32-year-old gay man with advanced leukemia, was being cared for by his primary nurse, Scott. Kevin had entered the hospital from home with shortness of breath, severe fatigue, and uncontrolled pain. Kevin's medical record had a do not resuscitate (DNR) order in place. Before leaving for the evening, Scott communicated closely with the interdisciplinary team to ensure intensive treatment of Kevin's physical symptoms. Overnight, Kevin's breathing became more labored, his oxygen saturation decreased, and he was placed on a high-flow nasal cannula.

Scott started the next day's shift and administered the medications ordered for symptoms of shortness of breath and then sat with Kevin. Scott had noticed that Kevin's same-sex partner, Alex, was never present when Kevin's parents were in the room. With Kevin's breathing less labored, Scott began asking Kevin about his values and relationships. Kevin explained that his parents were not accepting of Alex and refused to acknowledge their 7-year relationship. This was a source of distress for Kevin as he struggled to reconcile his love for both his parents and Alex.

Scott expressed his concern about Kevin's emotional suffering and offered referrals for social work and chaplaincy. Kevin accepted both, explaining his parents were deeply religious and did not recognize the validity of Kevin's long-term relationship with Alex.

Scott coordinated a chaplain visit when Kevin's parents were visiting, having notified chaplaincy of the distress Kevin was experiencing due to his parents' refusal to accept Alex. The chaplain was able to meet with Kevin and his parents, discuss their values and beliefs, and focus his parents' actions on providing support and acceptance in the final days Kevin had left. Three days later, after Kevin had made the decision to remove the high-flow nasal cannula, Kevin's parents and Alex were all present at his bedside as he took his final breath.

References

1. National Cancer Institute. Cancer statistics. Updated September 25, 2020. Accessed May 7, 2022. https://www.cancer.gov/about-cancer/understanding/statistics
2. National Comprehensive Cancer Network. Distress during cancer care. Updated March 11, 2020. Accessed May 7, 2022. https://www.nccn.org/patients/guidelines/content/PDF/distress-patient.pdf
3. National Cancer Institute. Adjustment to cancer: anxiety and distress (PDQ®)-health professional version. Updated June 23, 2021. Accessed May 7, 2022. https://www.cancer.gov/about-cancer/coping/feelings/anxiety-distress-hp-pdq
4. Suk R, Hong Y, Wasserman RM, et al. Analysis of suicide after cancer diagnosis by US county-level income and rural vs urban designation, 2000-2016. *JAMA Netw Open.* 2021;4(10):e2129913. doi:10.1001/jamanetworkopen.2021.29913
5. Zaorsky NG, Zhang Y, Tuanquin L, Bluethmann SM, Park HS, Chinchilli VM. Suicide among cancer patients. *Nat Commun.* 2019;10(1):207. doi:10.1038/s41467-018-08170-1
6. National Cancer Institute. Depression (PDQ®)-health professional version. Updated April 19, 2022. Accessed May 31, 2022. https://www.cancer.gov/about-cancer/coping/feelings/depression-hp-pdq
7. Loeffler S, Poehlmann K, Hornemann B. Finding meaning in suffering? Meaning making and psychological adjustment over the course of a breast cancer disease. *Eur J Cancer Care.* 2018;27(3):1–10.
8. Lichtenthal W, Roberts K, Pessin H, Applebaum A, Breitbart W. Finding meaning in the face of suffering. *Psychiatric Times.* 2020;37(8):23–25.
9. Breitbart W. *Meaning-Centered Psychotherapy in the Cancer Setting: Finding Meaning and Hope in the Face of Suffering.* Oxford University Press; 2017.
10. Streeck N. Death without distress? The taboo of suffering in palliative care. *Med Health Care Philos.* 2020;23:343–351.
11. Saunders C. Into the valley of the shadow of death. A personal therapeutic journey. *British Medical Journal.* 1996;313:1599–1601.
12. Lentz R, Benson III AB, Kircher S. Financial toxicity in cancer care: prevalence, causes, consequences, and reduction strategies. *J Surg Oncol.* 2019;120(1):85–92.

13. Moss JL, Pinto CN, Srinivasan S, Cronin KA, Croyle RT. Persistent poverty and cancer mortality rates: an analysis of county-level poverty designations. *Cancer Epidemiol Biomarkers Prev.* 2020;29(10):1949–1954.
14. Ramsey SD, Bansal A, Fedorenko CR, et al. Financial insolvency as a risk factor for early mortality among patients with cancer. *J Clin Oncol.* 2016;34(9):980–986. doi:10.1200/JCO.2015.64.662012
15. Bestvina CM, Zullig LL, Rushing C, et al. Patient-oncologist cost communication, financial distress, and medication adherence. *J Oncol Pract.* 2014;10(3):162–167.
16. Yearby R. Racial disparities in health status and access to healthcare: the continuation of inequality in the United States due to structural racism. *Am J Econ Sociol.* 2018;77(3–4):1113–1152.
17. Meghani SH, Byun E, Gallagher RM. Time to take stock: a meta-analysis and systematic review of analgesic treatment disparities for pain in the United States. *Pain Med.* 2012;13(2):150–174.
18. Aazami S, Shamsuddin K, Akmal S. Assessment of work-family conflict among women of the sandwich generation. *J Adult Dev.* 2018;25:135–140. doi:10.1007/s10804-017-9276-7
19. Friedman E, Park S, Wiemers E. New estimates of the sandwich generation in the 2013 panel study of income dynamics. *Gerontologist.* 2017;57(2):191–196. doi:10.1093/geront/gnv080
20. Vlachantoni A, Evandrou M, Falkingham J, et al. Caught in the middle in mid-life: provision of care across multiple generations. *Ageing Soc.* 2020;40:1490–1510. doi:10.1017/S0144686X19000047
21. Boyczuk AM, Fletcher PC. The ebbs and flows: stress of sandwich generation caregivers. *J Adult Dev.* 2016;23:51–61. doi:10.1007/s10804-015-9221-6
22. Miller K, Fidler-Benaoudia M, Keegan T, Hipp H, Jemal A, Siegel R. Cancer statistics for adolescents and young adults, 2020. *CA Cancer.* 2020;70:443–459. doi:10.3322/caac.21637
23. National Cancer Institute. Adolescents and young adults with cancer. Updated September 24, 2020. Accessed February 25, 2022. https://cancer.gov/types/aya
24. Sung H, Siegel R, Rosenberg P, Jemal A. Emerging cancer trends among young adults in the USA: analysis of a population-based cancer registry. *Lancet.* 2019;4:137–147. https://dx.doi.org/10.1016/52468-2667(18)30267-6
25. Barnett M, McDonnell G, DeRosa A, et al. Psychosocial outcomes and interventions among cancer survivors diagnosed during adolescence and young adulthood (AYA): a systematic review. *J Cancer Surviv.* 2016;10:814–831. doi:10.1007/s11764-016-0527-6
26. de Boer AGEM, Griedanus MA, Dewa CS, Duijts SFA, Tamminga SJ. Introduction to special section on: current topics in cancer survivorship and work. *J Cancer Surviv.* 2020;14:101–105.
27. Schenker, Y. Primary palliative care. In: Post RA, ed. *UpToDate.* UpToDate; 2022. Accessed April 5, 2022. https://uptodate.com/contents/primary-palliative-care#H2957596467
28. Avery J, Geist A, D'Agostino NM, et al. "It's more difficult … ": clinicians' experience providing palliative care to adolescents and young adults diagnosed with advanced cancer. *JCO Oncol Pract.* 2019;16(1):100–108. https://doi.org/10.1200/JOP.19.00313
29. National Cancer Institute. Survivorship. Updated October 25, 2021. Accessed June 7, 2022. https://www.cancer.gov/publications/dictionaries/cancer-terms/def/survivor
30. Joshy G, Thandrayen J, Koczwara B, et al. Disability, psychological distress and quality of life in relation to cancer diagnosis and cancer type: population-based Australian study of 22,505 cancer survivors and 244,000 people without cancer. *BMC Med.* 2020;18:372. https://doi.org/10.1185/s12916-020-01830-4

31. Ueland V, Dysvik E, Hemberg J, Furnes B. Cancer survivorship: existential suffering. *Int J Qual Stud Health Wellbeing.* 2021;16(1):2001897. https://www.ncbi.nlm.nih.gov/pmc/artic les/PMC8592584/

32. Schmidt M, Hermann S, Arndt V, Steindorf K. Prevalence and severity of long-term physical, emotional, and cognitive fatigue across 15 different cancer entities. *Cancer Med.* 2020;9:8053–8061. doi:10.1002/cam4.3413

33. Siembida E, Wilder Smith A, Potosky A, Graves K, Jensen R. Examination of individual and multiple comorbid conditions and health-related quality of life in older cancer survivors. *Qual Life Res.* 2021;30:1119–1129. https://doi.org/10.1007/s11136-020-02713-0

34. Kamen C. Lesbian, gay, bisexual, and transgender (LGBT) survivorship. *Semin Oncol Nurs.* 2018;34(1):52–59. https://doi.org/10.1016/j.sonen.2017.12.002

35. Clarke M, Lewin J, Lazarakis S, Thompson K. Overlooked minorities: the intersection of cancer in lesbian, gay, bisexual, transgender, and/or intersex adolescents and young adults. *J Adolesc Young Adult Oncol.* 2019;8(5):525–528. https://doi.org/10.1089/jayao.2019.0021

36. Wickline MM, Berry DL, Belza B. Bearing witness in oncology nursing: sharing in suffering across the cancer care trajectory. *Clin J Oncol Nurs.* 2021;25(4):470–473.

37. Back AL, Bauer-Wu SM, Rushton CH, Halifax J. Compassionate silence in the patient-clinician encounter: a contemplative approach. *J Palliat Med.* 2009;12(12):1113–1117. doi:10.1089/jpm.2009.0175

38. McCracken C, McAndrew N, Schroeter K, Klink K. Moral distress: a qualitative study of experiences among oncology team members. *Clin J Oncol Nurs.* 2021;25(4):35–43. doi:10.1188/21.CJON.E35-E43

39. Schlak AE, Rosa WE, Rushton CH, Poghosyan L, Root MC, McHugh MD. An expanded institutional- and national-level blueprint to address nurse burnout and moral suffering amid the evolving pandemic. *Nurs Manage.* 2022;53(1):16–27. doi:10.1097/01.NUMA.0000805032.15402.b3

12

Bearing Witness to Suffering at End of Life

Stephanie Van Hope, Janet Booth, and William E. Rosa

We all need basic human kindness—the reliable presence and love of another person, someone willing to be in regular contact with us for the duration of our journey through suffering.

—Christine Longaker[1(p54)]

Introduction

Before the advent of modern medicine, most people died of infections or injuries,
at younger ages, at home with family caregivers, within a robust and involved community, and with little access to professional health care. The majority of Americans
now live longer, die more slowly of chronic diseases, and have access to life-extending
treatments. In addition, they commonly have unclear goals of care, they die within
health facilities, and families struggle to meet complex caregiving needs. Where death
was once considered a natural part of the lifecycle, the modern perspective is often
that death is a failure of medicine.

With a predominant cultural reticence to speak openly about dying and death, it is
hard for many people to recognize life's end as a meaningful stage of life. Many of the
rituals that have sustained communities in the past as ways to navigate dying, death,
and grief are no longer part of current practices and norms. When death is seen only
as a medical event by health practitioners, there is often less attention to psychospiritual exploration and existential support. These factors and shifts intersect and impact
the end of life for the seriously ill person, chosen family and friends, social networks,
the health care team, and society at large.

This chapter examines four approaches to end-of-life care, which overlap and build
on one another. The first approach to care focuses on *cure* until shortly before time of
death. These deaths often happen in acute care settings and the general perception
is: "Despite our best efforts, death is happening." Care in this paradigm focuses on
eliciting advance directives and incorporating palliative care for symptom management with limited time and resources available to address the psychosocial needs of
the patient and family.

The second approach to care centers on *comfort*, often with the support of hospice,
summarized as an attitude of: "Death is happening, but we can make it more comfortable." Here, the patient's and family's wishes to allow natural death have been established, and more substantial time and resources can be devoted to psychosocial needs

Stephanie Van Hope, Janet Booth, and William E. Rosa, *Bearing Witness to Suffering at End of Life* In: *The Nature of Suffering and the Goals of Nursing*. Second Edition. Edited by: William E. Rosa and Betty R. Ferrell, Oxford University Press.
© Oxford University Press 2023. DOI: 10.1093/oso/9780197667934.003.0012

and symptom management as clinical priorities. A patient's spiritual and existential needs may also be supported, often with the assistance of pastoral care, but death is still often lamented as an unfortunate event, rather than a rite of passage.

The third approach, nascent but developing, is one that centers on *consciousness*. This type of care requires a patient who has a willingness to prepare for their death ahead of time with a general sentiment of: "Death is a teacher. Dying is our last developmental act." Within this approach, death is treated as one of the most sacred and important moments in one's life. Here, palliative care might be integrated throughout the serious illness trajectory, sometimes in conjunction with disease-directed treatment, to mitigate suffering. Depending on patient preferences, physical or other types of suffering are sometimes embraced and supported as a part of the human experience that can provide teaching and insights.

The final approach incorporates *culture* and involves reclaiming caregiving and death care practices from the professional realm back to family and community, acknowledging: "There is value in honoring death together." This movement, which can involve home caregiving, home wakes, and green burials, can be seen as akin to the natural birth movement, in which suffering is reconceptualized and reclaimed from pathological to empowering, from dehumanizing service provision to human-centered relationship-based care, and from the health care setting to a home environment, potentially supported by health care professionals but recentered around family and community culture. Caring for dying and deceased loved ones can provide a vehicle for working with grief through action and connection—a process known to all cultures worldwide that we are calling *participatory grieving* (see section on cultural approach).

From Curative to Palliative Care

According to 2020 mortality data from the Centers for Disease Control and Prevention, 9 of the 10 leading causes of death are related to chronic, progressive diseases.[2] It is noteworthy that although most people will die slowly and have the opportunity to prepare, only half of all Medicare decedents are enrolled in hospice at the time of their death, with a median length of stay of only 18 days.[3] Additionally, only approximately one in three US adults completes any type of advance directive for end-of-life care.[4] Many studies have shown that, if possible, around 80% of Americans would prefer to die at home (though further understanding of the sociocultural demographics of these samples is needed).[5] Estimates suggest that around 35% of Americans die in acute care hospitals, 27% in nursing homes, and 31% at home.[6]

Nurses working in hospital settings will care for these patients and families before, during, and after these deaths. There are stressors that contribute to nurses' suffering when death occurs in an acute care setting. As outlined in Box 12.1, these include unclear goals of care, the lack of family preparation for death, nurses' cumulative grief from multiple losses, witnessing futile medical care, and the pace and demands of hospital nursing. In contrast to the hospice philosophy that allows for a natural death, hospital systems are designed to prevent death. Additionally, many nurses may feel unprepared for serious illness conversations, high-stakes medical decision-making,

---

Box 12.1 Factors Unique to the Suffering of Nurses Who Bear Witness to Deaths in an Acute Care Setting

- Cumulative losses and grief experienced over time
- Patients/families unprepared for death—more confusion, distress, and unexpressed grief
- Chaos and stress related to unclear patient goals of care
- Fast pace and demands of hospital nursing care
- Philosophical discrepancy between "allowing natural death" and "death as failure"
- Witness to medically futile care

---

ethical dilemmas, and complex psychosocial family dynamics that may occur at the end of life.[7]

"Dying well" is one of the eight trends noted in a recent global health summit report on the future of wellness.[8] There is also growing recognition of "successful dying" from a human developmental point of view. A systematic review of systematic reviews identified common themes that would inform a "good death," including dying in one's preferred place, alleviation of pain and psychological distress, loved ones' emotional support, autonomy in decision-making, effective communication with health professionals, and performance of desired rituals, among others.[9] What people typically want to experience at the end of life—emotional well-being, a sense of life completion or legacy, dignity in the dying process—are generally not quick fixes. Nurses need to engage in values-directed conversations over a period of months to years and not just in the days or weeks before a patient's death to position themselves as key practitioners within the continuity of end-of-life care. The American Nurses Association (ANA) states that all nurses benefit from basic palliative care skills to strengthen symptom management and serious illness communication.[10] Nurses are ideally positioned as a resource and support for patients and families in end-of-life decision-making, especially to advocate for care aligned with patient preferences. This process can involve collaboration with experts in decision-making, such as specialty palliative care teams or ethics committees.

Case Exemplar 12.1

A nurse on a hospital medical-surgical floor is caring for a 68-year-old man, Eddie, who has dementia, heart disease, and hepatic cirrhosis. Eddie is a Korean War veteran whose eldest daughter describes him as self-reliant, private, and having a "fighting spirit." He adamantly wants to be back in his home with his older caregiver spouse, Doris. There is occasional broader family caregiving support, but it is complicated by years of estrangement among the four adult children. Doris appears hesitant to speak up to either her husband or the medical team about her husband's condition. There are unclear advance directives, as Eddie refuses to talk about his illnesses with anyone and there are different ideas among family members about what Eddie wants and what end-of-life decisions he would make.

Eddie has had several recent hospital admissions for infections. He is now admitted for pneumonia. His condition is unstable. The medical team needs Doris to decide Eddie's code status, but the children are not in agreement about what Eddie would want. The nurse caring for Eddie feels uneasy about both the medical team pressure and the family indecisiveness.

Complicating the nurse's work is constrained time to spend with the family due to the high census and acuity on the floor. She knows that she has a role in helping the family work toward clarity in the goals of care, but she doesn't feel empowered or confident enough to have those conversations. She decides to call the nurse on the palliative care service and consults with her about initiating and guiding a family discussion about what Eddie would want.

It is a challenging family meeting characterized by strong emotions. Eddie's children direct their anger at the specialist palliative nurse. The palliative nurse models clear boundaries by redirecting aggressive communication instead toward the grief and confusion they might be feeling. When the nurse acknowledges that Eddie didn't want to die in the hospital, Doris speaks up: "He didn't want to be on any machines. He just wanted to die in peace." As the patient's medical power of attorney, Doris's words change the trajectory of the next 18 hours. Due to his rapid decline, Doris decides Eddie should remain in the hospital rather than transfer home while honoring Eddie's desire for privacy, comfort, and dignity.

The bedside and palliative nurses both work with the primary team to complete a do not resuscitate (DNR) order and create a home-like environment in the patient's room, and—collaborating closely with the team social worker and chaplain—have found ways to actively include family members in Eddie's care. One of his daughters brings in a small battery-powered candle for his bedside, and they turn the lights down in the room. Two of the siblings speak with the hospital chaplain, who support them to express their grief over years of complicated family dynamics. These conversations allow them to say things to their father that express love and forgiveness. Doris is able to sleep in a recliner chair next to his hospital bed, which allows her to be with Eddie when he dies peacefully in the early hours of the following morning.

Advocacy for patients and their end-of-life decision-making is challenging when goals of care are unclear and decisions need to be made quickly. The nurse—experiencing prolonged, direct contact with patients and families—is witness to the particular kind of suffering that emerges when families are unprepared and conflicted. The nurse is often challenged by the competing values of quality versus quantity of life, the benefit versus burden of disease-directed treatments, and patient/family control versus lack of control throughout the process. The weighing of these competing values offers a potent area for discussion with patients and families when discerning direction and priorities at end of life.

Nurses can play a critical role to help shift a person's experience away from the anxiety and uncertainty of an immediate crisis toward the bigger picture of "what matters most." This shift requires a kind of pause—an opening—and a chance to breathe more easily as patients and families reflect and recalibrate the path forward. This ability to focus and pause is a skill that supports the nurse's well-being within a sometimes chaotic and intense acute care setting.

Part of the intensity for nurses is the amount of grief—expressed or unexpressed—that they witness. Just as stress can be cumulative over time, so can exposure to the intense emotions of grief and loss. Nurses may be unaware of their own grief in bearing witness to patient and family suffering. Another piece of well-being in this work is the examination of one's own beliefs/experiences/feelings about serious illness, death, loss, and grief. Some say that normalizing grief and grieving with self-compassion can cultivate "grief literacy."[11] Understanding one's own history with end-of-life care and grief can ease the emotional weight a nurse carries, which may free them to be more present for others in their grief. In addition, bereavement-conscious care can be fostered by prioritizing bereavement considerations long before the death of a patient, focusing concerns on loved ones' needs, worries, and fears; ensuring clear and compassionate communication pathways with care teams; facilitating family presence and opportunities to have important conversations with the dying one; leading bereavement risk screening; advocating for proper supports for family members at risk for complicated grief; and providing condolence calls following the death to minimize abandonment.[12,13]

Types of physical suffering that can be easily prevented or relieved with nursing interventions include mild to moderate pain, nausea, sleeplessness, anxiety, constipation, skin breakdown, and others. In an acute care setting, palliative trained clinicians are often better able to anticipate and recognize common symptoms, elevate their priority, suggest a range of pharmacological and nonpharmacological interventions, administer multimodal medication regimens, and reassess symptom burden toward achieving a patient's goals.

There are some physical symptoms, however, that are difficult to fully relieve or are accompanied by side effects or trade-offs. A skilled palliative nurse is honest with patients and through active listening and inquiry helps patients identify their values and where they are willing to make trade-offs (e.g., drowsiness for pain relief). Some patients want full relief of symptoms even if it requires sedation; others are willing to live with some discomfort if it means they can be lucid enough to have meaningful interactions with family, complete important business, and maintain awareness of the many layered changes that are happening within them; while other patients do not want any kind of pharmacological intervention. These priorities can shift and change at any time.

Nurses working in care settings have an important opportunity for initiating conversations with patients about advance care planning (e.g., identifying a surrogate decision maker), quality of life (e.g., what makes life meaningful?), and patient priorities (e.g., dying at home, aggressive symptom management). The more normalized these conversations can become in all the places where people receive health care, the more likely that patients will have the time and support needed to complete the important practical, relational, and spiritual work of preparing for dying.

Comfort-Focused Care Approach

The hospice movement, which began in England and took root in the United States in the 1970s, transformed care for dying people, primarily by de-pathologizing death, prioritizing comfort and value-concordant care, recognizing death as a lifecycle event, and putting patients and families at the center of the experience. In disease-focused care, suffering can be seen as a potentially necessary side effect of treatment, whereas in hospice care, tending to suffering itself is the goal of care—hospice is often synonymous with comfort-focused care.

The process of adopting hospice itself can be one that introduces or relieves certain types of suffering. For some patients and families, recognizing that the patient is likely to die from their condition may be perceived as a defeat against the illness accompanied by feelings of disappointment, desolation, and anticipatory grief. For others, once this outcome is imminent, it is a relief not to have to use physical and emotional energy fending it off, and the shift to a focus on quality of life in the time remaining may enrich joy and meaning. Many patients and families experience a mix of these reactions. And sometimes an admission to inpatient hospice care for someone whose needs for food, shelter, and medical care are not adequately addressed at home can mean the alleviation of suffering by meeting basic needs.

In the original edition of this volume, Ferrell and Coyle write that "nurses diagnose sources of suffering and identify those that can and should be relieved, and they recognize the aspects of illness and suffering that should be witnessed and supported."[14(p21)] Though many people fear pain at the end of life, other types of suffering that cannot be medicated can also cause substantial levels of distress. Records from Oregon's implementation of the Death with Dignity Act reveal that most participating patients are motivated by nonphysical suffering. Loss of autonomy (90.6%), decreased ability to enjoy life (89.9%), loss of dignity (73.6%), and perceived burden on friends and family (47.5%) are more prominent end-of-life concerns than actual or potential inadequate pain control (27.4%).[15] A dying person must let go of everything they have and know—abilities, independence, roles and identities, relationships—whether slowly or quickly. The dying person's loved ones are simultaneously being challenged to adapt and let go at a fundamental level.

Anticipatory grief—also known as predeath grief, predeath or anticipatory loss, anticipatory bereavement, and anticipatory mourning—plays a role in this process of "letting go." This is grief that happens before the death occurs and is a natural response to that anticipated loss. It is commonly experienced by the loved ones as well as by the person who is dying, and it can include signs and symptoms of grief. Although this experience of grief might be confusing for some people—"Is it wrong that I'm feeling these things before he dies? How can I feel this and still have hope?"—it can also be an impetus for personal growth and closure.[16] It gives the dying person and their loved ones an opportunity to begin the grieving process together, to have hard conversations that could lead to authentic closeness and healing moments. Nurses have an important role in educating and supporting people experiencing anticipatory grief—naming it, normalizing it, and focusing on what opportunities might be available for healing and closure.[17]

Conversations that bring in aspects of life review and life completion have been shown to improve a sense of well-being for seriously ill people. Research conducted by Steinhauser and colleagues has shown that discussion of life completion may improve important health outcomes—decreasing suffering and increasing quality of life—for patients at the end of life.[18] Their interview questions covered three areas: life story, forgiveness/regret, and legacy. The outcomes included improvements in functional status, anxiety, depression, and preparation for end of life. Their model of skillful questions and deep listening was designed to help with the role transitions that occur during serious illness, with a goal of allowing people to go beyond the "patient" role by integrating their whole-person resources and taking the time to ask questions like "What do I cherish most about my life? Is there someone I need to ask forgiveness from? What are the most valuable life lessons I learned?" Physician and author Atul Gawande refers to this perspective as one of bringing a *coherent view* to managing the complexity of medical decision-making.[19] Coherence can be understood as inviting the possibility that our dying might fit into the unified whole of who we are, continuing the values we've lived by throughout our life.

While there is no medication for a patient's perceived loss of dignity, a nurse can offer the intervention of "presence, listening, and communication that enables patient expression."[14(p15)] The last chapter of a novel can reframe the entire story. Patients at the end of their life may struggle to reinterpret their life story when the end comes while they are unprepared. Active listening provides a space for meaning making. And even when a patient dies with unresolved existential anxiety, the experience of being witnessed and sharing that suffering with others creates opportunity for a rarely felt level of connection and tenderness.

Conscious Dying Approach

The Lancet Commission on the Value of Death report declared a paradigm shift to "bring death back into life" and create pathways across health and death systems to rehumanize living, dying, death, and grief.[20] The commission called for a "realistic utopia" where the social determinants of death, dying, and grief were tackled; dying could be understood as a relational/spiritual process instead of a mere physiological event; networks of care endeavor to support people who are dying, caring, and grieving; conversations and stories about everyday dying, death, and grief are normalized; and death is recognized as having value.[20]

For the last 40 years, the hospice movement has improved care for the dying by offering the possibility of "a good death." A conscious dying approach goes further to acknowledge the value of death itself and recognize the imminence of death throughout one's life as a teacher—if one can be awake to it. Acknowledging that death can come at any moment naturally leads to better preparation for death, increased connection with and appreciation for loved ones and community, and considerations for after-death care and legacy.

Conscious dying as a nursing framework "strives to deepen the nurse healer's awareness in tending to a patient's dying and death, returning death to its sacred place in the cycle of life."[21] Conscious dying principles include creating caring-healing environments; increasing opportunity for beauty, caring, tenderness, and love; and acknowledging mysteries and miracles. Conscious dying practitioners must deeply acknowledge, reflect upon, and confront their own mortality and beliefs about dying to serve as coaches and guides for others. In addition, they can reflect on the capacities of their health systems to cultivate human-centered end-of-life care and advocate for needed changes.[21]

Beyond recognizing the value of death, a conscious dying approach acknowledges the value of suffering. Religions and cultures worldwide recognize suffering as an inevitable part of life and often encourage its direct approach through rituals and rites of passage such as fasting, intensive prayer, pilgrimage, vision questing, and coming-of-age rituals that confront a person with the opportunity to suffer consciously in order to transcend a certain part of themselves and step into a new sphere of existence.

An emerging paradigm of treating end-of-life existential anxiety through such a rite of passage is psychedelic-assisted therapy (PAT). Research in the use of psilocybin in serious illness, though still only in phase II trials with small sample sizes, shows promising outcomes, including rapid, significant, and sustained improvements in anxiety and depression; enhanced quality-of-life and spiritual well-being; and marked decreases in hopelessness and demoralization.[22,23] Often, patients in PAT trials have described an experience of the mystical that seems to engender feelings of wholeness, love, the divine, and transcendence over the fear of death. If phase III trials deliver similar results that lead to rescheduling of these medicines, nurses will have key roles to play in providing thoughtful and competent care to PAT patients during preparation, journeying, and integration.[24–27]

Nursing theorist Pamela Reed argues that self-transcendence is "a developmental imperative, meaning that it is a human resource that demands expression, much like other developmental processes such as walking in toddlers, abstract reasoning in adults, and grieving in those who have suffered a loss. These resources are a part of being human and of realizing one's potential for well-being ... and nursing has a role in facilitating this process."[28(p111)] The multitude of losses a dying person is faced with—loss of identity, relationship, capability—can be opportunities to disidentify with the temporal parts of oneself and to search for connection to who one is beneath social masks and identities. While these losses may bring suffering, a prepared person may take the attitude of "I am suffering, and that is as it should be. Stay with it and see what it has to offer." It may be difficult for nurses to abandon an aspect of their training that demands that every symptom presented be eliminated or at least ameliorated. But indeed, many experiences of suffering that come at the end of life cannot be fixed, only deeply witnessed, accepted, and supported as a natural process.

In a response to the modern body of work around suffering related to Eric Cassell's work, philosopher Govert den Hartogh argues that suffering is a response to very real threats to a person's life and well-being, and that in these circumstances "it would rather be a pathological symptom not to be sad and not to suffer. Suffering, therefore, is sometimes and to some extent a condition to be respected."[29(p413)] Den Hartogh, while recognizing that the alleviation of suffering is a primary aim of palliative care, argues it should not be absolute. A beneficial approach by a nurse or palliative specialist could be to first understand the patient's experience as they experience it and *accept it as it is*, without judging any part of it as bad, wrong, or "shouldn't be happening."

From that ground of acceptance, a nurse can move forward with the patient to determine what changes in their plan of care they may desire and what may be possible.

While opportunities for great strides in personal and relational growth are available at the end of life, it is more likely that a person will "die as they lived." A person wanting to die with full consciousness and embrace dying as a last developmental act may have to learn to live with a greater degree of consciousness. Thus, living with more presence becomes a desirable side effect of contemplating one's death ahead of time, including being present to suffering.

Case Exemplar 12.2

Marian is a late middle-aged woman, mother of four and grandmother of five, and retired schoolteacher living with her husband, Sam, in a rural community. Marian was diagnosed with early-stage breast cancer in her early 50s that was treated with a lumpectomy and radiation. The experience awakened her to the reality that death can come at any moment. She began exploring spiritual teachings on death, using her own Methodist faith as a starting point. She attended local death cafes—community meetings where people get together and discuss death—which were organized by a hospice nurse and death doula, where she became familiar with ideas such as home wakes and green burials. Marian started considering the concept of being cared for at the time of death at home by her family. The idea of limiting the amount of medical involvement as much as possible appealed to her given dissatisfying experiences with the health system and clinicians during her cancer care.

Despite her desire to speak about her death, her family (especially her husband) was unwilling to entertain these conversations, insisting her death seemed unlikely and distant, and accusing her of being "morbid and paranoid." Marian could feel that thinking of losing her, their rock, caused suffering for them. Her daughter June was supportive of Marian, hiring the death doula that Marian had encountered at the death cafe to help guide them through the difficult and meaningful conversations needed to establish Marian's end-of-life goals and preferences. Marian and June found that, though sometimes uncomfortable, these conversations led both of them to value their time together more. And for Marian, she found her contemplation of death helped strengthen her spiritual life, be closer to God, and prioritize how she wanted to spend the time she had left on this earth, which led her to create a local community garden. The garden gave her great comfort as she realized it would exist beyond her death, offering a place of comfort for many.

Marian maintained a high level of function and quality of life throughout her breast cancer treatment. However, 3 years later, Marian died in a car accident. Amid the shock and grief, her daughter June felt cheated out of the opportunity to care for her mom at the end of life in the way they had envisioned, though she was able to provide the after-death care that her mom wanted—organizing friends, family, and church members to hold a wake in their home for 3 days and burying Marian in a wicker casket she had already selected in the green burial section of a regional cemetery. Though June's siblings and father were unable to participate in discussions about her death when Marian was alive, June was now able to share with them her mother's beliefs about death and her wishes for how the family could carry her legacy forward, which helped to provide some guidance through their grief process.

Cultural Approach and Participatory Grieving

Cultures since time immemorial have created rituals around caring for the dead, many involving the entire community connected to the dying person and their family in all aspects of caring, from practical to spiritual. These rituals have largely been outsourced to death professionals in Westernized settings. In many places in the world these rituals are still robust, and in others they are intact but fragile.[20] In a beautiful video testimony of the power of participatory rituals around death, an American family describes coming together to weave their mother's casket ahead of her death, caring for her at home (with the help of professional caregivers), anointing her body with oil and prayer after the moment of death, keeping her body at home (supported by dry ice) for 3 days as family grieved together and visitors paid their respects, carrying the casket by hand through town to the burial site, and together covering her body with dirt at the gravesite.[30] All these practices were common for families to perform until less than a century ago. This family describes the gifts that they received by being engaged with their grief, physically through their very hands, and together as a family system. We refer to this involvement with active and communal death and after-death care as *participatory grieving*.

Contemplative author Francis Weller proposes that we collectively experience grief not only for personal losses of loved ones but also for cultural losses, such as the loss of the old ways of community, what he refers to as "what we expected in this life and did not receive."[31] Weller speaks to how we might locate ourselves in the bigger picture of our communities, the natural world, and the cosmos—our sense of belonging on a deeper level. Without that sense of knowing we belong, there can be a widespread feeling of loneliness and disconnection. This loss of community, ritual, and connectedness may be related to the mental health and substance abuse crises unfolding in America, perhaps more indicative of social and cultural suffering. The loss of community death-tending skills robs us of our ability to engage in participatory grief. The key understanding put forward by the Lancet Commission on the Value of Death is:

> Our relationship with death and dying has become unbalanced, and we advocate a rebalancing. At the core of this rebalancing must be relationships and partnerships between people who are dying, families, communities, health and social care systems, and wider civic society.[20(p1)]

A cultural approach to dying recognizes sources of suffering within systems and society that deny the value of death and the ripple effects this denial has on the way we live. Some nurses working from this perspective may shift emphasis from working with dying people to working with well people long before their death and from health care to community settings to provide leadership in this essential rebalancing.

In the last decade or so, many small, interwoven movements around community death care have begun to gain traction. Community death care is a grassroots movement that educates and supports families to care for their dying loved ones. It serves to normalize death and dying and to guide people in caregiving skills that many have forgotten. Interest is growing for death cafes, end-of-life doulas, creative resources for advance care planning, green burials, home funerals, new forms of cremation, and awareness of the significant role of spirituality and consciousness. The compassionate care community movement empowers communities in which everyday people play a stronger role in the care and support of people as they age and at the end of life. It is an approach to improving the end-of-life experience for people by mobilizing local networks, groups, and services to be more conscious, aware, and equipped to offer support.[20] This public health education approach to death and dying is proposed to both upstream and normalize the conversation about advance care planning in the domain of a broader death education context.[32] Nurses can reimagine their role from caregiver/care coordinator (either inpatient or at home) to educator, coach, and community organizer.

Responses to Suffering

There has been a strong emergence within the general American culture of resources and education that support emotional and spiritual well-being, especially related to mindfulness, self-compassion, and compassionate presence. For instance, as part of the Being with Dying program, nurses and other health practitioners learn the skills and practices of compassionate presence. It can be seen as an integration of three parts: not knowing, bearing witness, and acting compassionately.[33] As nurses, we bear witness to suffering on all levels. Bearing witness calls us to be present with the suffering and joy inherent in our nursing practice, without judgment or any attachment to outcome—which can be challenging while working within fragmented and often resource-constrained health systems. A key concept is the practice of being present with what is. Suffering is increased for many of us when we feel things "should" be different (i.e., the suffering in front of us should not be happening). The acceptance of what is in the present moment helps free us from the worries or anxieties about the past and the future.

A nurse accompanying a suffering patient can acknowledge first the difficulty they are experiencing and extend compassion for self. Kristin Neff, who first clinically conceptualized self-compassion, defines it as "ways that individuals emotionally respond to suffering (with more kindness and less judgment), cognitively understand suffering (as part of the human experience rather than as isolating), and pay attention to suffering (in a more mindful and less overidentified manner)."[34(p122)] Self-compassion in hospice health professionals has been associated with increased capacity for self-care, mindfulness, and professional quality of life, as well as a decrease in perceived burnout risk and secondary traumatic stress.[35]

With self-compassion engaged, a nurse could then respond to the suffering of the patient, family member, coworker, community, or system, first by acknowledging that suffering is present, without immediately trying to fix or eliminate it. The existence of suffering often feels like failure to a health care professional. A nurse can relieve themselves of this feeling of failure by understanding suffering as a part of the human experience. The nurse, by allowing themselves to be touched by this human experience of another's suffering while also not taking it on as their own, can make an authentic connection with the patient. From this perspective a nurse can then determine a course of action—for example, teaching patients nonpharmacological symptom management techniques that transform a patient's relationship to discomfort, such as noticing the shifting qualities and borders of pain in order to experience oneself as the more spacious witness of suffering rather than as the sufferer.

A nurse working from a conscious dying/participatory grieving perspective can also accept suffering *as it is* on a systems level. While a nurse may feel frustrated that our systems are not designed to help patients face their mortality through human-centered approaches, they can accept that this is indeed the case and ask what possibilities are available for a certain patient/family/community/system in the situation. Engaged nurses can work to make changes inside institutions to normalize dying and help patients to approach the reality of death earlier.

Conclusion

There has been a substantive evolution in how communities and systems care for the dying and their loved ones, with multiple and iterative shifts from curative and comfort-focused care to conscious dying and cultural/participatory approaches. The nurse is a constant presence throughout the wellness-illness-dying-death-bereavement expanse. Learning to bear witness to suffering—to be with, empathize with, appreciate, and respond compassionately to the other—is a lifelong process. In addition, nurses are now being called to work as an integral part of networks, teams, and communities as societies relearn how to bear witness to suffering together.

References

1. Longaker C. *Facing Death and Finding Hope: A Guide to the Emotional and Spiritual Care of the Dying*. Broadway Books; 1998.
2. Leading causes of death. Centers for Disease Control and Prevention. Published January 13, 2022. Accessed March 20, 2022. https://www.cdc.gov/nchs/fastats/leading-causes-of-death.htm
3. Hospice facts and figures. National Hospice and Palliative Care Organization. Published October 28, 2021. Accessed March 24, 2022. https://www.nhpco.org/hospice-care-overview/hospice-facts-figures/
4. Yadav KN, Gabler NB, Cooney E, et al. Approximately one in three US adults completes any type of advance directive for end-of-lifecare. *HA*. 2017;36(7):1244–1251.

5. Aldridge MD, Bradley EH. Epidemiology and patterns of care at the end of life: rising complexity, shifts in care patterns and sites of death. *Health Aff (Millwood)*. 2017;36(7):1175–1183. doi:10.1377/hlthaff.2017.0182

6. QuickStats: percentage of deaths, by place of death — National Vital Statistics System, United States, 2000–2018. *MMWR*. 2020;69(19):611.

7. Croxon L, Deravin L, Anderson J. Dealing with end of life—new graduated nurse experiences. *J Clin Nurs*. 2018;27(1–2):337–344.

8. 2019 Global wellness trends report. Global Wellness Summit. Published January 28, 2019. Accessed February 17, 2022. https://www.globalwellnesssummit.com/2019-global-wellness-trends/

9. Zaman M, Espinal-Arango S, Mohapatra A, Jadad AR. What would it take to die well? A systematic review of systematic reviews on the conditions for a good death. *Lancet Healthy Longevity*. 2021;2(9):e593–e600.

10. American Nurses Association. Nurses' roles and responsibilities in providing care and support at the end of life (position statement). Published 2016. http://www.nursingworld.org/MainMenuCategories/EthicsStandards/Ethics-Position-Statements/EndofLifePositionStatement.pdf

11. Breen L. Grief literacy: a call to action for compassionate communities. *Death Stud*. 2022;46(2):425–433.

12. Roberts KE, Lichtenthal WG, Ferrell BR. Being a bereavement-conscious hospice and palliative care clinician. *J Hosp Palliat Nurs*. 2021;23(4):293–295. doi:10.1097/NJH.0000000000000775

13. Lichtenthal WG, Roberts KE, Ferrell BR. Bereavement care: walking the walk. *J Palliat Med*. 2021;24(6):805–806. doi:10.1089/jpm.2021.0195

14. Ferrell BR, Coyle N. *The Nature of Suffering and the Goals of Nursing*. Oxford; 2008.

15. Oregon Health Authority Public Health Division. *Oregon Death with Dignity Act 2020 Data Summary*. 2021.

16. Allard E, Genest C, Legault A. Theoretical and philosophical assumptions behind the concept of anticipatory grief. *Int J Palliat Nurs*. 2020;26(2):56–63. doi:10.12968/ijpn.2020.26.2.56

17. Corless IB, Meisenhelder JB. Bereavement. In: Ferrell BR, Paice JA, eds. *Oxford Textbook of Palliative Nursing*. 5th ed. New York, NY: Oxford University Press; 2019:390–404.

18. Steinhauser K, Alexander S, Byock I, et al. Seriously ill patients' discussions of preparation and life completion: an intervention to assist with transition at end of life. *Palliat Support Care*. 2009;7:393–404.

19. Gawande A. *Being Mortal: Medicine and What Matters in the End*. Metropolitan Books; 2014.

20. Sallnow L, Smith R, Ahmedzai SH, et al. Report of the Lancet Commission on the Value of Death: bringing death back into life. *The Lancet (Br ed.)*. 2022;399(10327):837–884. doi:10.1016/S0140-6736(21)02314-X

21. Rosa W, Estes T, Hope S, Watson J. Conscious dying: human caring amid pain and suffering. In Rosa W, Horton-Deutsch S, Watson J, eds. *A Hand Book for Caring Science: Expanding the Paradigm*. Springer Publishing; 2018:145–161.

22. Ross S, Bossis A, Guss J, et al. Rapid and sustained symptom reduction following psilocybin treatment for anxiety and depression in patients with life-threatening cancer: a randomized controlled trial. *J Psychopharmacol*. 2016;30(12):1165–1180. doi:10.1177/0269881116675512

23. Agin-Liebes GI, Malone T, Yalch MM, et al. Long-term follow-up of psilocybin-assisted psychotherapy for psychiatric and existential distress in patients with life-threatening cancer. *J Psychopharmacol*. 2020;34(2):155–166. doi:10.1177/0269881119897615

24. Rosa WE, Sager Z, Miller M, et al. Top ten tips palliative care clinicians should know about psychedelic-assisted therapy in the context of serious illness [published online ahead of print, Mar 14, 2022]. *J Palliat Med.* 2022. doi:10.1089/jpm.2022.003625.

25. Penn A, Dorsen CG, Hope S, Rosa WE. Psychedelic-assisted therapy: emerging treatments in mental health disorders. *Am J Nurs.* 2021;121(6):34–40. doi:10.1097/01.NAJ.0000753464.35523.2926.

26. Rosa WE, Dorsen CG, Penn A. Fostering nurse engagement in psychedelic-assisted therapies for patients with serious illness. *J Palliat Med.* 2020;23(10):1288–1289. doi:10.1089/jpm.2020.024127.

27. Penn AD, Phelps J, Rosa WE, Watson J. Psychedelic-assisted psychotherapy practices and human caring science: toward a care-informed model of treatment. *J Human Psychol.* April 2021. doi:10.1177/00221678211011013

28. Reed P. Theory of self-transcendence. In: Smith MJ, Liehr PR, eds. *Middle Range Theory for Nursing.* 4th ed. Springer Publishing Company; 2018:109–139.

29. Den Hartogh G. Suffering and dying well: on the proper aim of palliative care. *Med Health Care Philos.* 2017;20(3):413–424. doi:10.1007/s11019-017-9764-3

30. Sturmann J. *Taking Back the Process: The Handmade Funeral of Loie Knowles* [Video]. Vimeo; April 2, 2019.

31. Weller F. *The Wild Edge of Sorrow: Rituals of Renewal and the Sacred Work of Grief.* North Atlantic Books; 2015.

32. Prince-Paul M, DiFranco E. Upstreaming and normalizing advance care planning conversations—a public health approach. *Behav Sci (Basel).* 2017;7(2):18.

33. Rushton C, Halifax J, Dossey B. Being with dying-practices for compassionate end-of-life care. *Am Nurse Today.* 2007;2(9):16–18.

34. Neff KD, Tóth-Király I, Knox MC, Kuchar A, Davidson O. The development and validation of the state self-compassion scale (long- and short form). *Mindfulness.* 2020;12(1):121–140. doi:10.1007/s12671-020-01505-4

35. Mesquita Garcia AC, Domingues Silva B, Oliveira da Silva LC, Mills J. Self-compassion in hospice and palliative care: a systematic integrative review. *J Hosp Palliat Nurs.* 2021;23(2):145–154. doi:10.1097/NJH.0000000000000727

13

Suffering of Caregivers, Loved Ones, and the Community

Tamryn F. Gray

Introduction

Within medicine and health care more broadly, the alleviation of suffering is a key goal, particularly as patients and families are impacted by serious illnesses. Despite improvements in serious illness and end-of-life care, some unrelieved suffering persists for patients with advanced illness and their family members. Suffering is defined as an unpleasant or even anguishing experience that severely affects a person at a psychophysical and an existential level. Moreover, suffering is personal, individual, and commonly expressed as a narrative,[1,2] meaning that it engenders a crisis of meaning and is perceived as a threat, fear, or concern about the future. While suffering is often considered synonymous with pain, it can happen independently of pain and other physical symptoms. Suffering arises from perceptions of impending destruction of an individual's personhood and continues until the threat of disintegration has passed or the integrity of the person is restored. While suffering is most often attributed to patients, family caregivers also experience significant suffering as they serve as witnesses of the patient experience and struggle with their own grief.[3,4]

As understood in its fundamental sense as a response to suffering, palliative care has a critical responsibility to those who suffer the greatest morbidity and mortality, particularly the poor. Palliative care is intended for people living with serious illness, and preventing and alleviating suffering continues to be an important priority area within palliative and end-of-life care. Palliative care has been defined as "the active holistic care of individuals across all ages with serious health related suffering due to severe illness and especially of those near the end of life. It aims to improve the quality of life of patients, their families and their caregivers."[4(p755)] Particularly within palliative care, an individual's suffering must be heard and accepted, as the denial of the person's story of suffering and sacrifice is a denial of their identity as a sufferer.[5]

The purpose of this chapter is to (1) define suffering of caregivers, loved ones, and the community; (2) discuss consequences related to suffering; (3) identify evidence-based ways to respond to suffering; and (4) outline the possible benefits of suffering including meaning making, personal growth, and introspection and reflection.

Tamryn F. Gray, *Suffering of Caregivers, Loved Ones, and the Community* In: *The Nature of Suffering and the Goals of Nursing*. Second Edition. Edited by: William E. Rosa and Betty R. Ferrell, Oxford University Press. © Oxford University Press 2023. DOI: 10.1093/oso/9780197667934.003.0013

Manifestations of Suffering

Suffering is a specific state of severe distress associated with events that threaten the intactness of a person. It is the result of an imbalance between perceived threats and regulatory processes, leading to exhaustion. The experience of exhaustion, physical and emotional, is common in family caregivers. There are many different dimensions of suffering, including physical, psychological, social, and spiritual, and there is some indication that much suffering comes from nonphysical sources.[5,6] Suffering can be seen from an existential perspective for family caregivers, known as existential suffering, that is focused on suffering events such as feeling a loss of control in caring for the patient, changes in the relationship, social isolation, and facing the patient's death and anticipatory grief. Suffering can also be seen from an experiential perspective that examines the actual suffering experiences, known as experiential suffering, including sensory, emotional, cognitive, and spiritual experiencing of suffering events.[7]

Suffering has the potential to lead to significant deterioration in well-being and quality of life (QOL) and comprises a unique, complex, and multidimensional experience. Observing a patient in pain is a common experience causing suffering for caregivers. Caregivers may feel helpless in relieving the pain or even wish for death in order to see the patient suffering end.[8] Suffering may also have effects on various desires, priorities, relationships, and character.

Measuring Suffering in Palliative Care

The first step in reducing suffering is to measure it.[9] While suffering should be assessed subjectively, its subjectivity also creates challenges as the experience varies between individuals,[9,10] and suffering is often compounded in family caregivers who are experiencing chronic illnesses of their own or who have other life challenges. A suffering assessment instrument should be (1) able to measure subjective elements over a concrete period of time, (2) understandable and replicable, (3) simple and fast to administer, (4) noninvasive to the individual, and (5) unlikely to suggest new problems. While not used regularly in the palliative care setting and none constitutes a gold standard, there are many assessment tools available to measure suffering. Table 13.1 describes the available instruments to assess suffering. Most were created to assess patient suffering but may also be useful to assess family caregiver suffering.

In addition to administrating evidence-based instruments, there are clinical signs to assess suffering among patients and their families. For example, health care professionals need to listen to what is said and unsaid, watch face and body for expression and actions, learn to listen without interpreting or judging, and practice silence to allow the individual to share their experiences related to suffering in the context of serious illness. As in Case Exemplar 13.1 with Tom's family, the palliative care team will need to listen intently to understand the experience of both a wife and a mother as they face his death and imagine life without him.

Table 13.1 List of Available Instruments to Measure Suffering

Instrument	Description
Initial Assessment of Suffering (IAS)[11]	20 items Assesses the initial experience of suffering in patients who are dying from advanced cancer 0–5 Likert scale
Pictorial Representation of Illness and Self-Measure (PRISM)[12]	Measures the perceived burden of suffering due to illness Using a white colored board representing one's life at present, with a yellow disc representing "self" in the bottom right corner, patients are asked to place a red disc representing their illness anywhere on the board. Depending on the patient, other colored discs are available. The distance between the "self" and illness disc is a quantitative measurement of self-illness separation representing the patient's perception of burden and control of the illness.
Suffering Assessment Tool (SAT)[13]	10 items Measures physical, spiritual, personal, and familial suffering 0–10 scale (0 = none, 1–3 = mild, 4–6 = moderate, 7–10 = severe)
Mini-Suffering State Examination (MSSE)[14]	10 items Assesses severity of the patient's condition and level of suffering for patients with end-stage dementia. Additionally, clinician and family perception of the patient's illness are included. Each item is scored as a 0 (no) or 1 (yes). Higher total scores reflect higher levels of suffering.
Structured Interviews for Symptoms and Concerns (SISC)[15]	13 items Structured interview measuring severity levels of symptoms and concerns 0–6 scale (0 = none, 6 = extreme)
State of Suffering (SOS-V)[16]	69 items Measures the nature and intensity of unbearable suffering in end-stage cancer patients 1–5 scale (1 = not at all, 5 = very seriously) Open-ended questions are asked when a score of 4 or 5 on any item is given and the patient explains the higher score experience.
Suffering Pictogram[9]	A pictogram is used to measure suffering in palliative care evaluating discomfort, worry, fear, anger, sadness, hopelessness, difficulty in acceptance, and emptiness. Current experience of suffering: 0–4 scale (0 = none, 4 = a lot) Overall suffering: 0–10 scale (0 = none, 10 = worst possible suffering)
FACT-G Caregiver vs. 4[17]	27 items Assesses the physical, social/family, emotional, and functional well-being of those caring for cancer patients 0–4 scale (0 = not at all, 4 = very much)

Case Exemplar 13.1

Tom is a man in his mid-30s who is admitted to an oncology unit after a recent diagnosis of a late-stage incurable cancer. For the past 5 years, he has been living with his wife, 3-year-old daughter, and newborn son. Since his diagnosis, his mother has been staying most nights to assist in caring for him and her grandchildren. Lately, Tom has been experiencing increased dyspnea, drowsiness, pain, and decreased mobility as a result of disease progression. After Tom's recent admission to the intensive care unit, the palliative care team meet with Tom's wife and mother and sense their intense suffering as they describe their anguish in observing his pain as well as their sense of helplessness and intense grief.

One of the first responses by the care team is to witness and acknowledge the suffering and create an environment for Tom's family caregivers to openly share their emotions and concerns. The palliative care team provides care on a daily basis and includes one psychologist, two nurses, one palliative care physician, and the hospital chaplain. Each care team member is well poised to meet the physical, existential, and psychosocial needs of Tom and his family.

Members of the care team initiate a conversation to further assess the needs for support for Tom's wife, mother, and young children. They develop a plan for care at home after his discharge and also schedule a meeting with Tom and his wife to discuss hospice care.

The Suffering of Caregivers, Loved Ones, and the Community

Providing care to a loved one with serious illness can put a significant burden on family caregivers, who must balance their caregiving tasks, work responsibilities, family duties, and financial responsibilities.[18,19] Disease-related suffering, such as related to symptoms of the disease and the impact on the patient and family, is among the most commonly identified by clinicians. Another gap is the focus in most literature only on care during the end of life or preparing caregivers for the death itself, but studies have not extended into the time of bereavement.[20] Caregivers who provided care for a long time or whose loved ones had a prolonged illness often have some understanding of what to expect during bereavement, but during this time, more interventions are needed to support caregiver suffering. Family caregivers experience suffering due to a variety of circumstances, including when they bear witness to the patient suffering, face the reality of poor prognosis or imminent patient death, acknowledge the patient's death during bereavement, observe the patient experiencing worsening symptoms, experience exhaustion from caregiving, feel obligated to neglect their own life, and worry about other family and child-rearing responsibilities outside of their caregiver role.[7]

In addition, caregiver suffering is often exacerbated when the care situation becomes unmanageable, with demands exceeding resources and arising from diverse facets of the illness experience. Another form of suffering can occur when caregivers perceive a threat to their sense of self and identity that arose from their experiences of illness and caregiving. When caregivers, loved ones, and other members of the patient's community experience suffering from the patient's illness, feelings of exhaustion, anger, guilt, uncertainty, and hopelessness can manifest.[21]

Family caregivers are often a part of a larger community support network, wherein individuals are also struggling with the patient's illness and/or death. Others in the community may also withdraw to avoid the negative emotions of the one suffering, which may impact individual friendships and relationships as well as broad community engagement. Reengagement with community members has the potential to alleviate suffering through the empathy of others and can assist with processing and understanding the situation.[22]

Suffering and the Human Experience

Suffering is inherent in the human experience. Each person suffers to some degree, but the extent of suffering will vary considerably across persons, place, and time. Given that loss is inevitable in this life, suffering cannot be eliminated, only alleviated and responded to. While the alleviation of suffering is an important goal, it should be viewed as secondary to that of the promotion of human flourishing. In response, humans should demonstrate empathy toward one another as an important way to alleviate suffering in palliative care, particularly as it focuses on seeing the world from the perspective of others. In addition, compassion is the cornerstone of all therapeutic relationships and is a key characteristic of most health care providers. Using components of the mindfulness-based supportive therapy (MBST) framework, patients, health care providers, and family caregivers can become fully aware of what to say and what not to (compassionate communication) and aware of what to do and what not to (compassionate action) in addressing suffering. To fully understand the human experience during suffering, health care providers may find it beneficial to demonstrate curiosity by seeking to understand the stories, narratives, and perspectives of patients and their family caregivers and other loved ones as well as ask questions to invite their concerns related to an illness.[6,7,10] In the case of Tom's family, an important initial step in responding to the family suffering will be to hear their stories. What is it like for this wife to see her husband's suffering? What is this experience like for a mother to witness her son die before her life ends? How must it feel to be responsible for his comfort? How is this death experienced by the children?

Ethical Perspectives on Suffering

From an ethical perspective, suffering is a concept related to an individual's whole experience of life, health, and illness in a physical, mental, and spiritual sense.[23] Suffering violates human dignity and implies loss and dying, but also the possibility of new life and reconciliation. According to the international code of ethics by the International Council of Nurses,[23] it is the responsibility of nurses to promote health, prevent illness, restore health, and alleviate suffering. This responsibility to alleviate suffering resonates within the philosophy of hospice and palliative care with the goal of alleviating suffering and optimizing quality of life for patients, their families, and communities for whom they provide care. Feminist ethics can be applied to understand the impact of suffering on patients, family caregivers, and members of the patient's community, specifically in relation to concepts such as relationship, compassion, and respect. It is essential that health care providers establish a trusting relationship with patients and families in the illness experience, use compassion and respect to affirm the presence of suffering, maintain human dignity, and use hope and growth in understanding the meaning of life, illness, and suffering. Family caregivers make many important ethical decisions regarding care such as withdrawing life support, changing a code status, and balancing relief of symptoms with fear of potentially hastening death. Nurses play a critical role in supporting families with these decisions.[23,24]

Responses to Family Suffering

Listening intently is a simple yet effective way for health care providers to respond to suffering experienced by family caregivers. As health care providers, it is the nurse's responsibility to maintain a high level of awareness to the presence of suffering among families and individuals within the patient's community, especially in the presence of serious illness. All health care professionals must be equipped with skills to understand patients' and family members' responses to bad news and respond to their experience of suffering. The commitment to nonabandonment and to listening openly to the family members is necessary to accompany them through serious illness and end-of-life care.[6,10] Building trust, clarity of communication, and confidence between patients, their families, and health care professionals is essential for reducing suffering. Health care professionals should also seek to understand the resiliency family caregivers bring to the care experience to transform understanding of the suffering that exists.[6,19]

In addressing suffering, traditional approaches that deal with the threat are combined with cognitive methods to target the three cognitive appraisals of threat, damage, and coping as well as whole-person care or healing to find a new sense of integrity, independent of illness, recovery, or death. To help patients and families achieve growth through suffering, health care professionals may find it helpful to ask two fundamental questions: (1) Even though there are some things you can no longer do, what activities can you still enjoy? (2) Are there things about your life that this experience does not affect?

Social support is another potential response to suffering. In some cases, social support helps to reduce suffering, while in other cases it may be burdensome and may intensify suffering.[2,6] In the context of palliative care, mindfulness has also been shown to be a potential strategy to reduce suffering. Mindfulness is a nonjudgmental awareness of the present moment, cultivated by paying attention to being as openhearted as possible and simply noticing what is taking place. Mindfulness-based interventions, such as mindfulness-based stress reduction (MBSR) and mindfulness-based cognitive therapy (MBCT), have been shown to improve pain acceptance, insomnia, stress, anxiety, depression, and caregiver stress, among other outcomes. Key mechanisms of mindfulness include the process of paying attention on purpose, paying attention in the present moment, and paying attention nonreactively. Table 13.2, developed by Beng et al.,[25] describes some mindfulness-based interventions to ameliorate suffering for both patients and caregivers. These interventions were derived from the development of the MBST framework, which consists of five components: (1) presence, (2) listening, (3) empathy, (4) compassion, and (5) boundary awareness.

For both patients and family caregivers, there may also be disenfranchised suffering for those whose experience is overlooked, ignored, dismissed, or invalidated.

Suffering Gives Rise to New Opportunities

Suffering gives rise to new opportunities related to meaning making, personal growth, introspection, and reflection. Figure 13.1 describes strategies for clinicians to help patients and their family caregivers transcend suffering. Many caregivers have shared that their experiences of caring for a loved one at the end of life was a time of personal growth or finding new strengths and meaning.

Table 13.2 Examples of Interventions in the Palliation of Suffering

Type of Suffering	Intervention
Patient-centered suffering	
Dependent suffering	Mobilizing support and resources
Differential suffering	Rehabilitation
Empathic suffering	Care of caregivers
Emotional suffering	Supportive listening, emotional processing, and relaxation techniques
Terminal suffering	Disease-modifying treatment
Interactional suffering	Communication training of health care providers
Environmental suffering	Patient-centered hospital design
Sensory suffering	Symptom control
Cognitive suffering	Supportive listening, cognitive restructuring, and hope fostering
Caregiver-centered suffering	
Spiritual suffering	Spiritual support, pastoral care, and nonabandonment

Finding Meaning in Suffering

Suffering, to some extent, may offer an opportunity to find greater meaning through illness. Relatedly, religious beliefs themselves can provide resources for understanding and finding meaning in the context of suffering and may lead to an embrace of suffering to attain higher ends.[10] For instance, suffering can lead to a clarification of and a purifying of one's desires for that which is most important. Many caregivers have found great meaning in providing care. Caring for a loved one, especially at the end of life, may also be a time to seek or offer forgiveness.

Personal Growth

As author David Brooks has previously said, "Suffering drags you deeper into yourself ... and gives people a more accurate sense of their own limitations, what they

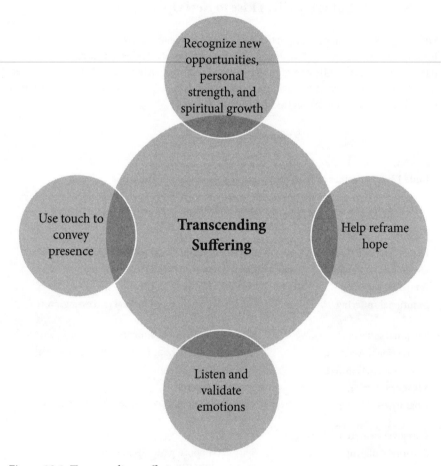

Figure 13.1 Transcending suffering.

can control and cannot."[22] Suffering has the potential to give rise to individual personal growth and lead to a deepening of self, a profound connectedness to life, and an awareness beyond self. More specifically, those who endure suffering may experience posttraumatic growth or the experience of positive change that occurs as a result of the challenging life crisis. As in Case Exemplar 13.1, Tom's wife may experience tremendous growth in recognizing her ability to care for her husband and to assume the role of single parent.

Introspection and Reflection

There is potential for introspection and reflection in response to suffering. While suffering may alter how a person views themselves and their identity following a threat, cognitive processing may occur as a result to introspect, reflect, and reevaluate their values, desires, goals, emotions, and circumstances. Cognitive responses to suffering may help clarify the loss or threat, adjust to it, or determine what is needed for the restoration of some good.

Conclusion

In summary, supportive care interventions to address human suffering should be tailored to the individual patient, caregiver, and community needs. Within the clinical setting, suffering should be assessed using validated and reliable measures and throughout the care trajectory. To better support family caregiver suffering during the illness and bereavement, health care providers must develop a trusting relationship with caregivers and equip them with tools and resources to reduce their own suffering during this phase. Relatedly, it is critical that health care providers are trained on appropriate screening and assessment of suffering among their patients and family caregivers and identify ways to respond effectively and empathically. Responding to suffering often means simply being with, witnessing, providing care for, listening to, and supporting the person who is suffering.

Reference

1. Borneman T, Brown-Saltzman K. Meaning in illness. In: Ferrell BR, Paice JA, eds. *Oxford Textbook of Palliative Nursing*. 5th ed. Oxford University Press; 2019:456–466.
2. Ferrell B, Coyle N. *The Nature of Suffering and the Goals of Care*. Oxford University Press; 2008.
3. Bassola B, Cilluffo S, Lusignani M. Going inside the relationship between caregiver and care-receiver with amyotrophic lateral sclerosis in Italy, a grounded theory study. *Health Soc Care Community*. 2021;29(4):1083–1090.
4. Radbruch L, De Lima L, Knaul F, et al. Redefining palliative care—a new consensus-based definition. *J Pain Symptom Manage*. 2020;60(4):754–764.

5. Benites AC, Rodin G, de Oliveira-Cardoso ÉA, dos Santos MA. "You begin to give more value in life, in minutes, in seconds": spiritual and existential experiences of family caregivers of patients with advanced cancer receiving end-of-life care in Brazil. *Support Care Cancer*. 2022;30(3):2631–2638.

6. Limonero JT, Maté-Méndez J, Gómez-Romero MJ, et al. Family caregiver emotional distress in advanced cancer: the DME-C scale psychometric properties. *BMJ Support Palliat Care*. 2022;12(e4):e585–e591.

7. Oh J, Kim J-A, Chu MS. Family caregiver suffering in caring for patients with amyotrophic lateral sclerosis in Korea. *Int J Env Res Public Health*. 2021;18(9):4937.

8. Spatuzzi R, Vespa A, Fabbietti P, et al. Elderly helping other elderly: a comparative study of family caregiver burden between patients with dementia or cancer at the end of life. *J Soc Work End-of-Life Palliat Care*. 2022;18(1):96–108.

9. Beng TS, Ann YH, Guan NC, et al. The suffering pictogram: measuring suffering in palliative care. *J Palliat Med*. 2017;20(8):869–874.

10. VanderWeele TJ. Suffering and response: directions in empirical research. *Soc Sci Med*. 2019;224:58–66.

11. MacAdam D, Smith M. An initial assessment of suffering in terminal illness. *Palliat Med*. 1987;1(1):37–47.

12. Buchi S, Sensky T. PRISM: pictorial representation of illness and self measure: a brief nonverbal measure of illness impact and therapeutic aid in psychosomatic medicine. *Psychosomatics*. 1999;40(4):314–320.

13. Baines BK, Norlander L. The relationship of pain and suffering in a hospice population. *Am J Hosp Palliat Care*. 2000;17(5):319–326.

14. Aminoff BZ, Purits E, Noy S, Adunsky A. Measuring the suffering of end-stage dementia: reliability and validity of the Mini-Suffering State Examination. *Arch Gerontol Geriatr*. 2004;38(2):123–130.

15. Wilson KG, Graham ID, Viola RA, et al. Structured interview assessment of symptoms and concerns in palliative care. *Can J Psychiatry*. 2004;49(6):350–358.

16. Ruijs KD, Onwuteaka-Philipsen BD, van der Wal G, Kerkhof AJ. Unbearability of suffering at the end of life: the development of a new measuring device, the SOS-V. *BMC Palliat Care*. 2009;8:16.

17. Cella DF, Tulsky DS, Gray G, et al. The Functional Assessment of Cancer Therapy scale: development and validation of the general measure. *J Clin Oncol*. 1993;11(3):570–579.

18. Ferrell BR, Kravits K, Borneman T, Pal S, Lee J. A support intervention for family caregivers of advanced cancer patients. *J Adv Pract Oncol*. 2019;10(5):444–455.

19. Ferrell BR, Kravitz K, Borneman T, Taratoot Friedmann E. Family caregivers: a qualitative study to better understand the quality-of-life concerns and needs of this population. *Clin J Oncol Nurs*. 2018;22(3):286–294.

20. Hartogh GD. Suffering and dying well: on the proper aim of palliative care. *Med Health Care Philos*. 2017;20(3):413–424.

21. Bovero A, Vitiello LP, Botto R, Gottardo F, Cito A, Geminiani GC. Demoralization in end-of-life cancer patients' family caregivers: a cross-sectional study. *Am J Hospice Palliat Med*. 2021;39(3):332–339.

22. Brooks D. What suffering does. *New York Times*. April 8, 2014, A25.

23. The ICN code of ethics for nurses. International Council of Nurses. Published October 20, 2021. Accessed July 5, 2022. https://www.icn.ch/system/files/2021-10/ICN_Code-of-Ethics_EN_Web_0.pdf

24. Bueno-Gómez N. Conceptualizing suffering and pain. *Philos Ethics Human Med.* 2017;12(1). https://doi.org/10.1186/s13010-017-0049-5
25. Beng TS, Chin LE, Guan NC, et al. Mindfulness-based supportive therapy (MBST): proposing a palliative psychotherapy from a conceptual perspective to address suffering in palliative care. *Am J Hosp Palliat Care.* 2015;32(2):144–160.

14

Social Suffering, Biopower, and the Naturalization of Inequality

Alic G. Shook, Robin A. Narruhn, and Christine R. Espina

Introduction

Since its onset in late 2019, the global COVID-19 pandemic caused by severe acute respiratory syndrome-coronavirus 2 (SARS-CoV-2) has revealed long-standing and historically rooted inequities in the US health care system that drive the disproportionate burden of suffering, disease, debility, and economic deprivation for people subjected to structural injustice.[1] The pandemic has unequally impacted people of color, older individuals, and those in the lowest power strata of society.[2-5] Marginalized communities (e.g., people of color; immigrants; individuals experiencing homelessness; people with disabilities; the lesbian, gay, bisexual, transgender, and queer [LGBTQ+] communities; individuals with mental illness; the incarcerated; people who use drugs; and sex workers) have also been disproportionately impacted by the residual effects of the pandemic—the global economic downturn, social isolation, and movement restriction measures.

Beginning in late May of 2020, following the brutal murder of George Floyd, a 46-year-old African American man, by former Minneapolis police officer Derek Chauvin, communities took to the streets worldwide to protest structural racism and the persistent violence inflicted on Black and African American men by the US policing system.[6] Protesters frequently chanted, "I can't breathe," a slogan associated with the Black Lives Matter movement that originates from the last words of Eric Garner, who, like George Floyd, was suffocated to death in 2014 after being put in a chokehold by a New York City police officer. Preliminary data at the time of the protests demonstrated that Black and African American people living in the United States were at disproportionately high risk for COVID-19 infection and death compared to their White counterparts.[7] Shortly after the protests erupted worldwide, social scientist Brett Bowman, in reflecting on this moment, wrote, "Pitting the risk of infection against the drive to protest against the violence of systemic racism encapsulated in the slow suffocation of George Floyd brings into relief the calculus underpinning exactly what sort of life is deemed worth living."[8(p313)] The COVID-19 pandemic and widespread protests against police brutality have highlighted interwoven threads of inequality and health, particularly as health and economic inequities disproportionately impact US communities of color.[9,10]

By June of 2020, 20 US cities and counties and three states had declared racism a public health crisis.[11,12] Since then, public social discourse about the systemic and structural

Alic G. Shook, Robin A. Narruhn, and Christine R. Espina, *Social Suffering, Biopower, and the Naturalization of Inequality*
In: *The Nature of Suffering and the Goals of Nursing*. Second Edition. Edited by: William E. Rosa and Betty R. Ferrell,
Oxford University Press. © Oxford University Press 2023. DOI: 10.1093/oso/9780197667934.003.0014

conditions that produce suffering from unequal power systems has rightfully intensified. In response, public health organizations, schools of medicine, major nursing organizations, and nursing schools in the United States have put forth position statements on racism and health.[13] Position statements—such as those issued by influential nursing organizations—are helpful in as much as they influence nursing practice and health policies and have the potential to influence social discourse that shapes and guides the provision of health resources. In 2021, Knopf et al. reviewed position statements issued by national professional nursing organizations (the American Nurses Association [ANA], American Academy of Nursing, American Association of Colleges of Nursing) and found consistent themes, including condemnation of police brutality, acknowledgment of the effects of racism on health, and calls to action to end systemic racism.[13]

Notably, the role of structural racism—defined here as macro-level systems, social forces, institutions, and ideologies that coalesce to produce and maintain racial inequities[14]—in creating unequal burdens of suffering among US communities of color was well documented before the COVID-19 pandemic and the killing of George Floyd. It has been confirmed, for example, that US police kill upwards of 1,000 people per year, disproportionately Black Americans.[9] Moreover, before June of 2020, it was well documented that structurally mediated physical and psychological violence enacted by law enforcement systems results in deaths, injuries, trauma, and stress that disproportionately affects marginalized populations more generally.[15] How has such tremendous suffering been naturalized and mainly rendered invisible until recently?

This chapter argues that suffering not apprehended as such (i.e., that goes overlooked, naturalized, systematically excluded) is a particular kind of suffering that cuts across multiple aspects of experience and identity and is produced by inequitable arrangements of power. Medical anthropologist Arthur Kleinman termed this "social suffering," which "results from what political, economic, and institutional power does to people."[16] The production of social suffering is rooted in systems of oppression that penetrate all aspects of everyday life in individual, interpersonal, and institutional contexts. Examples of systems of oppression that sustain imbalances in power, wealth, and opportunity are racism, colonialism, sexism, heterosexism, transphobia (e.g., cissexism), and ableism. Social suffering is directly linked to inequity in health and social systems. It drives health inequities (e.g., maternal mortality, average life expectancy, disease burden, COVID-19 infection and death rates, injury and death from police brutality, etc.) within and between communities and populations.[17] Because social suffering is rooted in the creation of norms that govern the distribution of life chances and make some more vulnerable to violence, exclusion, harm, and death than others, recognizing and responding to social suffering requires an understanding of the political dimensions of suffering—aspects of which are embedded throughout every part of society, including the US health care system, and codified in nursing values such as social justice and advocacy in the ANA Code of Ethics.[18]

The chapter begins by exploring how nurses have analyzed the politics of suffering in historical and contemporary times, with a focus specifically on Jane Georges' attention to the politics of suffering and her work to illuminate how suffering and biopolitics are entangled. Then it looks more closely at the relationship between biopower and nursing, focusing on Foucault's original conception and later how Italian political philosopher Giorgio Agamben theorized biopower, which has particular significance for nursing and nurses' abilities to apprehend social suffering. The chapter describes the role that discourse plays in naturalizing inequality and rendering some suffering invisible and explores three related concepts: the biopolitics of disposability, slow violence, and necropolitics. It ends by summarizing three specific strategies, previously outlined by Espina and Narruhn,[10] that nurses can utilize in response to social suffering in their practice, scholarship, and teaching: critical conscientization, structural competency, and advocacy, activism, and allyship.

Nursing and the Politics of Suffering

Drawing on emergent conceptualizations of suffering from the social sciences in the late 1990s and early 2000s, over a decade, Jane Georges utilized a critical-feminist, self-reflective approach to reconceptualize suffering as we make sense of it within nursing. Like Kleinman, Georges argued that suffering "must be conceptualized as a causal web in a global political economy in which political factors such as sexism and racism play complex roles."[19(p251)] Georges' work was, in part, a response to increased attention to suffering as a prominent theme in a broad array of academic disciplines (e.g., anthropology, theology, psychology) and a response to the dominant conception of caring as the essence of nursing. Georges argued that because their work as nurses is saturated in power relations, they must pay particular attention to the relationship between relations of power and the mechanisms via which suffering is produced. Additionally, she encouraged nurses to reconsider "the 'invisible' suffering all around [them] as more than just 'health disparities.'"[19(p255)] Notably, her work is part of a broader genealogy of nursing scholarship that foregrounds the critical role of power relations in shaping nursing practice and scholarship and locates nurses as agents embedded within systems of power.

Georges was initially interested in exploring the nature of suffering as an avenue for rethinking compassion in nursing, which she defined as "a sympathetic consciousness of others' distress with a desire to alleviate it."[20(p59)] Notably, in Georges' formulation of compassion in nursing, compassion is not static but rather "grows as individual[s] develop the capacity for connectedness with others and [are] the recipient[s] of compassion."[20(p59)] She argued that suffering and biopower are entangled with the presence and absence of compassion in the practice setting; furthermore, compassion has been radically reduced—if not rendered impossible—in contemporary practice settings that have been fundamentally altered by market forces.[19] More recently, nurse scholars have introduced the concept of the Capitalocene—which names capitalism as a system of power[21]—to analyze the central role of capitalism in reshaping nursing identity and politics.[22]

Georges' early attention to the biopolitical spaces in nursing practice was an important divergence from Eurocentric accounts of suffering as individual, apolitical occurrences. White dominant cultural portrayals of suffering have frequently conceptualized suffering as a response to discreetly identifiable events or situations rather than the result of social and political forces such as racism, colonialism, and militarism.[23] Based on a reading of Bronwyn McFarland-Icke's work in *Nurses in Nazi Germany: Moral Choices in History*,[24] Georges demonstrated how, in an apolitical framing of the suffering encountered by nurses, particular discursive themes are present: (1) *the use of psychological distancing*, which allows nurses to cast people as "inferior," "undeserving," or "other" and renders suffering "natural," "normal," or "just the way it is,"[19(p241)] and (2) *free-floating responsibility*, which shifts the burden to account for suffering from individuals to more amorphous forms of authority that are frequently imagined to be lawful. When suffering happens on a large scale or to specific populations "in the past" (such as in the cases of settler-colonialism and the transatlantic slave trade), it is often thought of as a distant or past atrocity rather than the effect of ongoing relations of power of which nurses are a part, and which continue to produce suffering in ways that nurses are connected to.

Biopower

Foucault's Conception of Biopower

Biopower generally refers to power over life, "an explosion of numerous and diverse techniques for achieving the subjugation of bodies and the control of populations."[25] It is foundational to understanding both the politics of suffering and the nature of any kind of suffering that is normalized, rendered invisible, and systematically relegated to the margins of society. Initially coined by French philosopher Michel Foucault in volume 1 of *The History of Sexuality*,[25] many scholars have since theorized biopower. All of them have a concern with the intersection of politics and life, or politics and "the living." Foucault was primarily concerned with power, specifically how power, discourse, and social identities—what he termed "subject positions"—are constructed. In Foucault's view of power, "power is not something that people possess—instead, it circulates throughout social relations and constitutes people into certain kinds of subjects suitable to the prevailing political order."[26] Power is pervasive, productive, socially distributed, and discursively managed. The authors discuss discourse and the nature of suffering in more detail shortly. But first, they explore biopower as Foucault originally conceived it; the relationship between biopower, nursing, and governmentality; and how Italian political philosopher Giorgio Agamben later theorized biopower, which has particular significance for nursing.

Foucault's conception of biopower characterized a new form of power that first appeared in the 18th and 19th centuries. He argued that biopolitics is a "matter of taking control of life and the biological processes of man-as-species and of ensuring that [people] are not disciplined, but regularized."[27(p256)] These new relations of power—*biopolitics*, which refers to the style of government that regulates populations through biopower—were concerned less with the body as an object of disciplinary techniques (e.g., punishment) and more with the body as a site to be systematized. This is to say, biopolitics is a reference to the processes via which life—specifically at the level of the population—is managed, and it requires experts (e.g., physicians, nurses, psychologists) to make determinations about, for example, what is normal versus what is abnormal, who is a good and deserving patient versus who is a malingerer, etc. While there are biopolitical implications at the level of the body, biopower is targeted at managing entire groups or populations. For example, Foucault suggests that government surveys of population health to eradicate sexually transmitted diseases and incest among the working class were intended to improve the population's health and had the effect of controlling the population more tightly.[28] Biopower operates as a form of bioregulation (i.e., regulation of biological or living processes) administered across institutions throughout a society (e.g., medicine, nursing, insurance, etc.) that treats the individual as an economic subject and sees the subject in terms of their "productive" capacities as human capital.[29] It is a kind of analysis of the interaction between the body—or *bodies*—and institutions where biopower is fundamentally about establishing the value of human lives or stratifying the value of human life.

Case Exemplar 14.1

Biopower and Anti-Trans Legislation

In thinking about how biopower operates to create and distribute norms that establish and regulate the value of human lives, consider the recent wave of anti-transgender legislation sweeping the United States, particularly legislation targeted at transgender youth (i.e., youth under age 18). In 2021 alone, lawmakers across 35 states brought forth 127 anti-transgender bills and 9 states passed some form of anti-transgender legislation, including barring or criminalizing health care for transgender youth. The majority of these bills target transgender youth by preventing them from participating in athletics and making it illegal for them to access particular types of health resources. Other bills make it difficult, if not impossible, to change the sex designation on one's birth certificate, thus subjecting transgender youth to ongoing vulnerability, violence, and exclusion. Biopower operates via both health care and the law as norms are created and debated about what is normal versus abnormal with regard to gender, what types of health and legal resources an individual can access related to gender, and the degree to which transgender individuals are afforded basic privileges that allow individuals to participate in everyday life as full human beings. These bills convey powerful messages that transgender people do not really exist and perpetuate false ideas about both sex and gender. A 2020 survey of LGBTQ+ youth mental health found that 21% of transgender youth have attempted suicide and 52% have seriously considered it. Notably, negative mental health outcomes among transgender youth have recently been exacerbated in response to increased anti-trans discourse that appears in the news. The American Psychiatric Association has found a direct connection between the discrimination transgender people face, their lack of equitable civil rights, and the harmful impact of anti-trans hate (including in health care and the law) on their mental health.

Biopower, Nursing, and Governmentality

Nursing is charged with the responsibility for labeling, coding, organizing, and moving individual bodies—and sometimes entire populations or groups of individuals—through a for-profit health care system that rationalizes and organizes life and death and that frequently makes determinations about the value of human life. This includes attending to those who are suffering and frequently ascertaining "real" suffering and making decisions or recommendations about what resources should be leveraged on behalf of those who suffer. This also includes participation in the systematic disregard, production, and maintenance of "not knowing"—or an epistemology of ignorance—concerning particular expressions of pain and suffering. This is a function of nursing's task in what Foucault termed "governmentality." Governmentality describes the elaborate and often subtle ways a society shapes and manages individuals and populations.[30] Holmes and Gastaldo have theorized nursing as a means of governmentality, and they argue that nurses both help the state to govern at a distance *and* are a critical body that challenges the status quo and works for more equitable systems of care.[31] Foucault's conception of governmentality links both constructive and repressive ways of exercising power (i.e., emancipatory versus oppressive expressions of power). This is particularly important for nurses to consider when critically reflecting on their roles as biopolitical "experts" within a fundamentally inequitable health care system that places a higher value on some lives over others and that legitimizes some forms of suffering while invalidating others.

> Working at the junction of the individual and collective body within power relations that promote and recuperate life, nurses are able, through their interventions, to mold, conduct, or affect people as well as construct, with the help of other health professionals, people's subjectivities.[31(p563)]

What does it mean to construct another's subjectivity? Foucault argued that the subject, or subject positioning, results from relations of power rather than something that precedes those relations.[28] This was a divergence from the White-dominant focus on the individual. Within this frame, for example, it becomes possible to reconsider what Georges termed "discursive themes deeply ingrained in the European metanarrative" that "assure us that suffering is perpetuated by distant people who are separate from us"[19(p254)] to appreciate suffering as the result of social and political forces of which all people are *a part*. Nurses are, in effect, often tasked with producing "the suffering subject" in ways of which they are both aware and unaware. This is a function of their social position as nurses and their role as "experts."

Agamben and Biopower

In her work on compassion in nursing and the politics of suffering, Georges relied heavily on Giorgio Agamben's formulation of biopower. Agamben's seminal work *Homo Sacer: Sovereign Power and Bare Life*[32] carries forth Foucault's study of biopolitics. He asserts that all power—or "sovereignty," as he termed it—is by nature biopower. This includes having power over another, which involves the power of life or death.[32] This might be thought of as an *administration* of life and death. Like Foucault, Agamben argues that biopower is state sanctioned, and in Agamben's conception, it involves the administration of what he termed "bare life," "zoe," or "non-person." Any individual who fails to comply with socially constructed norms (e.g., obey the law) begins to descend within the social strata (i.e., loses power), with the extreme being the point at which an individual's very humanity is erased or occluded to the point that it makes them particularly vulnerable to violence, exclusion, and death. Importantly, this is a *normalizing* process, meaning it is a taken-for-granted socio-structural process embedded in institutions and everyday life. It is perceived to be the "natural" order of things.

Conversely, Agamben uses the term "bios" to refer to individuals who possess social agency or power and occupy a "real" person status.[32] According to Agamben, one is either "bios," meaning they are granted political agency by the prevailing order and are protected by social norms, or "zoe," meaning they are stripped of political agency and vulnerable to violence, exclusion, and death. While this zoe-bios dichotomy is systematically concealed via normalizing processes, "it has its most visible forms in biopolitical spaces such as prisons and hospitals, where the zoe-bios divide is so prominent and all-encompassing that participants inside these locations perceive it as 'natural.'"[20(p54)]

Discourse and the Unspeakable

Both nurses and those we work with are caught up in the zoe-bios divide. In many cases, people may be assigned a "zoe" status because of a given socially constructed difference (e.g., race, class, gender, sexual orientation, immigration status, ability, etc.).[33] An essential aspect of how these assignments—these distributions of the value of human life—operate is that they have, until recently, not been spoken about in dominant public social dialogue. This is a function of discourse, which makes it possible to think some thoughts and not others, empower some speakers, and disqualify or negate others.[34] Discourses are systems of thought that construct social reality and are enacted and contested at the site of the body.[35] Dominant discourses—such as Whiteness, or the normalization of White racial identity,[36] for example—promote viewpoints and uphold ideologies that codify existing power relations, hierarchies, and social structures.[37]

Feminist scholars have used the term "Unspeakable" to describe any event or experience so threatening to the power structure that no language exists to describe it.[38] Others have used it to describe patterns of discourse that are so profoundly normalized and taken for granted that they disappear from an individual's consciousness.[39] Georges developed a definition of the Unspeakable in her work on biopower and compassion in nursing. She writes, "The Unspeakable in nursing is the creation/maintenance of biopolitical spaces in which compassion—for oneself or one's patients—is rendered severely diminished to nearly impossible."[40(p131)] This is a kind of uncritical acceptance of routinized, normalized, taken-for-granted suffering such that it motivates no action. Nurses may see this type of suffering as normal or not see it at all.

Examples of the Unspeakable include the common practice of withholding necessary treatment for patients living with a history of substance use disorder[41] or being accused of drug-seeking behaviors while Black.[42]

The frames through which nurses view "the Other" are saturated in relations of power and are themselves operations of power.[43] Acts of inclusion and exclusion—what nurses see and don't see, what nurses say and don't say—are politically saturated. Nurses' work occurs at the confluence of discourse, culture, life, and death, and thus nurses are "necessarily connected to normative frames that exclude certain parts of populations."[44(p285)] When an individual—or a "patient," as the case may be—is not recognized as human in the full sense (i.e., is dehumanized and rendered invisible—what Agamben termed "zoe" or "non-person"), their life is not apprehended as life and becomes what Butler calls "a living figure outside the norms of life."[43(p8)] Drawing on Butler's work, critical nurse scholar Thomas Foth has argued in his work on care and biopolitics that "dehumanization first occurs within discourses and then gives rise to physical violence 'that in some sense delivers the message of dehumanization that is already at work in the culture.'"[44(p291)] For example, in clinical spaces when a person with a substance use disorder suffers because they're denied appropriate treatment for withdrawal, this may not be seen as suffering but as something they "deserve." This framing and these ideas have material implications. Foth argues that the frames through which we view others are less about individual choice and are restricted by norms and culture. "Questions arise then," he writes, "as to whose face makes an ethical demand on me."[44(p289)]

Related Concepts: The Biopolitics of Disposability, Necropolitics, and Slow Violence

Before specific strategies for responding to social suffering in nursing practice, education, and policy are discussed, a few related concepts are explored: the biopolitics of disposability, necropolitics, and slow violence.

Biopolitics of Disposability

American Canadian scholar and cultural critic Henry Giroux introduces the politics of disposability in his works *Stormy Weather: Katrina and the Politics of Disposability*[45] and "Reading Hurricane Katrina: Race, Class, and the Biopolitics of Disposability."[46] Giroux argues that government neglect in the wake of Hurricane Katrina—a Category 5 hurricane that caused over 1,800 fatalities and $125 billion in damage in late August 2005—revealed the emergence of a new kind of politics, "one in which entire populations are now considered disposable, an unnecessary burden on state coffers, and consigned to fend for themselves."[46(p174)] Utilizing biopolitical concepts and in a critique of postwelfare neoliberalism, Giroux's work illustrates how the new biopolitics of disposability both justifies and obscures state-sanctioned violence and relegates entire populations of people to "spaces of invisibility and disposability"[46(p181)]—most often poor people of color. This notion of the biopolitics of disposability adds to an understanding of suffering that is rendered invisible by highlighting how the politics of suffering are structured mainly around racial and class inequities. Foucault's conception of biopower holds that biopower "inscribes a kind of racism into mechanisms of the state,"[44(p290)] which sanctions differentiation between races and allows for racial hierarchization (i.e., at its core, biopower characterizes some races as superior to others).

> When you have a normalizing society, you have a power which is, at least superficially . . . biopower, and racism is the indispensable precondition that allows someone to be killed, that allows others to be killed. Once the State functions in the biopower mode, racism alone can justify the murderous function of the State.[27(p256)]

Importantly, Foucault underscores the idea that to kill someone can mean both physically putting to death and indirect forms of murder, such as placing certain subjects in positions whereby their risk of death is increased or where they are rendered politically dead (i.e., expulsion, exclusion, rejection, displacement, marginalization, etc.). A recent example is the disproportionate COVID-19 deaths in the United States among poor communities of color (who have fewer choices to reduce their exposure risks). Yet policies were developed that restricted COVID-19 testing and treatment and supported premature lifting of COVID-19 protections.[47]

Necropolitics and Slow Violence

Achille Mbembe's concept of necropolitics is entwined with the Foucauldian conception of biopolitics. Importantly, Mbembe argued that Foucault's biopower/biopolitics could not fully explain contemporary forms of subjugation, such as slavery and colonialism, resulting in the bodily suffering and death of people living under exceptional violence and brutality. Mbembe describes how enslaved people's bodies were "kept alive but in a state of injury"[48(p75)] and that enslaved people were "treated as no longer existing except as mere tool[s] and instrument[s] of production."[48(p75)] They were devalued to the point of being seen as "non-persons," their lives, Mbembe argues, "a form of death-in-life."[48(p75)] Mbembe's conception of necropolitics, or necropower, accounts "for the various ways in which, in our contemporary world, weapons are deployed in the interest of maximally destroying persons and creating *death-worlds*."[48(p92)] He argues that these death-worlds are "new and unique forms of social existence in which vast populations are subjected to living conditions that confer upon them the status of the *living dead*."[48(p92)] These forms of violence do not necessarily result in immediate death. Still, they involve the permanent wounding of entire populations via exposure to repeated, everyday forms of violence (e.g., environmental racism and climate change) and the naturalization of persistent suffering that results from these exposures. This violence is consistent with Agamben's *homo sacer*.

Slow violence was originally coined by literary theorist Rob Nixon and is frequently used interchangeably with necropolitics.[49] Nixon described slow violence as "a violence of delayed destruction that is dispersed across time and space, an attritional violence that is typically not viewed as violence at all."[50(p2)] Slow violence highlights the association of time and environmental harm. It interacts with marginalization in that it is disproportionately suffered by dispossessed people, whom Nixon called "casualties of accumulative environmental injury."[50(p144)] The distribution of environmental injustice is highly racialized and is "predicted by an entrenchment of long-standing social inequalities, rendering some groups more vulnerable than others."[49(p1541)]

Like the biopolitics of disposability, both necropolitics and slow violence add to an understanding of invisible and naturalized forms of suffering by drawing attention to the reality that the politics of suffering are structured largely around long-standing racial and class inequities. The concepts of slow violence, biopower, and the Unspeakable are all evident in the history of the United States' destruction of the Marshall Islands,[51] for example (Case Exemplar 14.2).

Case Exemplar 14.2

Slow Violence, Biopower, and the Unspeakable and the Republic of the Marshall Islands

For one decade (1948–1958), the Republic of the Marshall Islands (RMI) was a nuclear test site for the United States. Sixty-seven tests were conducted to study large-scale weapons of mass destruction. The largest of these was equal in force to 1,000 Hiroshima-sized bombs. In 1956, the Atomic Energy Commission declared the RMI as the most contaminated place in the world. People from the RMI were exposed to enormous amounts of radiation, and those living on nearby atolls suffered immediate and long-term injuries and illnesses from exposure to nuclear fallout. This vast exposure—which exceeds Chernobyl and Fukushima—is not well known. The United States' destruction of the RMI and its people is not found in our history books and contributes to the erasure of these communities, such as the Marshallese, who were medically experimented on, dehumanized, and called nuclear savages.[51] This erasure from public consciousness is consistent with Agamben's biopower and Georges's the Unspeakable. RMI soil and marine ecosystems remain contaminated, severely impacting food sources. Radiation rendered food sources inedible, affecting the health of people living on the RMI. The impact of this contamination persists today and is demonstrated in disproportionate cancer rates, loss of sustainability, and poverty among the Marshallese. Worse, the social and economic fabric of communities has suffered from the loss of the previous way of life.

In 1986, the Compact of Free Association (COFA) Treaty between the United States and the RMI promised public benefits to Marshallese nationals such as health care access and educational loans in exchange for the militarization of the largest island Kwajalein, now known as the Ronald Reagan Ballistic Missile Defense Test Site. The Marshallese began to immigrate to the United States in the 1990s because of the ecological destruction and pursuit of economic opportunity, education, and access to health care. As of the 2010 census, approximately one-third of the entire population of the RMI had migrated to the United States. Marshallese are not considered US citizens, nationals, or immigrants and do not have the status of lawful permanent residents, placing them in a precarious position comparable to biopower and Agamben's homo sacer. The COFA benefits were inexplicably removed during Clinton's Personal Responsibility and Work Opportunity Act in 1996, breaking the United States' end of the treaty, yet the United States maintained access to Kwajalein. COFA benefits were not reinstated until 2021, and ironically, the original COFA Treaty is set to expire in 2023. Despite migrating in pursuit of increased opportunity, the health of the Marshallese people has not improved, and they face disproportionate burdens of cancer, diabetes, COVID-19 infection, and death. The nuclear bombings and their generational impacts and the broken COFA Treaty leading to early mortality are akin to the mechanisms of slow violence.[51] The Marshallese were and are treated as less than human and unworthy of basic human needs (biopower) despite the culpability of the United States in the disparate rates of cancer due to nuclear exposure.[51]

Responses to Suffering

There are a number of ways that nurses can meaningfully engage with the politics of suffering and mitigate the impact of inequitable burdens of suffering on the most vulnerable populations. Nursing is an inherently political practice saturated in relations of power; thus, nurses are instruments of power, and they "have the capacity to both exercise and resist power."[52(p111),53] If nurses wish to live up to their commitment to social justice and responsibility to integrate principles of justice into nursing practice, policy, and the provision of health resources more generally, they must not only be capable of installing "new frames"[43(p12)] (i.e., new ways of seeing the world that apprehend suffering, especially when it is obscured by inequitable relations of power) but also able to critically self-reflect on their roles in the production of suffering and deconstruct the normative frames that render some lives more valuable than others. Espina and Narruhn[10] offer three strategies nurses can use to mitigate these injustices, summarized next: critical conscientization, structural competency, and advocacy, activism, and allyship.

Critical Conscientization

Critical approaches to education in the health professions (i.e., those that teach skills for examining unquestioned assumptions at the individual, institutional, and cultural levels of health care) have been recommended in response to concerns that competency-based education falls short of fostering compassion and social responsibility among health care providers, particularly concerning raising providers' awareness of the conditions under which the most marginalized live and experience health and illness (i.e., making known what has been obscured regarding the inequitable distribution of suffering).[54,55] Critical consciousness is an educational concept that arises from emancipatory work with marginalized communities, particularly the work of Paulo Freire as he worked to transform education among the poor in Brazil in the 1970s.[56] Freire argued that for education to be transformational, "learners needed to connect with their own personal, cognitive, and emotional experience, to engage with others through dialogue (an engaged discussion that includes affective and experiential knowledge) and to emancipate themselves and others through praxis (the realization of theory within action)."[57(p13)] This type of transformational education requires that teachers and learners engage in critical self-reflexivity and be willing to challenge their position(s) of power and privilege. *Conscientization* involves a "reflective reading of the world,"[57(p13)] focusing on taken-for-granted and socially embedded inequities. A critical stance allows nurses to pay attention to the underlying sociopolitical nature of both education and health care, recognize opportunities for challenging unexamined assumptions that perpetuate systems of oppression, and implores them to act as agents of change.[56] Adopting a critical stance is foundational to apprehending the politics of suffering. Therefore, nursing should integrate conscientization into the profession's definition of critical thinking. Content focused on understanding the distribution of wealth, health, and opportunity (i.e., social justice content) should be given equal weight in nursing education curriculum as biomedical content.[10]

Structural Competency

Structural competency as a concept was initially introduced in Metzl's 2010 book *The Protest Psychosis: How Schizophrenia Became a Black Disease.*[58] In 2014, Metzl and Hansen proposed structural competency as a paradigm for medical education[59] and it has since been utilized and advanced in multiple educational settings.[60–62] In their original conception, Metzl and Hansen define structural competency as the capacity of trained health professionals to recognize how "a host of issues defined clinically as symptoms, attitudes, or diseases"[59(p128)] are frequently the downstream consequences of broader economic and sociopolitical forces (i.e., upstream factors). Structure refers not only to environmental infrastructure (e.g., buildings, transportation, water, sewage, food and waste systems, electronic communication systems, etc.) but also to the "diagnostic and bureaucratic frameworks that surround biomedical interactions" (e.g., health care access)[59(p128)] and the "assumptions embedded in language and attitude that serve as rhetorical social conduits for some groups of persons, and as barriers to others."[59(p128)] In other words, "structural" denotes not only social and economic policies, including those that regulate the distribution of health and social resources, but also social stratification based on race, ethnicity, immigration status, ability, gender identity, sexual orientation, etc. Competency, in this formulation, does not suggest mastery of structural forces. Rather, it is grounded "in the belief that conceptualizing and intervening into abstract social formations is a skill that requires study and practice over time"[59(p128)] as well as the humility to recognize that nurses' work as health care professionals is saturated in relations of power.

Structural competency has been utilized in nursing education as a pedagogical framework intended to help prepare nurses to understand health inequities in the context of macro-level systems/structures and recognize the status and privilege conferred on them as health care workers.[62] Woolsey and Narruhn,[62] for example, have used a graduate nursing–level course grounded in biopower and structural competency that connects the structural causes of suffering among marginalized communities via critical concepts such as "Othering," epistemic injustice, historical trauma, intersectionality, embodiment, and internalized oppression. Students explore how these concepts show up across various public health issues such as mass incarceration, substance use, and homelessness and are encouraged to critically self-reflect on how their own biases and privileges impact their abilities to recognize how inequitable burdens of suffering among the most marginalized are frequently the result of inequitable arrangements of power.[62] Structural competency is an innovative pedagogical method congruent with Freire's conscientization[10] and Giroux's critical pedagogy.

Advocacy, Activism, and Allyship

Provisions 1, 3, 5, 8, and 9 in the ANA Code of Ethics[18] charge nurses to advocate for vulnerable individuals and communities and promote social justice. This professional obligation applies to the instances of injustice arising from biopower, slow violence, structural racism, and other mechanisms of injustice.[10] Because of the nature of their work and the proximity to the suffering of others that their role affords, nurses frequently assume the role of advocate when they wish to "tell the narratives of suffering [they] have witnessed."[20(p60)] Without critical awareness of existing power differentials, taking on advocacy roles may exacerbate these power imbalances, impede patients' capacity for agentic self-determination, and perpetuate the notion that nurses always know what is "in the best interest" of the individuals they serve.[63] "Solutions" that arise from such an individualistic focus frequently perpetuate paternalistic practices in health care and are often short term and ineffective at making long-term, systems-level change.[52] Given what is known about power and the inequitable distribution of suffering, upstream strategies rooted in community knowledge and self-determination and that focus on establishing concrete social policy in areas such as shelter, work, food, health care, and legal status may be more effective for both ensuring that suffering among the most marginalized is apprehended as such and establishing systems-level change that genuinely transforms the conditions under which the marginalized suffer. Additionally, systems-level advocacy strategies and participation in "movements that seek to redress experiences of oppression"[52(p108)] may also help to repair and heal existing distrust between nurses and marginalized populations who have historically been harmed by inequitable distributions of health resources and pathologized via normalizing practices within systems of "care."[52]

Conclusion

In accordance with nurses' ethical responsibility and mandate for social justice, they must commit to ongoing processes of critical self-reflection and recognize their responsibility in apprehending social suffering, particularly when it is not popular or palatable. A central part of their responsibility in apprehending social suffering is in naming and deconstructing the role that systems of oppression play in driving disproportionality in the distribution of suffering, disease, debility, and economic deprivation for people subjected to structural injustice and in recognizing the processes by which some lives are rendered more valuable than others. As the largest segment of health care workers globally, nurses have a tremendous capacity to leverage their collective political power in service of movements for social justice, centering "the voices of the most marginalized to ensure that their voices also inform health care practice and policy."[52(p109)] This involves fundamentally altering their orientation—from experts to allies—acknowledging how power operates in and through their work as nurses and committing themselves to a more liberatory vision of health and healing for all.

References

1. Pilkington E. As 100,000 die, the virus lays bare America's brutal fault lines—race, gender, poverty, and broken politics. *The Guardian*. Published 2020. Accessed March 23, 2022. https://www.theguardian.com/us-news/2020/may/28/us-coronavirus-death-toll-racial-disparity-inequality.

2. Millett GA, Jones AT, Benkeser D, et al. Assessing differential impacts of COVID-19 on black communities. *Ann Epidemiol*. 2020;47:37–44. doi:10.1016/j.annepidem.2020.05.003

3. Holden TM, Simon MA, Arnold DT, Halloway V, Gerardin J. Structural racism and COVID-19 response: higher risk of exposure drives disparate COVID-19 deaths among Black and Hispanic/Latinx residents of Illinois, USA. *BMC Public Health*. 2022;22(1):1–13. doi:10.1186/s12889-022-12698-9

4. Salisbury-Afshar EM, Rich JD, Adashi EY. Vulnerable populations: weathering the pandemic storm. *Am J Prev Med*. 2020;58(6):892–894. doi:10.1016/j.amepre.2020.04.002

5. Chotiner I. The interwoven threads of inequality and health. *New Yorker*. Published 2020. Accessed March 23, 2022. https://www.newyorker.com/news/q-and-a/the-coronavirus-and-the-interwoven-threads-of-inequality-and-health

6. Galofaro C. Voices of protest, crying for change, ring across US, beyond. Associated Press. Published June 17, 2020. Accessed March 23, 2022. https://www.voanews.com/a/usa_voices-protest-crying-change-ring-across-us-beyond/6191284.html

7. Yancy CW. COVID-19 and African Americans. *JAMA*. 2020;323(19):1891–1892.

8. Bowman B. On the biopolitics of breathing: race, protests, and state violence under the global threat of COVID-19. *South African J Psychol*. 2020;50(3):312–315. doi:10.1177/0081246320947856

9. Krieger N. ENOUGH: COVID-19, structural racism, police brutality, plutocracy, climate change-and time for health justice, democratic governance, and an equitable, sustainable future. *Am J Public Health*. 2020;110(11):1620–1623. doi:10.2105/AJPH.2020.305886

10. Espina CR, Narruhn RA. "I can't breathe": biopower in the time of COVID-19: an exploration of how biopower manifests in the dual pandemics of COVID and racism. *Adv Nurs Sci*. 2021;44(3):183–194. doi:10.1097/ANS.0000000000000355

11. Singh M. "Long overdue": lawmakers declare racism a public health emergency. *The Guardian*. Published June 12, 2020. Accessed March 23, 2022. https://www.theguardian.com/society/2020/jun/12/racism-public-health-black-brown-coronavirus

12. Vestal C. Racism is a public health crisis, say cities and counties. Pew Stateline. Published June 15, 2020. Accessed March 23, 2022. https://www.pewtrusts.org/en/research-and-analysis/blogs/stateline/2020/06/15/racism-is-a-public-health-crisis-say-cities-and-counties

13. Knopf A, Budhwani H, Logie CH, Oruche U, Wyatt E, Draucker CB. A review of nursing position statements on racism following the murder of George Floyd and

other Black Americans. *J Assoc Nurses AIDS Care*. 2021;32(4):453–466. doi:10.1097/JNC.0000000000000270

14. Powell JA. Structural racism: building upon the insights of John Calmore. *North Carol Law Rev*. 2008;86(3):791–816.

15. Addressing law enforcement as a public health issue. American Public Health Association. Published November 13, 2018. Accessed March 23, 2022. https://www.apha.org/policies-and-advocacy/public-health-policy-statements/policy-database/2019/01/29/law-enfo rcement-violence

16. Kleinman A, Das V, Lock M, ed. *Social Suffering*. University of California Press; 1997.

17. Harvard Global Institute. Systems of oppression. Published 2022. Accessed March 24, 2022. https://globalhealth.harvard.edu/domains/systems-of-oppression/

18. American Nurses Association. Code of ethics. Published 2015. Accessed May 21, 2022. https://www.nursingworld.org/practice-policy/nursing-excellence/ethics/code-of-ethics-for-nurses/coe-view-only/

19. Georges JM. The politics of suffering: implications for nursing science. *Adv Nurs Sci*. 2004;27(4):250–256.

20. Georges JM. Compassion, biopower, and nursing. In: Kagan PN, Smith MC, Chinn PL, eds. *Philosophies and Practices of Emancipatory Nursing: Social Justice as Praxis*. Routledge; 2014.

21. Moore JW, ed. *Anthropocene or Capitalocene?: Nature, History, and the Crisis of Capitalism*. PM Press; 2016.

22. Dillard-Wright J, Walsh JH, Brown BB. We have never been nurses: nursing in the Anthropocene, undoing the Capitalocene. *Adv Nurs Sci*. 2020;43(2):132–146. doi:10.1097/ANS.0000000000000313

23. Georges JM. Suffering: toward a contextual praxis. *Adv Nurs Sci*. 2002;25(1):79–86. doi:10.1097/00012272-200209000-00009

24. McFarland-Icke B. *Nurses in Nazi Germany: Moral Choices in History*. Princeton University Press; 1999.

25. Foucault M. *The History of Sexuality, Volume 1: An Introduction*. Random House; 1978.

26. Sutherland O, LaMarre A, Rice C, Hardt L, Jeffrey N. Gendered patterns of interaction: a Foucauldian discourse analysis of couple therapy. *Contemp Fam Ther*. 2016;38(4):385–399. doi:10.1007/s10591-016-9394-6

27. Foucault M. *Society Must Be Defended: Lectures at the College De France 1975-1976*. (Bertani M, Fontana A, Ewald F, eds.). Picador; 2003.

28. Mills S. *Routledge Critical Thinkers: Michel Foucault*. London: Routledge; 2003.

29. Foucault M. *The Birth of Biopolitics: Lectures at the College de France 1978-1979*. (Ewald F, Fontana A, eds.). Picador; 2004.

30. Focault M. Governmentality. In Burchell G, Gordon C, Miller P, eds. *The Foucault Effects: Studies in Governmentality*. Harvester Wheatsheaf; 1991:87–104.

31. Holmes D, Gastaldo D. Nursing as means of governmentality. *J Adv Nurs*. 2002;38(6):557–565. doi:10.1046/j.1365-2648.2002.02222.x

32. Agamben G. *Homo Sacer: Sovereign Power and Bare Life*. Stanford University Press; 1995.

33. Georges JM. Bio-power, Agamben, and emerging nursing knowledge. *Adv Nurs Sci*. 2008;31(1):4–12.

34. McHoul A, Grace W. *A Foucault Primer: Discourse, Power and the Subject*. Routledge; 2015.

35. Foucault M. *The Archaeology of Knowledge*. Tavistock; 1972.

36. Puzan E. The unbearable whiteness of being (in nursing). *Nurs Inq*. 2003;10(3):193–200. doi:10.1046/j.1440-1800.2003.00180.x

37. van Dijk TA. Ideology and discourse. In: Freeden M, Stears M, eds. *The Oxford Handbook of Political Ideologies*. Oxford University Press; 2013:1–27.

38. Lacey N. *Unspeakable Subjects: Feminist Essays in Legal and Social Theory*. Hart Publishing; 1998.
39. Tyler SA. *The Unspeakable: Discourse, Dialogue, and Rhetoric in the Postmodern World*. University of Wisconsin Press; 1987.
40. Georges JM. Evidence of the unspeakable: biopower, compassion, and nursing. *Adv Nurs Sci*. 2011;34(2):130–135. doi:10.1097/ANS.0b013e3182186cd8
41. Renbarger K, Draucker C. Nurses' approaches to pain management for women with opioid use disorder in the perinatal period. *J Obstet Gynecol Neonatal Nurs*. 2021;50(4):412–423.
42. Dyal B, Abudawood K, Schoppee T, et al. Reflections of healthcare experiences of African Americans with sickle cell disease or cancer: a qualitative study. *Cancer Nurs*. 2021;44(1):E53–E61.
43. Butler J. *Frames of War: When Is Life Grievable?* Verso; 2009.
44. Foth T. Understanding "caring" through biopolitics: the case of nurses under the Nazi regime. *Nurs Philos*. 2013;14(4):284–294. doi:10.1111/nup.12013
45. Giroux HA. *Stormy Weather: Katrina and the Politics of Disposability*. Paradigm Publishers; 2006.
46. Giroux H. Reading Hurricane Katrina: race, class, and the biopolitics of disposability. *Coll Lit*. 2006;33(3):171–196. doi:10.1353/lit.2006.0037
47. Andrasik MP, Maunakea AK, Oseso L, et al. Awakening: the unveiling of historically unaddressed social inequities during the COVID-19 pandemic in the United States. *Infect Dis Clin North Am*. 2022;36:295–308. doi:10.1016/j.idc.2022.01.009
48. Mbembe A. *Necropolitics*. Duke University Press; 2019.
49. Davies T. Toxic space and time: slow violence, necropolitics, and petrochemical pollution. *Ann Am Assoc Geogr*. 2018;108(6):1537–1553. doi:10.1080/24694452.2018.1470924
50. Nixon R. *Slow Violence and the Environmentalism of the Poor*. Harvard University Press; 2011.
51. Narruhn RA, Espina CR. "I've never been to a doctor": healthcare access for the Marshallese in Washington State [published online ahead of print, 2022 Sep 9]. *ANS Adv Nurs Sci*. 2022;10.1097/ANS.0000000000000456. doi:10.1097/ANS.0000000000000456.
52. Weitzel J, Luebke J, Wesp L, et al. The role of nurses as allies against racism and discrimination. *Adv Nurs Sci*. 2020;43(2):102–113.
53. Gastaldo D, Holmes D. Foucault and nursing: a history of the present. *Nurs Inq*. 1999;6(4):231–240. doi:10.1046/j.1440-1800.1999.00042.x
54. Kumagai AK, Lypson ML. Beyond cultural competence: critical consciousness, social justice, and multicultural education. *Acad Med*. 2009;84(6):782–787. doi:10.1097/ACM.0b013e3181a42398
55. Jarvis-Selinger S, Pratt DD, Regehr G. Competency is not enough: integrating identity formation into the medical education discourse. *Acad Med*. 2012;87(9):1185–1190. doi:10.1097/ACM.0b013e3182604968
56. Freire P. *Pedagogy of the Oppressed*. Continuum; 1993.
57. Halman M, Baker L, Ng S. Using critical consciousness to inform health professions education: a literature review. *Perspect Med Educ*. 2017;6(1):12–20. doi:10.1007/s40037-016-0324-y
58. Metzl JM. *The Protest Psychosis: How Schizophrenia Became a Black Disease*. Beacon Press; 2010.
59. Metzl JM, Hansen H. Structural competency: theorizing a new medical engagement with stigma and inequality. *Soc Sci Med*. 2014;103:126–133.
60. Metzl JM, Hansen H. Structural competency in the U.S. healthcare crisis: putting social and policy interventions into clinical practice. *J Bioeth Inq*. 2016;13(2):179–183.

61. Woolsey C, Narruhn R. Structural competency: a pilot study. *Public Health Nurs.* 2020;37(4):602–613.
62. Woolsey C, Narruhn R. A pedagogy of social justice for resilient/vulnerable populations: structural competency and bio-power. *Public Health Nurs.* 2018;35:587–597.
63. Spenceley SM, Reutter L, Allen MN. The road less traveled: nursing advocacy at the policy level. *Policy Polit Nurs Pract.* 2006;7(3):180–194. doi:10.1177/1527154406293683

15

Suffering in the Face of Humanitarian Crises and Emergencies

Sheila Davis and Marc Julmisse

> Bearing witness surely has a certain value, especially if it is linked to good-will efforts to prevent unnecessary suffering caused by war or disease or insufficient preparation for natural disasters.[1]

Background

There is no one definition of a humanitarian crisis or emergency. A crisis can be one single event or a series of events that threaten a large number of people's health, security, or survival. The distinction of "man-made" versus "natural" disasters is becoming less relevant as we see that the climate crisis, undeniably man-made, has dramatically increased the number of hurricanes, cyclones, and other "natural disasters."[2] Humanitarian crises are becoming increasingly prevalent in the world, with the United Nations estimating the need for global humanitarian aid in 2022 to be 274 million people, an increase from 235 million people in 2021.[3]

Political instability, ongoing conflicts, and war are major drivers of crisis situations affecting millions of people. The World Bank describes fragility, conflict, and violence (FCV) as a set of substantial challenges that are impacting the developmental efforts to end extreme poverty in both low- and middle-income countries, stating that "by 2030, up to two-thirds of the world's extreme poor could live in FCV settings. Conflicts also drive 80% of all humanitarian needs."[4] Similarly, populations in low-income countries where a large percentage of the population lives in extreme poverty are more vulnerable to the effects of natural disasters.[5] Therefore, it must be acknowledged that there is a disproportionate impact of humanitarian crises of any type on low- and middle-income countries (LMICs).

Beyond the consequences of conflict, the impact of climate change on humanitarian crises leads to serious implications for health, economy, and security, including direct effects from the increase in temperature and changes in the frequency and strength of heatwaves, storms, floods, and droughts. There are also changes in food production, increases in infectious diseases, climate-induced population displacement, and resultant conflict. As noted above, LMICs are disproportionately impacted by humanitarian crises, which will continue to exacerbate existing global health challenges and inequalities.[6] The Global Assessment Report (GAR2022), released by the

Sheila Davis and Marc Julmisse, *Suffering in the Face of Humanitarian Crises and Emergencies* In: *The Nature of Suffering and the Goals of Nursing*. Second Edition. Edited by: William E. Rosa and Betty R. Ferrell, Oxford University Press.
© Oxford University Press 2023. DOI: 10.1093/oso/9780197667934.003.0015

United Nations Office for Disaster Risk Reduction (UNDRR), reveals that between 350 and 500 medium- to large-scale disasters took place every year over the past two decades, and this number of disaster events is projected to reach 560 per year—or 1.5 disasters per day—by 2030.[7]

Disparities become more pronounced during crisis. Women and girls are at higher risk of violence during the acute and ongoing responses to any humanitarian crisis. Those most vulnerable prior to a crisis become most impacted in the aftermath. On average, natural disasters are more likely to be the cause of death for women when compared to men and cause death at a younger age for women than men.[8] Furthermore, relief policies are biased to the needs of men, and relief resources are also largely controlled and managed by men, which leads to the needs of women being ignored following a disaster. This, coupled with the fact that women are more likely to experience poverty, suggests unequal access to resources, which leads to higher rates of death and disenfranchisement of women following a natural disaster. In the aftermath of a crisis, women and girls are also increasingly at risk of maternal death. According to the United Nations, "Some 60 percent of all preventable maternal deaths in the world take place in conflict, displacement or disaster settings." One example of this unsettling phenomenon comes from the 1994 Rwandan genocide, in which it is estimated that 250,000 women were raped throughout the conflict. Of these rapes, an estimated 20,000 babies were born. This violence affect not only the women themselves but also the children born of these assaults. Data from support groups in Rwanda found that these children are often "disparaged, tend to live in poverty, fac[ing] higher rates of HIV, and domestic abuse than their peers."[9]

Conflict, climate-induced disasters, and humanitarian crises can force people to flee their homes. According to the UN High Commissioner for Refugees (UNHCR), as of mid-2021 there were over 84 million forcibly displaced people globally,[10] which includes refugees, internally displaced people, and asylum seekers. Many suffer from insufficient hygiene and sanitation facilities, creating conditions conducive to the spread of disease, food insecurity, and a lack of access to basic medical care. These conditions drive the profound vulnerability for displaced populations and increased illness, compounding dehumanizing conditions and inadequate palliative care. For instance, Rohingya refugees in Bangladesh with advanced illness are facing substantial physical, emotional, and social suffering due to a lack of symptom relief.[11,12] Additionally, Ukrainians in need of pain management confront barriers at the intersection of inadequate opioid access and war.[13]

Humanitarian aid, although lifesaving, is flawed, and colonialist history led to deeply entrenched policies and systems that have perpetuated gross global inequity. Racism is clearly impacting global response to crises. Journalist Maher Mezahi reflected on the difference in the global response to European versus African war and conflict and the clear differences in who is welcomed into surrounding countries.[14] The role of the media cannot be ignored. Various news outlets were forced to apologize for their coverage of the conflict in Ukraine versus many conflicts in the Middle East or on the African continent.[15] Every human life is of equal value, but one cannot ignore the correlation between varied gradients of skin color and who is deemed worthy of compassion and intervention. In the United States, as recently as July 2020, evidence shows that Black and Brown individuals make up 23% of deaths related to the COVID-19 pandemic despite making up only 13% of the US population. Black and Brown people are expected to be resilient, and the reality of who is worthy of the acknowledgment of suffering is disturbingly evident.[16] Suffering is normalized for Black and Brown people.

In addition to the personal and familial impact of a natural disaster or conflict, health care workers are also at risk. According to a World Health Organization (WHO) report on the impact of COVID-19 on health and health care workers, "In 2019, WHO recorded 778 attacks on health care workers from 10 countries and territories, resulting in 156 deaths and 895 injuries."[17] These numbers report only documented cases, and the full extent of violence against health care workers in natural disasters is unknown.

Acute-on-Chronic Emergency

The inequitable impact of humanitarian crises on LMICs is the result of acute disaster confounded by chronic emergency. There is no guaranteed access to quality health care globally. High-quality health systems are better able to withstand disasters of any type, but sustained enthusiasm and investment in building quality health systems remain elusive. In the words of Bill Gates, "Strengthening health care systems not only improves our ability to deal with epidemics, but it also promotes health more broadly. Without a functioning health system, it is very hard for a country to end the cycle of disease and poverty."[18]

Despite the repeated assaults on precarious health systems, there is minimal investment in strengthening health systems to promote resilience. From a 2021 report on philanthropic spending in 2019, $352 million was funded by foundations and public charities for disasters and humanitarian crises. Natural hazards and severe weather events accounted for 55% of disaster funding, and of the 51% of dollars that were allocated for response and relief efforts, 17% of funding went toward disaster preparedness, 6% went toward reconstruction and recovery, and only 4% supported resilience measures.[19]

Even before the COVID-19 pandemic, the world would not reach the United Nations' Sustainable Development Goal (SDG) health targets by 2030 or the goal of providing universal health coverage to 1 billion more people by 2023. The provision of essential health services is challenged in many places, and the additional patient load caused by the pandemic has strained already weak health systems.[20] The long-term impact of the pandemic on achieving universal health care is unknown, but with the challenge of the emergence of a new pathogen, our global health response effort has failed.

Humanitarian crises cause suffering. People in crisis, regardless of the cause, suffer physically, mentally, and emotionally. The accelerated pace of news media, paired with unprecedented access to the internet and the ability to upload footage from around the world, has given all of us a front seat to global suffering. Post–natural disaster immediate response includes stories of heroism, makeshift operating rooms, and working around the clock to save those impacted by an earthquake, hurricane, flood, or drought. Less known, less researched, less of interest to the frenzied news media is: What is the impact on the nurses and family caregivers who are responding to these extraordinary events? What is the impact of not just one disaster, but a series of simultaneous and ongoing emergency response situations compounded daily? What is the impact of suffering on the health care workers who themselves are victims of natural disasters and humanitarian crises, both acute and chronic? This chapter will explore these issues with a focus on how nurses respond to suffering and the impact on care.

Haiti and Humanitarian Crises

In August 2021, a 7.2 magnitude earthquake in Haiti occurred approximately 150 miles west of Port-au-Prince, largely affecting the cities of Les Cayes, the capital of the South, or Sud, and Jérémie, the capital of Grand Anse in the southern part of the country. At least 2,248 deaths were reported, and an additional 12,763 people were injured with at least 650,000 people in need of humanitarian support.[21] Although the impact was not as large as the devastating January 2010 earthquake that destroyed the city of Port-au-Prince and caused massive destruction and casualties, it came on the heels of a tumultuous time for the country with the unsolved assassination of President Jovenel Moïse in July of 2021.

Haiti is the poorest nation in the Western Hemisphere, suffering from a treacherous history of foreign exploitation and structural violence including decades of both the occupation by the United States and detrimental political instability. It was in the context of long-standing social, political, and economic conditions that these earthquakes struck and resulted in catastrophic acute-on-chronic disaster. These were not the first, nor last, humanitarian crises for Haiti in the 21st century. Frequently battered by tropical storms, situated on seismic fault lines, and enduring centuries of exploitation and the additional catastrophic impact of the pandemic, Haiti has weak public infrastructure and an overwhelmed health system that is ill-prepared to serve its 11 million inhabitants.

It is well noted that natural disasters disproportionately affect communities where there is an unstable government, weak infrastructure, and inadequate health services, particularly mental health services.[22] Researchers acknowledge the lack of studies identifying the adoption of long-term mental health and psychosocial support following a disaster.[23] Long-term support is often not planned, even though the link between the development of mental health issues and psychosocial issues in a post-disaster setting has been well established.[24] Immediate postdisaster crisis counseling is sometimes provided to the survivors and health care providers. Unfortunately, the duration of the services is limited and scale-up of interventions is difficult due to multiple barriers such as lack of oversight, lack of support provided to trained service providers, lack of ongoing technical assistance, lack of policy promoting integration, lack of political will, noncontextualized curricula, and lack of financial and human resources.[25]

Nursing Burnout

Clinical practices and specialties are experiencing an alarming rate of burnout. Fifty-nine percent of the global health care workforce consists of nurses.[26] In a profession that is demanding physically and emotionally, burnout rates and compassion fatigue have been steadily increasing.[27] Several terms have been used interchangeably to describe the negative transformations that occur in clinicians because of ongoing occupational stress.[28] One of these terms is "burnout," which is defined as the gradual process of increasing physical and mental fatigue or the "exhaustion of physical or emotional strength or motivation usually as a result of prolonged stress of frustrations."[29] Compassionate care, which is at the moral center of the nursing profession, can be at risk when the caregiver is overwhelmed from the witnessed suffering of patients. The idea may be true that "the process of caring for a suffering person is painful for the nurse and requires exceptional effort on the nurse's part, but the very act that drains the nurse can also create the fuel for compassionate care."[30] However, in cases where the nurse is exposed to repeated suffering without psychological intervention and support, the development of compassionate fatigue (CF) is imminent. Compassion is described as "a virtuous response that seeks to address the suffering and needs of a person through relational understanding and action."[31,32] CF, sometimes described as the *cost of caring,* is the emotional and physical fatigue that progressively develops in professionals when repeatedly exposed to traumatized individuals.[25,33] The practice that some nurses develop, erecting barriers and distancing themselves from patients suffering as a protective measure, may be the beginnings of CF, as evidenced by the comment made by Haitian nurses working at a tertiary level hospital (Case Exemplar 15.1).

Case Exemplar 15.1

"Nurses, when faced with a patient's suffering, must not become emotionally attached to a patient. Nurses have to maintain a professional relationship with the suffering patient. It is not recommended to interact with a lot of sympathy. Between human beings, there are images that haunt you when you think of a particular case, even unconsciously." (Medical-surgical nurse in Haiti)

"In a family fold, the nurse's family members do not understand how she can take a case with such delicacy. Why is the nurse so calm? Well, it is because we—the nurses—see so many cases in front of us day-to-day, so we do not show any concern about a case in the community or/and in the family. As an oncology nurse, death means the end of all suffering. Due to our experiences, knowing a person is dead does not affect nurses nowadays. However, they feel much more helpless when they cannot ease a patient's suffering.... The nurse does not develop too much intimacy and/or sensitivity because she considers that this can make her weak and can divert her care to support the patient." (Oncology nurse in Haiti)

In the Global North, nursing burnout is well documented, and it is known that "many nurses who care for suffering patients burn out."[30] In the United States, a Joint Commission survey identified that more than 15% of nurses surveyed reported burnout.[34] Another survey conducted in 2019 by the Joint Commission identified that "burnout is among the leading patient safety and quality concerns in health care organizations."[34] Furthermore, the article highlighted the Joint Commission's finding that the "negative effect of these stressors can affect the ability of the health care professionals to care for others."[34] A policy brief published by the International Council of Nurses (ICN) indicated that 20% of nurses in the national nurses associations (NNAs) connected to the ICN are reporting their intention of leaving the nursing profession, citing the "emotionally and physically draining" environment, the increase in critical patients, and the inadequate staffing for the volume of patients as reasons.[35] In the 2021 ICN COVID-19 update, data collected by the ICN showed that nurses reporting mental health distress increased by 20% during the first wave of the pandemic. Several countries are reporting elevated levels of stress and anxiety. The United States reported that 93% of health care workers were suffering from stress and 76% reported burnout. In Africa, a survey conducted over 13 countries showed an 18% increase in symptoms of depression and anxiety; 80% of nurses in Spain are reporting symptoms of anxiety and burnout; 90% of nurses in China are reporting anxiety; and in Brazil 49% of nurses are reporting anxiety and 25% are reporting depression.[36] A multitude of research exists providing insight into the effects of burnout and the supportive measures and interventions necessary to reduce the burnout rate in health care professionals in the global north,[37] and the same is required in the Global South.

In the majority of LMICs, where the global burden of disease is higher and where acute traumatic events are often combined with chronic events and chronic systemic gaps such as lower staffing ratios, lack of materials to intervene even when clinical knowledge exists, lack of space to provide care, and inadequate staff and salaries, there continues to be a significant lack of research and documentation on the impact that these systemic issues, chronic traumas, and primary exposure to traumatic events and secondary traumatic stress have on the long-term health and mental health of the health care provider. In LMICs, literature evaluating the burnout rate in clinicians, and more specifically in nurses, is difficult to find. In one study in sub-Saharan Africa the burnout rate is estimated to be between 51% and 87%.[38] Protracted exposure to traumatic events is known to increase the burden of mental health disorders.[25] It is widely noted in LMICs that face a scarcity of resources in the mental health sector that services provided often focus on postdisaster crisis counseling in the immediate aftermath.

As noted earlier, psychological support for existing trauma in LMICs where there are ongoing humanitarian crises in the presence or absence of an acute disaster is difficult to find in practice or in available research. With the dearth of supportive mental health services for clinical providers in many LMICs for acute and chronic trauma, the term "resilient" is often applied to describe these communities or individuals as they begin the process of recovery.[38] In such cases, the term "resilience" requires further investigation in both the definition and its application.

Resilience

Sometimes Haitian people resign themselves to life. They know pain very well and it allows them to be very resilient in the face of many things. Haiti, everything you do there, even the simplest thing, you do in suffering. Suffering is second nature to Haitians. This is the very theme of Haiti, "PAIN." (Interview with an intensive care unit nurse in a Haitian hospital)

A well-known Haitian proverb says "Sa ki pa touyeou, li angrese ou." Translation: What does not kill you fattens you. Concept: You are resilient. In the wake of a disaster or in the midst of a protracted crisis, communities or persons are sometimes described as resilient and are often commended for their ability to return to "normal" or a version of a new normal. Resilience has been described as the "human capacity to adapt swiftly and successfully to stressful and traumatic events and manage to revert to a positive state."[39] The textbook definition of resilience is the "ability to recover from or adjust easily to misfortune or change." Gang Wu further describes resilience as the "capacity and dynamic process of adaptively overcoming stress and adversity while maintaining normal psychological and physical functioning."[37] Two words often define resilience: "recover" and "adjust." These are key terms that are foundational to the concept of resilience. The prevailing thought is that either one recovers, returning to a previous state of normalcy, or adjusts, continuing life with modifications to establish a new normalized pattern of life. There is not one common or agreed-upon definition of resilience. In the study of resilience in the psychobiological construct as it relates to mental health disorders, researchers define resilience as both a protective factor preventing the development of mental health issues and a risk factor to developing certain clinical conditions.[39]

Pathological Resilience

Cénat and Derivois noted that between 30% and 50% of the population suffered from posttraumatic stress disorder (PTSD) and depression in an evaluation conducted of several postdisaster studies.[40] In society, resilience is often celebrated, and the survivors are often made out to be heroes. In countries such as Haiti where acute disasters occur with increasing frequency and chronic traumas are unresolved, and where there is difficulty obtaining positive global development or recovery, should the term that is used to describe a "resilient" population actually be referred to as a population that is "coping"? Would it make sense to refer to this population as having the mindset of "survival"? Is resilience culturally pathological?

Cénat and Derivois described pathological resilience as "a form of resilience that sublimates setback and makes it easy to roll with the punches."[40] In several studies there is documentation and evidence of people's ability to manage in the aftermath of the disaster; however, that is not always an indication of "positive development."[40] Are the systemic failures and inequalities inadvertently normalized by labelling them as "resilience"[41] and ignoring the invention of "paradoxical coping strategies"?[40]

Haitians are resilient, but it quickly becomes an expectation to be resilient and to accept the next disaster or atrocity that comes along, leaning toward patronization and reminiscent of colonial exploitation. It has soured the possibility of resilience as a positive. Nurses in communities where chronic trauma exists are expected to be strong and commended for their resilience. This is the pathological side of resilience.

Resilience Reimagined

The definitions that are widely accepted for resilience are regulated to major catastrophic external events. Some scholars propose that this trauma can be slow and chronic, undetectable to external observation.[42] To formulate a more accurate description of resilience, the concept of time should be acknowledged. "Resilience is dependent upon a state of uncertainty and shows no clear deadline and no time frame of resolution of the threat."[42] Take into consideration the following: duration of care (short- and long-term postdisaster crisis counseling); addressing chronic trauma; recognizing secondary trauma; incorporating environmental factors; discussing systemic failures; and developing supportive strategies that address burnout, compassion fatigue, and other mental health disorders at the individual and organizational level with the goal of promoting the development of true resilience and not pathological resilience, where a community is not functioning in a state of uncertainty.

Partners In Health (PIH) is an international nongovernmental organization that works in 12 countries providing a preferential option for health care for the most impoverished. PIH has worked in Haiti since 1987 in partnership with its sister organization Zanmi Lasante (ZL) supporting the Ministry of Health to provide health care. As of 2022, ZL provides a comprehensive model of health care for over 1.3 million people and has become Haiti's largest health care provider outside of the government, working closely with the Haitian Ministry of Health. ZL employs more than 6,300 staff, including 2,500 community health workers, to provide primary care, maternal and child health care, HIV and tuberculosis services, and more advanced secondary and tertiary care. PIH refuses to accept that the resilience of the Haitian people is a necessary byproduct of the challenges that the country has encountered in its history and instead works to create systems that break the cycle of harm being done within these communities.

Suffering and Leadership

The largest clinician cadre among PIH staff are nurses and midwives—affirming the global reality that quality care cannot be delivered without nurses and midwives. Nurses serve as the foundation and overall support, and without them, health systems and quality of patient care would suffer immensely. There is also profound responsibility that comes with the title of "nurse." Nurses at leadership levels are not exempt from burnout and its associated suffering.

Numerous studies focus on frontline clinicians and the factors that cause nurse burnout. What has not been studied widely is the development of burnout in nursing leadership, who potentially have the same or higher risk for burnout as that of nurses in nonleadership positions.[43] Factors that contribute to nursing burnout include clinical load, work environment, career growth, secondary trauma, and compassion fatigue. The nurse leader has the responsibility of ensuring employee satisfaction, improving staff retention and motivation, ensuring patient safety, and advocating for patients and staff in addition to setting a vision for the team—all while fostering professional identity and lifelong learning across settings.[43]

Nurse leaders are often not direct care clinicians. For those who engage in direct patient care, their time in the clinical setting is limited. The exposure nursing leadership has to patient suffering is less than that of a direct care nurse; however, that does not negate the risk the nurse leader has for secondary trauma. In one research study, four themes emerged in their findings as risk factors for nursing leadership burnout: (1) emotional drain, (2) every interaction tells a story, (3) managing one's psychological capital, and (4) work-life balance juggle.[43] Emotional drain is experienced by nurse leaders providing disciplinary measures and firing employees in addition to providing coaching and supporting hospital policy even when at odds with its implementation. Furthermore, the article identified the challenges encountered by nurse leaders such as maintaining work-life balance as they achieved higher leadership levels, insufficient resources, lack of peer support, and lack of executive leadership support, among others.[43]

Nursing leadership has the triple burden of disciplinary, organizational, and operational stress.[43] Being removed from frontline clinical care does not exclude the nurse leader from burnout. As there is extremely limited research studying burnout in nursing leadership, it is important to underscore the need for more research in that area.

Responses to Suffering

As leaders working amid humanitarian crises, it is important to acknowledge suffering in our patients, communities, staff, and ourselves. All crises and disasters are stressful, but the acute-on-chronic emergencies described in the case studies in Haiti above are particularly challenging. Pragmatic solutions that are used by PIH/ZL leaders in Haiti include providing direct operational support, teaching, accompaniment, funding, methods of data collection, and additional procurement of supplies to support mobile clinics and optimize health care delivery. Embedded within PIH's health systems approach is the idea that every individual deserves full access to health care, and yet without providing direct support to our nurses and staff in a comprehensive model, delivering such quality care is impossible; every human being is deserving of dignity and respect, and that includes the workplace, regardless of location and access to resources.

Nurses and those who are relied upon to deliver quality health care services are part of the ecosystem of global health delivery that is inextricably linked to their quality of life. Many live and work in the same environments they serve. At PIH/ZL, the workforce, which includes cooks, drivers, medical doctors, nurses, midwives, community health workers, and many other professions, is 88% Haitian and also living and working in their country of origin. With this comes the recognition that it is difficult to separate work and home environments and this can cause suffering, particularly when major humanitarian crises occur. If there is no separation of work and home, how is it possible to live free of the burden of exhaustion, burnout, and despair? If it is assumed an individual should be capable of living a fully human existence (as more than one identity)—for example, a nurse and a mother, a nurse and a brother, a nurse and a cook, a nurse and a friend, etc.—then how does one show up wholly and bear the weight of patient care daily? It is time to recognize that the profession of nursing is one that requires not only immense empathy and compassion but also strength, and to shift from mere survival mode to comprehensive care for the nursing workforce. Nurses need to feel supported and seen by the world they work to comfort every day. They must be treated with dignity and respect.

Grieving the work environment one had hoped for and envisioned is also important. Finding trusted colleagues to talk to without fear of impunity is essential. Modeling stepping away from the chaos, even for short periods of time, is useful, and as a leader, normalizing that you may need to step away from the work for longer periods is also crucial. To make a paradigm shift for change, it is crucial to resist viewing resilience as a virtue. Even among the chaos, it is important to make the deliberate decision to stay in the moment with a staff member and listen in solidarity. Consulting mental health professionals and engaging in transparent communication from the beginning and as an ongoing practice can help mitigate problems.

In 2021, a nurse in Haiti who had already had two warning letters for extremely aggressive behavior toward patients, family members, and other staff members was placed on temporary suspension. The nurse was strong clinically but had anger issues. Compassionate care directed at the nursing staff was needed rather than only issuing disciplinary measures. After meeting with the nurse and sharing with her the negative aspects repeatedly demonstrated in her actions, she was informed she would be placed on a temporary suspension with the condition that she would follow up with the psychosocial team. The team met with her again and she shared some of the unresolved trauma discovered during her consultations. Trauma is not limited to disasters, nor is compassionate care limited to patients.

Peer support practice may also be beneficial, with the relationship focused on creating a supportive caring environment versus a supervisory environment. Finding tangible ways of supporting each other in the patient care area is also encouraged and valued and can decrease the feelings of isolation that nurses may experience. Intentional listening with copious training on people management, conflict resolution, and workplace distress is essential to longevity in the field. The approach toward quality patient care must also be the approach toward self-care.

The most important thing that can be done as nurses is to work to strengthen health systems. Any true leader understands that health systems are built by changemakers—those who can see around corners and envision a brighter future. It is easy to claim to be committed to values of honesty, integrity, humility, accompaniment, and respect, but it is a challenge to the status quo to embody these values as nurse leaders and to uplift and amplify future nurse leaders who exemplify these qualities. It is imperative that nurses work together to build health systems that sustain the test of time—health systems that are built by the individuals who are living in the communities served. These community members are more than capable of building the future because they know what it is like to live without access to resources, to be overlooked and feel unimportant by the media, and to be treated as "the Other."

Conclusion

It is essential to show up first as a human being, as a global citizen, and as an advocate and be willing and eager to listen to the people who are so often silenced. Forming lasting partnerships and working to disrupt the cycle of suffering while challenging funding streams and advocating for integrated mental health services and programs for both formal and informal caregivers that are established as part of the core package of routine health care is not only needed but also critical. The approach must be to develop health care systems that support staff, provide quality access to care and resources, and hire and train educators and leaders in the field of nursing. Political instability and poverty intrinsically impact weakened health systems, and it is imperative to integrate the perspective of the world's leading medical and academic institutions with the lived experience of those living in poverty to build robust and sustainable health systems. It is time to listen to both patients and their caregivers and be bold, passionate, and compassionate. It is essential that care be provided during times of humanitarian crises, but most importantly, comprehensive quality care must always be provided for all.

References

1. Farmer P, Mukherjee J. *Haiti After the Earthquake*. PublicAffairs; 2012.
2. Climate change is the defining crisis of our time and it particularly impacts the displaced. United Nations High Commissioner for Refugees. Accessed May 4, 2022. https://www.unhcr.org/en-us/news/latest/2020/11/5fbf73384/climate-change-defining-crisis-time-particularly-impacts-displaced.html
3. United Nations Office for the Coordination of Humanitarian Affairs. Global humanitarian overview. Published 2022. Accessed May 2, 2022. https://gho.unocha.org/
4. Fragility, conflict, and violence. World Bank. Published 2022. Accessed May 2, 2022. https://www.worldbank.org/en/topic/fragilityconflictviolence/overview#1
5. Ritchie H, Roser M. Natural disasters. Our World in Data. Published 2014. Accessed May 2, 2022. https://ourworldindata.org/natural-disasters#link-between-poverty-and-deaths-from-natural-disasters
6. Watts N, Amann M, Ayeb-Karlsson S, et al. The Lancet Countdown on health and climate change: from 25 years of inaction to a global transformation for public health. *Lancet*. 2018;391(10120):581–630. doi:10.1016/s0140-6736(17)32464-9

7. Global assessment report on disaster risk reduction 2022. UNDRR. Published 2022. Accessed May 2, 2022. https://www.undrr.org/publication/global-assessment-report-disaster-risk-reduction-2022

8. Neumayer E, Pluemper T. *The Gendered Nature of Natural Disasters*. Blackwell Publishing; 2007:551–566.

9. Paquette D. Thousands of women were raped during Rwanda's genocide. Now their kids are coming of age. *Washington Post*. Published June 11, 2017. Accessed June 3, 2022. https://www.washingtonpost.com/sf/world/2017/06/11/rwandas-children-of-rape-are-coming-of-age-against-the-odds/

10. *Global Humanitarian Overview 2019*. United Nations; 2019:17.

11. Figures at a glance. UNHCR. Published 2021. Accessed May 3, 2022. https://www.unhcr.org/en-us/figures-at-a-glance.html

12. Doherty M, Power L, Petrova M, et al. Illness-related suffering and need for palliative care in Rohingya refugees and caregivers in Bangladesh: a cross-sectional study. Semantic Scholar. doi:10.17863/CAM.51173

13. Rosa WE, Grant L, Knaul F, et al. The value of alleviating suffering and dignifying death in war and humanitarian crises. *Lancet*. 2022;399(10334):1447–1450. doi:10.1016/S0140-6736(22)00534-7

14. Viewpoint on Ukraine: why African wars get different treatment. BBC News. Published 2022. Accessed May 3, 2022. https://www.bbc.com/news/world-africa-60603232

15. Europe's treatment of Ukrainian refugees is starkly different from what Syrians experienced, say some. CBC. Published 2022. Accessed May 3, 2022. https://www.cbc.ca/news/world/europe-racism-ukraine-refugees-1.6367932

16. Cohen L. "Our system is not built to serve everyone equally": doctors push for an end to racial discrimination in health care. CBS News. Published July 6, 2020. Accessed June 3, 2022. https://www.cbsnews.com/news/health-care-system-racial-discrimination-equality/

17. *The Impact of COVID-19 on Health and Care Workers: A Closer Look at Deaths* [ebook]. World Health Organization; 2021. Accessed May 4, 2022. https://apps.who.int/iris/bitstream/handle/10665/345300/WHO-HWF-WorkingPaper-2021.1-eng.pdf

18. Gates B. The next epidemic — lessons from Ebola. *N Engl J Med*. 2015;372(15):1381–1384. doi:10.1056/nejmp1502918

19. Candid and the Center for Disaster Philanthropy. Measuring the state of disaster philanthropy: data to drive decisions. Published 2021. Accessed May 3, 2022. https://www.issuelab.org/resources/38973/38973.pdf

20. World Health Organization and World Bank. Tracking universal health coverage: 2021 global monitoring report. Published 2021. Accessed May 3, 2022. https://cdn.who.int/media/docs/default-source/world-health-data-platform/events/tracking-universal-health-coverage-2021-global-monitoring-report_uhc-day.pdf?sfvrsn=fd5c65c6_5&download=true

21. International Medical Corps. *International Medical Corps Situation Update: Haiti Earthquake* [ebook]. 3rd ed. Published 2022. Accessed May 4, 2022. https://reliefweb.int/sites/reliefweb.int/files/resources/IntlMedCorps-HaitiEarthquake2021_SitRep03.pdf#:~:text=On%20August%2014%2C%202021%2C%20a%20devastating%207.2%20magnitude,least%202%2C248%20deaths%20and%20injuring%20some%2012%2C763%20people

22. Disaster Technical Assistance Center supplemental research bulletin: greater impact: how disasters affect people of low socioeconomic status. Published 2017. Accessed May 3, 2022. https://www.samhsa.gov/sites/default/files/dtac/srb-low-ses_2.pdf

23. Seto M, Nemoto H, Kobayashi N, et al. Post-disaster mental health and psychosocial support in the areas affected by the Great East Japan Earthquake: a qualitative study. *BMC Psychiatry*. 2019;19(1):261. Published 2019 Aug 27. doi:10.1186/s12888-019-2243-z

24. McFarlane AC, Williams R. Mental health services required after disasters: learning from the lasting effects of disasters. *Depress Res Treat*. 2012;2012:970194. doi:10.1155/2012/970194

25. Troup J, Fuhr DC, Woodward A, Sondorp E, Roberts B. Barriers and facilitators for scaling up mental health and psychosocial support interventions in low- and middle-income countries for populations affected by humanitarian crises: a systematic review. *Int J Ment Health Syst*. 2021;15(1):5. Published 2021 Jan 7. doi:10.1186/s13033-020-00431-1

26. The world still needs 6 million nurses. Public Services International. Published 2022. Accessed May 3, 2022. https://publicservices.international/resources/news/the-world-still-needs-6-million-nurses?id=10713&lang=en

27. Brennan E. Towards resilience and wellbeing in nurses. *Br J Nurs*. 2017;26(1):43–47. doi:10.12968/bjon.2017.26.1.43

28. Jaimes A, Hassan G, Rousseau C. Hurtful gifts? Trauma and growth transmission among local clinicians in postearthquake Haiti. *J Trauma Stress*. 2019;32(2):186–195.

29. Merriam-Webster. Burnout. Published 2022. Accessed May 3, 2022. https://www.merriam-webster.com/dictionary/burnout

30. Deal B. Finding the meaning in suffering. *Holist Nurs Pract*. 2011;25(4):205–210. doi:10.1097/HNP.0b013e31822271db

31. Sinclair S, Beamer K, Hack TF, et al. Sympathy, empathy, and compassion: a grounded theory study of palliative care patients' understandings, experiences, and preferences. *Palliat Med*. 2017;31(5):437–447. doi:10.1177/0269216316663499

32. Peters E. Compassion fatigue in nursing: a concept analysis. *Nurs Forum*. 2018;53(4):466–480. doi:10.1111/nuf.12274

33. Cocker F, Joss N. Compassion fatigue among healthcare, emergency and community service workers: a systematic review. *Int J Environ Res Public Health*. 2016;13(6):618. doi:10.3390/ijerph13060618

34. Palmer J. Joint Commission portal addresses nurse burnout. Patient Safety & Quality Healthcare. Published 2022. Accessed May 4, 2022. https://www.psqh.com/analysis/joint-commission-portal-addresses-nurse-burnout/?webSyncID=411a650a-6780-dccc-a9c1-c599b47b0caa&sessionGUID=09114cc4-e500-9e06-bec4-8164a561434d

35. The global nursing shortage and nurse retention. International Council of Nurses. Published March 11, 2021. Accessed June 3, 2022. https://www.icn.ch/system/files/2021-07/ICN%20Policy%20Brief_Nurse%20Shortage%20and%20Retention.pdf

36. Molina-Praena J, Ramirez-Baena L, Gómez-Urquiza J, Cañadas G, De la Fuente E, Cañadas-De la Fuente G. Levels of burnout and risk factors in medical area nurses: a meta-analytic study. *Int J Environ Res Public Health*. 2018;15(12):2800.

37. Wu G, Feder A, Cohen H, et al. Understanding resilience. *Front Behav Neurosci*. 2013;7:10. Published 2013 Feb 15. doi:10.3389/fnbeh.2013.00010

38. Owuor R, Mutungi K, Anyango R, Mwita C. Prevalence of burnout among nurses in sub-Saharan Africa: a systematic review. *JBI Evid Synth*. 2020;18(6):1189–1207. doi:10.11124/jbisrir-d-19-00170

39. Shrivastava A, De Sousa A, Lodha P. Resilience as a psychopathological construct for psychiatric disorders. *Adv Exp Med Biol*. 2019;1192:479–489. doi:10.1007/978-981-32-9721-0_23

40. Cénat JM, Derivois D. Assessment of prevalence and determinants of posttraumatic stress disorder and depression symptoms in adults survivors of earthquake in Haiti after 30 months. *J Affect Disord*. 2014;159:111–117. doi:10.1016/j.jad.2014.02.025

41. Jiha R. Haitian resilience is not a sign of strength, it's a sign of our betrayal. Medium. Published August 18, 2020. Accessed May 3, 2022. https://medium.com/@rjiha/haitian-res ilience-is-not-a-sign-of-strength-its-a-sign-of-our-betrayal-80b1ecfa49f3
42. Humbert C, Joseph J. Introduction: the politics of resilience: problematizing current approaches. *Resilience.* 2019;7(3):215–223.
43. Kelly LA, Adams JM. Nurse leader burnout: how to find your joy. *Nurse Leader.* 2018;16(1):24–28. doi:10.1016/j.mnl.2017.10.006

16

Suffering of Nurses

Cynda Hylton Rushton and Katie E. Nelson

Introduction

In his seminal work, Warren Reich defined suffering as "an anguish experienced as a threat to our composure, our integrity, the fulfillment of our intentions, and more deeply as a frustration to the concrete meaning that we have found in our personal experience. It is the anguish over the injury, or threat of the injury to self; and thus, the meaning of the self that is at the core of suffering."[1] When unpacking his definition, we begin to illuminate the context and nuances of nurse suffering. Given Reich's definition of suffering, the threat to one's wholeness is a particular kind of suffering that engages the moral aspects of our lives and the contours of integrity and conscience in clinical practice.[2] Nurses' suffering is not separate from their humanness. The ability to perceive the suffering of others and within oneself is fundamental to the commitment to relieve it.

Evidence of Nurse Suffering

Growing evidence of suffering among nurses and other health care professionals has led to an increased use of varying terms, which are often conflated but have distinct symptoms and consequences and should be addressed differently (Table 16.1). Each of these unique, interrelated terms illuminate a slightly different lens on the suffering nurses experience. Instead of using these terms interchangeably and giving suffering a seemingly unidimensional definition, it is prudent to examine how each contributes to understanding the complex dimensions of nurse suffering and the tools used to measure the effects and consequences. In short, suffering is not a one-size-fits-all phenomenon.

Sources of Suffering

Being at the forefront of caring for patients and families, nurses experience episodic, chronic, and cumulative occupational stress. Globally, 1 in 10 nurses have reported experiencing burnout and/or some degree of emotional and physical distress in carrying out their roles and responsibilities.[21] These statistics are the byproduct of individual- *and* organizational-level factors stemming from toxic work environments, ever-increasing nurse-patient ratios, lack of available resources, and decreased managerial support.[21,22] In a survey of frontline health care workers during COVID-19,

Cynda Hylton Rushton and Katie E. Nelson, *Suffering of Nurses* In: *The Nature of Suffering and the Goals of Nursing.* Second Edition. Edited by: William E. Rosa and Betty R. Ferrell, Oxford University Press. © Oxford University Press 2023. DOI: 10.1093/oso/9780197667934.003.0016

Table 16.1 Terms Used to Describe Nurse Suffering and Forms of Measurement

Term or Concept	Definition	Forms of Measurement
Compassion fatigue	"Diminished capacity to care as a consequence of repeated exposure to the suffering of patients"[3]	Professional Quality of Life: Compassion Satisfaction and Fatigue—Version V (ProQOL)[4]
Disenfranchised grief	"Grief experienced by those who incur a loss that is not socially acknowledged or supported (e.g., loss of a patient in a formal caregiving setting)"[5]	Brief Grief Questionnaire (BGQ) Inventory of Complicated Grief (ICG)[6]
Moral apathy	"When denial, lack of caring or willful ignorance makes it possible to ignore or not perceive the suffering of others"[7]	—
Moral disengagement	"A coping strategy to avoid self-condemnation and a sense of failure one might otherwise experience when one has acted in ways that violate or fall short of one's own moral standards"[8]	Currently there is no valid scale to measure moral disengagement in clinicians. See a general scale for adults[9]
Moral distress	"Anguish in response to a circumstance where one has 'violated a core value commitment, failed to fulfill a fundamental moral obligation, or in some other significant way fallen morally short under conditions of constraint or duress'"[10]	Moral Distress Scale—Revised[11]
Moral injury	"The profound psychological distress which results from actions, or the lack of them, which violate one's moral or ethical code"[12]	Moral Injury Symptoms Scale—Health Professionals[13]
Moral outrage	"Justifiable anger that arises after thoughtful reflection on values such as compassion, empathy, and discernment"[14,15]	—
Moral stress	"A state of arousal in response to a real or potential threat or challenge to one's integrity"[2]	—
Occupational burnout	"In a worker, occupational physical AND emotional exhaustion state or emotional burnout is an exhaustion due to exposure to problems at work"[16]	Burnout Assessment Tool (BAT)[17] Copenhagen Burnout Inventory[18]
Posttraumatic stress disorder	"A psychiatric disorder that can develop in people who have experienced or witnessed a traumatic event; previously referred to as 'shell shock' during World War I"[19]	Clinician Administered PTSD Scale (CAPS) Modified PTSD Symptom Scale (MPSS-SR) PTSD Checklist (PCL) Short PTSD Rating Interview (SPRINT)[19]
Secondary traumatic stress	"Natural behaviors and emotions resulting from exposure to patients' traumatic events; symptoms include intrusive thoughts, avoidant behavior, and hypertension"[4]	Secondary Traumatic Stress Scale[20]

one individual expressed, "We are not fine. We also know that PPE supplies are limited. Please don't insult me by telling me that we are safe as we should be right now."[22] Palpable organizational injustice, or the degree to which employees perceive being treated unfairly, led to heightened mistrust of institutions, workforce turnover, and lack of trust during the COVID-19 pandemic.[22,23]

Systems-level processes and guidelines have a trickle-down effect, which can inhibit nurses' ability to do their job in a way that makes them feel personally accomplished, bringing about symptoms of moral injury.[24,25] For instance, during COVID-19, limiting visitation opportunities for families greatly contributed to nurses' distress by placing them in the center of emotional and intense interactions day in and day out with little to no time for reprieve. One nurse lamented, "Having to watch patients who are completely mentally intact call their loved ones and tell them goodbye as they go on a ventilator, unsure if they will ever come off ... that has been the most haunting thing ... to watch that play out shift after shift."[26(p99)]

The ultimate pillar of the nursing profession is the provision of high-quality patient care; yet complex ethical and situational challenges left many nurses reporting statements like the following: "The patients are so sick that we are unable to make them comfortable ... seeing the struggle and decline is heartbreaking (273)"[26(p99)] or "They deserved a peaceful death, and yet many did not receive that."[22(p64)] Lack of support in the workplace can breach organizational trust and erode moral community, which then not only perpetuates individuals' personal suffering but also leaves organizations even more strapped for resources as nurses change jobs or leave the profession altogether.[21–23,25,27]

Responses to Suffering

Nurses, like all human beings, respond to their own suffering in a variety of ways. K. Turner's narrative (Case Exemplar 16.1) illustrates the range of responses to various situations one may experience, which can result in suffering that ranges from mild discomfort in isolated instances, to intense (yet manageable) responses, to accumulated, more recalcitrant forms of trauma or moral injury. Suffering may manifest through (1) physical symptoms, such as sleep disorders, gastrointestinal issues, headaches, etc.; (2) psychological symptoms, including depression, anxiety, and irritability; and (3) spiritual symptoms, like mourning the loss of moral and/or professional identity and meaning.

Case Exemplar 16.1

An Experience of Nurse Suffering

"I've watched patients' bodies become shadows of their former selves—their bodies degrading rather than healing under my own hands. I've watched clinical teams offer patients or their families unrealistic hopes when the evidence to the contrary seems so apparent. I get the sense from patients and families that surrendering part of their personhood is part of the price of ICU admission. We constantly trade off the quality of the person's life with the length of it. In reflective moments, I feel adamant that a person's dignity is not something we should ever ask to be traded away. I don't know if there is a moral or ethical difference between offering up your own dignity and having it unthinkingly chipped away at because of an unspoken, unexamined assumption that such is the price of the possibility of more time. I see myself begin to feel numb, going through the motions, and checking all the boxes during shifts without really engaging. The patient becomes a disintegrating body, not a person with a life story and people who love them. By depersonalizing our patients, do we add to or reinforce our own depersonalization and disconnection from our deepest values? I have thought for some time now that the similarities in adverse psychological outcomes among ICU patients, families, and nurses are because something is wrong in the ICU itself. You can say that patients have certain risk factors, families have their own risk factors, and staff have others. The experience that binds these parties is the ICU itself. We have figured out easy ways to capture specific big events—witnessing CPR, participating in withdrawal of life support, etc.—but what if the common risk factor that spans all entities is a harder one to pin down—the day-to-day insults to integrity and personhood?"(Turner K, personal communication, 2016)

There can be predictable patterns in responses to threats or violations of one's composure, personhood, identity, or intentions. Some individuals' initial response is to deny such threats, or to distract oneself from the experience by keeping busy or perceive something is wrong without a name to describe it. This inchoate awareness can become the pebble in one's shoe that causes continuous irritation or distress without a clear path for resolution. One nurse described, "You just put the blinders on, and you pretend ... pretend that it doesn't bother you." Another nurse stated, "We just ignore it. I have another patient to care for. And we just move on."[28(p238)]

Sometimes nurses have difficulty allowing themselves to connect to the reality of a given situation because it is just too painful to consider or acknowledge, or they are afraid of any consequences that might follow. Compounded by these feelings is a culture of shame and guilt that is widely prevalent in nursing, which encourages presenteeism—or coming to work while ill—and neglecting wellness practices.[29] These feelings and behaviors reflect attempts to protect oneself rather than representing and acknowledging what is typically thought of as denial. This is not a sign of stubbornness or weakness; it highlights how uncertain people can be about allowing themselves to perceive the suffering or to perceive something that feels wrong—especially when there is no name to sufficiently describe their feelings.

Nurses may either employ strategies that avoid the sources of their suffering or literally or figuratively abandon the source of their distress. Sometimes we become numb to the root causes of our suffering. One nurse reflected, "It starts a negative cycle specifically for the nurse because when you pretend the first time, it makes it easier to pretend the second time. And then it becomes a non-issue, and you stop thinking about it and you become numb."[28(p238)] Reflecting on the process of caring for sedated and ventilated patients with COVID-19, a nurse stated, "It was very easy to just treat their vital signs and treat their numbers, and almost detach from the situation, which emotionally I think made it easier to deal with. But when you sit down and think about it, it was very sad."[30(p7)]

Nurses' suffering can quite literally erode the caring and empathetic demeanor that encompasses nursing as the most trusted profession. A nurse working in the emergency department shared, "At one time I was so distressed I left the ED ... you don't want to come to work. You try to distance yourself from your patients. You try to be cold and uncaring, but you know you really aren't that way."[28] A nurse providing care during the COVID-19 pandemic said, "I feel I have lost some of my empathy. I feel like I'm just going through the motions, still providing excellent care but not with the feeling that I used to."[31a]

In resisting becoming numb or apathetic, nurses may at times rationalize suffering—"it's not *that* bad"—and instead can become angry, defensive, and outraged. In response to the COVID-19 pandemic one nurse stated, "People not realizing how serious COVID is makes me feel very angry. I'm very disgruntled and angry with the public ... they don't get it. It's just a frustration for me."[30(p5)] When nurses become overwhelmed and/or have resorted to all other feelings and emotions, it is not uncommon to lapse into moral apathy. It can keep people stuck in an endless cycle of despair, disappointment, resentment, and victimization. The nervous system then habitually remains in patterns of threat—fight, fright, or freeze—and the negative arousal pathways create disempowering narratives that continually reinforce the detrimental sequelae of suffering.

Consistent with Reich's definition, nurses' personal and professional identity can become eroded, dissonate, or corrupted by their experiences. This was a prominent theme during the COVID-19 pandemic, where commonly heard sentiments such as the following were heard: "People say we signed up for this. No, I never agreed to risk my life or my family to help others. I'm no soldier nor cannon fodder. I am a nurse (022)." Nurses also questioned the description of nurses as heroes: "Health care workers are NOT heroes. We are human and we are scared (075)."[26(p100)] Others reported regret regarding their career choice: "This has been the hardest it's ever been to be a nurse and I sincerely hope that we can change how nurses are treated. I would not encourage anyone to be a nurse, and this causes me great sadness because I love being a nurse."[31a] Loss of personal and professional identity is also a prominent feature of moral injury.[32] Concurrently, it is important to acknowledge that suffering can fundamentally and permanently change an individual. Critical care nurses disproportionately experienced this reality during the COVID-19 pandemic and made statements like "We can't unsee what we have witnessed. It stays with us (042)," and "I know I will never be the same person, nurse, mom or friend (194)."[26(p100)] Alongside this erosion of identity and wholeness, some nurses may blame themselves for the circumstances that caused the suffering or their own responses to them.

The Other Side of Suffering

> When we meet real tragedy in life, we can react in two ways—either by losing hope and falling into self-destructive habits, or by using the challenge to find our inner strength.
>
>   —H.H. Dalai Lama

Not all suffering results in detrimental consequences or experiences. Nurses' suffering can be a signal to pay attention. The same way that a fever alerts to the possibility of infection, the perception of suffering can also be a signal that important values, commitments, or intentions are being threatened or violated. Instead of seeing suffering as evidence of weakness or deficiency, it can also be understood as evidence of attunement and engagement in the complexity of life, and it reveals people's character, values, commitments, and integrity. It can be a raw experience that is undoubtedly difficult but necessary to build strength and resilience that can sustain wholeness, caring practices, clinical expertise, and well-being so that patients and their loved ones receive quality, safe, and compassionate care. As such, nurses' suffering can be a source of insight, growth, and restored integrity.[2,33]

During COVID-19, nurses found ways to maintain hope by celebrating patient outcomes. Hope, rather than optimism, is a stance that acknowledges challenges yet enables an individual to pivot toward the possibility that things will turn out well even when there is countervailing evidence that it might not. One nurse acknowledged that amid the COVID-19 pandemic they were transformed: "I believe it has made me a better nurse (109)," and it revealed their strength and determination: "I had emotional and physical strength that I didn't know I had (269)."[26(p101)]

From this perspective, suffering is not something that should be hidden or suppressed. Understanding the suffering of nurses demands that everyone engage in the dynamic process of learning to be with it, understand it, and potentially give meaning to it. Only through a commitment to a shared vision that embodies robust values of respect, compassion, and justice can clinicians and their institutions successfully impact the experience of suffering and its effect on patient care delivery. The other side of suffering can include the ability to transform suffering through the cultivation of compassion,[34] moral resilience,[2] posttraumatic growth,[35] moral courage,[36] or other means. Nurses must skillfully engage with personal suffering so that it can be transformed into integrity and compassion, rather than allowing it to disable basic human goodness and moral code. This requires letting go of a victimized narrative and meeting suffering with grace, integrity, and generosity. Ultimately, nurses must proactively harness inner strength, confidence, and agency to be able to choose how to respond and open themselves up to the possibility of discovering unseen or unknown resources and outcomes that are unimaginable.[30,36]

Equipping Nurses to Respond

There are a vast number of sources that can contribute to nurses' personal and professional suffering, suggesting a nuanced approach to responding is needed. However, in general, the strategies shown in Case Exemplars 16.2 through 16.4 may be helpful for nurses in restoring their wholeness, relieving some degree of suffering, and/or transforming it.

Case Exemplar 16.2

Recognize and Name Suffering

"I stepped into my shoes outside the zendo. They are my old work shoes, steeped in blood and propofol. I thought right away about what happened last summer during reflexology when, as the practitioner worked on my hands, images came up of all the harms and unpleasant things they had done at work in the service of trying to heal. I thought of the cries and begging for mercy. My throat was so tight that if someone had asked me what was wrong, no words would have come out. I felt like I was flailing inside, and my heart and brain were racing. I wanted my mom to give me a hug. I thought, if I can't soothe myself with the familiar balm of mother's love, I will do it with the familiar balm of one foot in front of the other and that's what I did. As I kept walking, I began to see that I am still the same me that was here before this overpowering wave and that it, too, would pass. The other thing I was thinking was that I must get rid of these shoes. They have served their purpose." (Turner K, personal communication, 2016)

Before nurses can work with or transform their suffering, they first need to notice its unique signature and *name it*. Through mindful awareness, they can notice the signals that indicate suffering is present and their responses to it. For example, K. Turner noticed tension in her throat, her heart racing, and her mind jumbled as she recalled images associated with her service as a nurse. These signals alert to potential threat or danger—whether it is physical, psychological, spiritual, or moral in nature. When they arise, there is an opportunity to inquire with mindful curiosity to notice the pattern of responses. She realized her need for support and the comforting "balm of her mother's love." Such insights can guide nurses to access available resources for enhancing well-being while also providing an opportunity to connect to personal essence, purpose, and values. Until nurses name the sources and consequences of our suffering, it is more likely to remain as what Reich refers to as "mute" suffering or become an unprocessed weight that further erodes health and well-being.

Case Exemplar 16.3

Restore Agency and Integrity

"I was in Mrs. C's bed doing CPR with the full blaze of code blue in progress when her daughter arrived and instructed us to stop resuscitation. 'Mom wanted to be DNR! What are you doing? Stop!' I flew off the bed in horror and shame. The ICU doctor flipped through the chart looking for an order and yelled over and over 'Keep going!' I told the other clinicians around the bed that they were welcome to continue, but that I would not go against the next-of-kin's refusal. No one moved. The doctor continued to press for the code to resume. It did not. This doctor followed me around the ICU for hours, venting his frustration and trying to convince me of his point. Finally, I turned around and said, 'It's not that I don't understand what you're saying; it's that I think you're wrong.'" (Turner K, personal communication, 2016)

Frequently, suffering renders feelings of powerlessness and helplessness in any given situation. As Reich highlights, situations like this one, that threaten composure (i.e., new information about a patient's code status), identity (e.g., advocating for the person who is unable to speak for themselves), meaning (i.e., how do I see myself as a good nurse under these conditions?), and purpose (e.g., to relieve suffering and promote well-being), can be at the crux of nurses' suffering.[1] In response, it is possible to leverage personal and professional values and courage to take integrity-preserving actions that restore agency and shield against involvement in unethical patient care encounters.

Case Exemplar 16.4

Cultivate Compassionate Awareness and Action

"Beth spent much of her first weeks in the ICU looking panicked. While visiting her on the floor, her partner Sam pulled me aside and said, 'Beth thinks that the whole ICU time, she was held in a train car, with no light and no air, and people would come in and hurt her.' A week later, Beth was back in the ICU, ventilated, restrained, and she and I were deep into a rocky shift. She would often wake up staring and trying to protect herself from things I couldn't see. Sam's words kept playing in my head, and it broke my heart to be one of the people she was afraid of. I became acutely overwhelmed and asked my co-worker Danielle if she would mind watching Beth so I could step off the unit to regroup. No hesitation, she did. I walked the halls, reciting over and over 'I feel this person's pain. I am not this person.' When I believed that, I resumed my post at Beth's side, ready for whatever." (Turner K, personal communication, 2016)

Compassion, understood as a state associated with perceiving the suffering of others and being motivated to act to potentially relieve another's suffering, is a complex, emergent process, involving noncompassion elements, that produces principled, wise, action(s).[3,7] Typical characterizations of compassion can be reduced to "being kind" or, when in limited supply, "compassion fatigue." Terms such as these are likely misapplied; studies suggest it is *empathy* rather than compassion that often becomes overwhelmed and fatigued.[3,4,7] Such characterizations of compassion have the potential to undermine the power of compassion to transform ourselves and others and the central role of compassion in healing ourselves and our relationships, systems, and society. Compassion is a key dimension of responding to the suffering of nurses. Without compassion, we may inadvertently cause more harm and disrupt, or undermine, healing and transformation.

The mnemonic GRACE was developed to engage the noncompassion components necessary for compassion to emerge.[7,37] The elements of GRACE can be used as a tool to explore our own suffering and cultivate necessary conditions for compassion to arise (Table 16.2). These simple, nonlinear, and emergent elements provide a scaffolding for application in different contexts, but developing the architecture to support compassion in action requires ongoing practice. These elements can be applied to situations that involve patients and their families, colleagues, leaders, or others where compassion will serve those involved and also to extend compassion to our own suffering.

Fostering Moral Resilience

Inevitably, our suffering is often multifaceted and rarely compartmentalized into physical, psychological, spiritual, or moral domains. We are whole integrated beings. When suffering includes threats to our values, commitments, and ultimately our integrity, we must accurately name its source and use strategies to restore our wholeness. Moral resilience, "the capacity of an individual to preserve or restore integrity in response to moral adversity,"[2(p68)] is a protective resource that can assist nurses in meeting moral and ethical challenges in a way that does not reduce their health or integrity.[23,26] The core elements of moral resilience are personal and relational integrity, buoyancy, self-awareness and self-regulation, moral efficacy, and self-stewardship.[38,39] As the case exemplars highlight, navigating ethical tensions or conflicts requires more than reasoning to create conditions for determining the path to preserve or maintain integrity. In Case Exemplar 16.4, K. Turner recognized signals of her distress and the source of it allowed the nurse space to engage in self-regulatory skills (mindfully walking and differentiating her suffering from her patient's pain). Additionally, repetition of the phrase "I feel this person's pain. I am not this person" helped calm her nervous system and shift her mindset and perspective in a way that supported her to continue to serve while avoiding detriment to herself or further depleting her energy. Repeating this phrase also helped her to differentiate the experience of the patient from her own experience, a key element in avoiding empathic overarousal.[37]

Table 16.2 Components of GRACE

G: Gathering your attention	Simple mindfulness practices such as soft belly breathing can stabilize the nervous system and focus attention on what is happening in your body, heart, and mind in this moment and help to regulate emotions and responses.
R: Recalling your intention	With stable attention, deliberately connect to your worldview, moral and ethical orientation, values, and intentions as a foundation to focus attention and to motivate aligned action.
A: Attuning first to one's own experience, then to another	Observe and connect to your body, heart, and mind before enlarging your perception to include another's experience. Staying grounded in your own experience supports differentiation, perspective taking, and balanced engagement with others.
C: Considering what will serve	A stable attention, awareness of one's experience, and connection with our intentions create the foundation to respond to complex situations with humility, curiosity, and openness to discover a path unseen or unknown that is aligned with who you essentially are, what you stand for, and what you seek to bring about.
E: Enacting, ethically, ending	Once you have considered what will serve, take principled, integrity-preserving steps to manifest the action in ways that are ethically grounded, transparent, and wise. Marking the ending of an interaction or process offers an intentional way to release the residue and prepare for the next encounter or step in the process.

Restoring Wholeness amid Suffering

Nurses, like other human beings, experience situations that cause suffering. It is inevitable that we all will bear witness to the suffering of others at some point, and in attempting to relieve it we may also experience suffering. Having specific strategies to rely on when we find ourselves in such situations can help restore agency, confidence, and wholeness (Table 16.3).

Nurses have an ethical obligation to invest in addressing their own well-being. The American Nurses Association Code of Ethics for Nurses[40] clearly states that nurses have the same obligations to self as to others, including preserving their own health, well-being, and integrity. COVID-19 has made visible the limits of nursing culture that view investments in one's own well-being as selfish or self-indulgent, and/or that self-sacrifice is a norm within the profession.[41] An elaboration of the meaning of this

Table 16.3 Restoring Wholeness amid Suffering (© Rushton, 2021)

Overarching Action	Small Steps or Strategies
Realistically appraise the situation without being swept away with fear, distraction, or dysregulated emotions	- Ground yourself by paying attention to your breath, feet on the floor, an object, or something else that helps ground your awareness and attention. - Stay focused on why you are here; connect to purpose, values, and intentions. - Apply the GRACE process to the situation or challenge.[7,34] - Ask yourself: "What part of this situation is mine to carry? What am I responsible and accountable for?"

Set realistic expectations of self and others	- Hard choices must be made.
	  ○ Tradeoffs of important values and consequences are predictable and inevitable.
	  ○ Assess what residue from the situation you can accept and live with.
	- Do the best you can with what you have.
	  ○ Recognize what is modifiable and what is not.
	  ○ Let go of expecting that you can fix unfixable situations.
	  ○ Bring your whole self to what is happening in front of you right now.
	- Accept limitations that are beyond your control.
	- Resist holding yourself responsible for things beyond your role or authority.
	  ○ Let go of unjustified shame, blame, guilt, and regret.
	  ○ Consider what you need to put down to lighten your burden(s).

Befriend uncertainty	- The landscape is rapidly changing, and uncertainty is expected and unavoidable in many circumstances. - Hold lightly to your position, assumptions, or agenda. ○ Welcome the unfolding process with curiosity. - Notice when fear or your need to control shows up. - Respond to these patterns of response with curiosity and kindness rather than judgment.

(continued)

Table 16.3 Continued

Overarching Action	Small Steps or Strategies

Resource yourself with tools, rituals, and practices	- Create rituals for coming to and leaving work.
	  o When arriving, set an intention for the day or take a breath to remember why you chose nursing as your profession.
	  o When leaving, pause as you wash your hands to consider your service and the good that was done, and to acknowledge you did the best you could with the resources that were available.
	- Regularly engage in intentional letting-go practices releasing what no longer serves from body, heart, and mind.
	- Use titration of exposure to distressing situations and use tools for internal and external resourcing to support well-being to maintain or restore stability.
	- Leverage tools like mindfulness, journaling, movement practices, or others that support well-being and resilience.

Increase social and relational connections	- Determine the people and relationships that nurture your well-being and integrity. - Support each other's personal and relational integrity. - Create opportunities for sharing experiences with colleagues in a safe, respectful environment. - Consider the intentions of leaders and colleagues when relationships become strained or complicated. - Create openness and space to be supported by others. - Practice giving and receiving support and resources.
Practice self-stewardship	- Comprehensively assess health and well-being. - Explore what nurtures your body, heart, and mind. - Conserve energy. o Take steps to reduce exposure to toxic situations, people, and environments. - Know your limits and honor them with compassion. - Establish boundaries and maintain them. - Create, refine, and implement a personalized self-stewardship plan. - Practice noticing and appreciating moments of integrity.

provision, in the context of the pandemic, offers nurses greater clarity about balancing their commitments to others and to themselves.[41] Turning toward humanity and suffering offers a pathway for personal and professional restoration.

Systemic Implications

The COVID-19 pandemic has underscored the irreplaceable role of nurses within health care systems and communities. Globally, we are experiencing a critical nursing shortage—largely due to nurses leaving the profession because of their suffering and distress. This has dire implications, as decades of research has proven that nursing shortages lead to decreased patient safety and increased patient morbidity and mortality.[42] The pandemic has highlighted the importance of holding institutions accountable for their ethical obligations to support clinicians' health and well-being.[43,44] Organizational leaders must take every opportunity to rebuild trust where it has been eroded and build in safeguards (i.e., clear policies and guidelines) for nurses (and all other staff) to report concerns, communicate ideas, and access resources to support their individual and team/department's well-being.[22,25,44] It is only through a shared commitment to addressing the modifiable systemic contributions to nurse suffering that real progress can be made.

Conclusion

Nurses are uniquely positioned to provide high-quality care for patients, families, and communities; yet this renders them at higher risk for suffering in their roles. Suffering can manifest in different ways based on the individual, the context, and their specialty within the nursing profession, and it can result in physical, psychological, spiritual, and moral consequences if not proactively acknowledged and addressed. Healing suffering requires patience, grace, and compassion toward oneself and others. Nurses and organizational leaders must be equipped to respond to suffering given the high-intensity, complex health care systems that nurses operate within. As the phrase goes, "You cannot pour from an empty cup," and as such, nurses must take the time to properly heal themselves so that—collectively—the profession can continue caring for all others.

References

1. Reich WT. Speaking of suffering: a moral account of compassion. *Soundings.* 1989;72:83–108.
2. Rushton CH. *Moral Resilience: Transforming Moral Suffering in Healthcare.* Oxford University Press; 2018.
3. Cavanagh N, Cockett G, Heinrich C, et al. Compassion fatigue in healthcare providers: a systematic review and meta-analysis. *Nurs Ethics.* 2020;27(3):639–665. 10.1177/0969733019889400

4. The Center for Victims of Torture. *ProQOL: Professional Quality of Life.* Published 2021. Accessed April 25, 2022. https://proqol.org/

5. Engler-Gross A, Goldzweig G, Hasson-Ohayon I, et al. Grief over patients, compassion fatigue, and the role of social acknowledgement among psycho-oncologists. *Psychooncology.* 2020;29(3):493–499. 10.1002/pon.5286

6. Igarashi N, Aoyama M, Ito M, et al. Comparison of two measures for complicated grief: Brief Grief Questionnaire (BGQ) and Inventory of Complicated Grief (ICG). *Jpn J Clin Oncol.* 2021;51(2):252–257. 10.1093/jjco/hyaa185

7. Halifax J. A heuristic model of enactive compassion. *Curr Opin Support Palliat Care.* 2012;6(2):228–235. https://doi.org/10.1097/SPC.0b013e3283530fbe

8. Bandura A. Selective moral disengagement in the exercise of moral agency. *J Moral Educ.* 2002;31:101–119. http://dx.doi.org/10.1080/0305724022014322

9. Moore C, Detert JR, Trevino LK, Baker VL, Mayer DM. Why employees do bad things: moral disengagement and unethical organizational behavior. *Pers Psychol.* 2012;65(1):1–48.

10. Carse A, Rushton CH. Harnessing the promise of moral distress: a call for re-orientation. *J Clin Ethics.* 2017;28(1):15–29.

11. Epstein EG, Whitehead PB, Prompahakul C, et al. Enhancing understanding of moral distress: the measure of moral distress for health care professionals. *AJOB Empir Bioeth.* 2019;10(2):113–124. 10.1080/23294515.2019.1586008

12. Williamson V, Murphy D, Castro C, et al. Moral injury and the need to carry out ethically responsible research. *Res Ethics.* 2021;17(2):135–142. https://doi.org/10.1177/174701612 0969743

13. Mantri S, Lawson JM, Wang Z, et al. Identifying moral injury in healthcare professionals: the moral injury symptom scale-hp. *J Relig Health.* 2020;59:2323–2340. 10.1007/s10943-020-01065-w

14. Jones-Bonofiglio K. *Health Care Ethics Through the Lens of Moral Distress.* Springer Nature; 2020. Accessed May 15, 2022. https://link.springer.com/content/pdf/10.1007/978-3-030-56156-7.pdf

15. Rushton C, Thompson L. Moral outrage: promise or peril. *Nurs Outlook.* 2020;68(5):P536–P538. https://doi.org/10.1016/j.outlook.2020.07.006

16. Canu IG, Marca SC, Dell'Oro F, et al. Harmonized definition of occupational burnout: a systematic review, semantic analysis, and Delphi consensus in 29 countries. *Scand J Work Environ Health.* 2021;47(2):95–107. 10.5271/sjweh.3935

17. de Beer LT, Schaufeli WB, De Witte H, et al. Measurement invariance of the Burnout Assessment Tool (BAT) across seven cross-national representative samples. *Int J Environ Res Public Health.* 2020;17(15):5604. 10.3390/ijerph17155604

18. Montgomery AP, Azuero A, Patrician PA. Psychometric properties of Copenhagen Burnout Inventory among nurses. *Res Nurs Health.* 2021;44(2):308–318. https://doi.org/10.1002/nur.22114

19. Hoffman V, Middleton JC, Feltner C, et al. *Psychological and Pharmacological Treatments for Adults with Posttraumatic Stress Disorder: A Systematic Review Update.* Agency for Healthcare Research and Quality; 2018. https://www.ncbi.nlm.nih.gov/books/NBK525132/pdf/Bookshelf_NBK525132.pdf

20. Bride B, Robinson M, Yegidis B, et al. Development and validation of the secondary traumatic stress scale. *Res Soc Work Pract.* 2004;14(1):27–35. https://doi.org/10.1177/1049731503254106

21. Jun J, Ojemeni MM, Kalamani R, et al. Relationship between nurse burnout, patient and organizational outcomes: systematic review. *Int J Nurs Stud.* 2021;119. 10.1016/j.ijnurstu.2021.103933

22. Nelson K, Hansen G, Boyce D, et al. Organizational impact on health care workers' moral injury during COVID-19: a mixed-methods analysis. *J Nurs Admin.* 2022;52(1):57–66. 10.1097/NNA.0000000000001103

23. Gimenez-Espert MD, Prado-Gasco V, Soto-Rubio A. Psychosocial risks, work engagement, and job satisfaction of nurses during COVID-19 pandemic. *Front Public Health.* 2020;8:566896. 10.3389/fpubh.2020.566896

24. Antonsdottir I, Rushton CH, Nelson KE, et al. Burnout and moral resilience in interprofessional healthcare professionals. *J Clin Nurs.* 2021;31(1–2):196–208. https://doi.org/10.1111/jocn.15896

25. Rushton CH, Thomas T, Antonsdottir I, et al. Moral injury, ethical concerns and moral resilience in health care workers during COVID-19 pandemic [online ahead of print]. *J Palliat Med.* 2022;25(5):712–719. https://doi.org/10.1089/jpm.2021.0076

26. Guttormson JL, Calkins K, McAndrew N, et al. Critical care nurses' experiences during the COVID-19 pandemic: a US national survey. *Am J Crit Care.* 2022;31(2):96–103. https://doi.org/10.4037/ajcc2022312

27. Bergman L, Falk AC, Wolf A, et al. Registered nurses' experiences of working in the intensive care unit during the COVID-19 pandemic. *Nurs Crit Care.* 2021;26(6):467–475. https://doi.org/10.1111/nicc.12649

28. Robinson R, Stinson CK. Moral distress: a qualitative study of emergency nurses. *Dimens Crit Care Nurs.* 2016;35(4):235–240. 10.1097/DCC.0000000000000185

29. Nelson KE, Rushton CH. Working while ill during COVID-19: ethics, guilt, and moral community. *AACN Adv Crit Care.* 2021;32(2):356–361. 10.4037/aacnacc2021342

30. Kelley MM, Zadvinskis IM, Miller PS, et al. United States nurses' experiences during the COVID-19 pandemic: a grounded theory [published online ahead of print]. *J Clin Nurs.* 2022;31(15–16):2167–2180. https://doi.org/10.1111/jocn.16032

31. University of Maryland School of Nursing. *Analysis of COVID-19's Impact on Maryland Nursing Workforce.* Published 2021. Accessed April 10, 2022. https://www.nursing.umaryland.edu/media/son/mnwc/MD-survey-of-post-COVID-workforce.pdf

31a.University of Maryland School of Nursing. *Analysis of COVID-19's Impact on Maryland Nursing Workforce.* Unpublished qualitative data. 2021.

32. Hall NA, Everson AT, Billingsley MR, et al. Moral injury, mental health and behavioural health outcomes: a systematic review of the literature. *Clin Psychol Psychother.* 2022;29(1):92–110. https://doi.org/10.1002/cpp.2607

33. Gray K, Dorney P, Hoffman L, et al. Nurses' pandemic lives: a mixed-methods study of experiences during COVID-19. *Appl Nurs Res.* 2021;60:151437. https://doi.org/10.1016/j.apnr.2021.151437

34. Halifax J. The precious necessity of compassion. *J Pain Manag.* 2011;41(1):146–153. https://doi.org/10.1016/j.jpainsymman.2010.08.010

35. Chen R, Sun C, Chen J-J, et al. A large-scale survey on trauma, burnout, and posttraumatic growth among nurses during the COVID-19 pandemic. *Int J Ment Health Nurs.* 2021;30(1):102–116. https://doi.org/10.1111/inm.12796

36. Khoshmehr Z, Barkhordari-Sharifabad M, Nasiriani K, Fallahzadeh H. Moral courage and psychological empowerment among nurses. *BMC Nurs.* 2020;19:43. https://doi.org/10.1186/s12912-020-00435-9

37. Halifax JS. G.R.A.C.E. for nurses: cultivating compassion in nurse/patient interactions. *J Nurs Educ Pract.* 2013;4:121. https://doi.org/10.5430/jnep.v4n1p121

38. Heinze KE, Hanson G, Holtz H, et al. Measuring health care interprofessionals' moral resilience: validation of the Rushton Moral Resilience Scale. *J Palliat Med.* 2021;24(6):865–872. https://doi.org/10.1089/jpm.2020.0328

39. Holtz H, Heinze K, Rushton C. Inter-professionals' definitions of moral resilience. *J Clin Nurs*. 2018;27(3–4):e488–e494. 10.1111/jocn.13989

40. American Nurses Association. *Code of Ethics for Nurses with Interpretive Statements*. Silver Spring, MD: American Nurses Association; 2015.

41. American Nurses Association. *Provision 5: Self-Care and COVID-19*. Published 2021. Accessed May 15, 2022. https://www.nursingworld.org/~4a1fea/globalassets/covid19/provision-5_-self-care--covid19-final.pdf

42. Yang YT, Mason DJ. COVID-19's impact on nursing shortages, the rise of travel nurses, and price gouging. *Health Aff*. 2022. 10.1377/forefront.20220125.695159

43. National Academy of Medicine. *Strategies to Support the Health and Wellbeing of Clinicians During the COVID-19 Outbreak*. Published 2020. Accessed May 15, 2022. https://nam.edu/initiatives/clinician-resilience-and-well-being/clinician-well-being-strategies-during-covid-19/

44. Rosa WE, Schlak AE, Rushton CH. A blueprint for leadership during COVID-19. *Nurs Manage*. 2020;51(8):28–34. 10.1097/01.NUMA.0000688940.29231.6f

17

Healing and Wholeness in the Face of Suffering

Mary Koithan and Mary Jo Kreitzer

Nurses are called to alleviate suffering by protecting, promoting, and restoring the health and well-being of individuals, families, groups, communities, and populations.[1] The American Nurses Association (ANA)[2] further refines the scope of nursing's responsibilities as the integration of the art and science of caring to optimize health and human functioning and alleviate suffering through compassionate presence and the treatment of human responses while recognizing the connection of all humanity.[2] Yet, the nature and origins of suffering and the strategies that are likely to mitigate the impact of suffering are elusive and poorly defined in the literature, and nurses are often left to wonder how they are to fulfill both the moral obligation to reduce suffering and the practice obligation to intervene effectively.[3]

Integrative nursing as a way of being-knowing-doing that advances the whole health of persons, families, and communities holds both theoretical and moral/ethical cues that facilitate our understanding of suffering.[4] Integrative nursing stresses that suffering is addressed not only by mitigating underlying causes of distress but also by bolstering a sense of wholeness, cocreating opportunities for healing, and nourishing well-being. In addition, the principles of integrative nursing practice suggest interventional techniques that nurses can employ to address whole-person and whole-system suffering. At the individual/family level of care, integrative nurses use caring/healing relationships, individualized person-centered care, and evidence-informed traditional and emerging therapeutics to alleviate both acute and chronic suffering. At the systems and planetary levels of engagement, integrative nurses use advocacy, political action, and leadership to address geopolitical and environmental suffering that threatens our very existence. While suffering appears to be a universal experience among living organisms, integrative nursing beliefs, values, and actions hold out hope and opportunity for healing, restoration, and promotion of well-being. Case Exemplars 17.1 and 17.2 highlight different expressions of suffering and integrative nursing approaches.

Case Exemplar 17.1

Matt
Matt is a 40-year-old male from northern Michigan who was diagnosed with schizophrenia in his early 20s. Additionally, he reports ongoing anxiety, depression, insomnia, posttraumatic stress disorder, and apathy. He is a musician and recently

Mary Koithan and Mary Jo Kreitzer, *Healing and Wholeness in the Face of Suffering* In: *The Nature of Suffering and the Goals of Nursing*. Second Edition. Edited by: William E. Rosa and Betty R. Ferrell, Oxford University Press. © Oxford University Press 2023. DOI: 10.1093/oso/9780197667934.003.0017 lost hearing in one ear due to a viral infection. Matt talks and writes often about the nature and depth of his suffering. Why, as a relatively young man who has tried so hard to manage his mental illness, is he facing once again a health challenge that is deeply impacting every aspect of his life? And, while Matt expresses deep gratitude for his health care team that includes a primary care provider, psychiatrist, and integrative mental health APRN/therapist, and for the antipsychotic drugs that reduce his hallucinations and delusions, they do little to address other symptoms that contribute to his deep suffering.

Case Exemplar 17.2

Planet

Planet Earth is a 4.5-billion-year-old ecological system in the Milky Way galaxy. She was diagnosed with environmental distress more than four decades, ago but recently the symptoms of planetary dis-ease have intensified, including unremitting drought, extreme temperature and climate fluctuations, rising greenhouse gases, and the loss of biodiversity. With the link between planetary and human health so obvious and the need for wise stewardship of our natural resources and flourishing natural systems so clear, she "questions" why the current inhabitants can't coalesce around global action that will heal both animate and inanimate components and reduce Earth's suffering. More importantly, she "asks" why they can't see that her deep suffering is ultimately tied to theirs. And she sighs.

The Nature of Suffering: An Integrative Nursing Perspective

Suffering is broadly defined as an experience of unpleasantness and aversion associated with the perception of harm or threat of harm.[5] Synonyms include distress, agony, and misery—implicating both physical and emotional aspects of health. Suffering has been described as a negative valence of the affective domain and appears in degrees of intensity from mild to intolerable.[6] Most literature describes suffering as a complex phenomenon that includes physical, mental, emotional, social, cultural, and spiritual components.[3,7-10] Although it is often ascribed only to sentient beings,[11] van Hooft[12,13] argues that suffering can occur in the absence of cognition or self-awareness and occurs when a physical entity's purpose is threatened. Based in Aristotelean philosophy, van Hooft rejects the notion of dualism and the claim that suffering occurs only at the emotional/psychological level of existence. Rather, van Hooft posits that suffering is a condition of the embodied whole and reflects the whole system's sense of well-being and potential for fulfillment. Therefore, van Hooft claims that suffering occurs within inanimate as well as animate objects, sentient as well as nonsentient living beings. From this perspective suffering is a universal phenomenon when telos or purpose in existence is threatened.

Therefore, both humans (animate living beings) and the natural environment that makes up planet Earth (an inanimate living being) have the capacity to suffer, consistent with the two case studies. While nurses clearly recognize their role in acknowledging and alleviating suffering that occurs in both human and animal beings, suffering experienced by the planet is often viewed as outside the scope of nursing practice. Yet, nurses are called to alleviate suffering and to optimize health broadly and to improve well-being through compassionate presence and healing actions. The theoretical concepts and meta-theoretical perspectives that inform integrative nursing provide additional insight into the nature of suffering from a systems perspective and clarify why attention to planetary, whole-system suffering is a moral obligation of the profession.

Integrative nursing aligns with complex systems science (CSS) as a meta-theoretical perspective and nursing grand theories by Martha Rogers, Margaret Newman, Rosemarie Rizzo Parse, and Jean Watson.[14] This perspective helps to situate suffering and define the scope and nature of an integrative healing approach to the experience of suffering. CSS identifies "how the parts of a system give rise to the collective behaviors of the system and how the system interacts with its environment."[15] Complex adaptive systems are (1) whole systems that (2) change over time. They are characterized by (3) emergence, connectivity, and mutual causation, which creates a global or holistic "order" that is (4) not predictable by the properties of the parts but is a function of the whole system. Emergence is often nonlinear; therefore, change can be exponential and potentially synergistic, driven by (5) self-organization. Change feeds back into the system across all levels of organization, allowing the system to self-tune for adaptive purposes, giving rise to a sense of an edge-of-chaos existence where (6) stability and flexibility are critically paired to create a continuously shifting or integrating system across all levels of existence (individual and collective).[16] These six basic tenets of CSS help us understand the nature of suffering as a manifestation of systems change.

The tenets of CSS are in full display in patient care and help to provide an explanatory framework for responses to illness that nurses witness on a daily basis. Consider the patient who makes a miraculous recovery, defying the odds of life-threatening conditions or perhaps the unexpected complication to a routine procedure, ending in the death of a young 23-year-old adult. Consistent with CSS, change is not necessarily linear and directly proportional to what might be considered "typical" and expected outcomes. Timing, system readiness, adaptability (plasticity), and sensitivity to treatment choice all conspire to create a possible future. Nurses, more than any other health care provider, understand that all systems—human, organizational, natural—are in perpetual transition where one transaction becomes the knowledge and input for subsequent change. Further, nurses understand the nuances of treatment choice, the individuality and specificity of intervention, and the importance of context or environment in the delivery of therapeutics. The subtleties of expert practice and deep understanding of the patient/family in the selection of treatment modalities have long been present in the profession's literature.[17-20]

Aligned with van Hooft's description of suffering, CSS also suggests that suffering is a dynamic pattern that is reflective of the undulating changes that occur over time. Responses to suffering (internal and external) feed back into the system and become part of the evolving pattern as the system adapts and learns. Internal feedback occurs at all levels of intrapersonal experience—physical, emotional, mental/cognitive, and spiritual. External feedback occurs through relationship with others—individually and collectively. Therefore, the degree of suffering decreases and increases over time based on reinforcing and extinguishing messages, giving rise to the observation that the degree of suffering manifests individually in response to similar situations. In some, grief from losing a loved one is transitory, while in others it is incapacitating and enduring. CSS also helps to explain what appears to be exponential and nonlocal suffering responses. As whole systems, a small change or perturbation in the system (e.g., musculoskeletal pain associated with overexertion) can create either local/physical suffering that is brief and easily relieved or distal/psychic suffering based on timing of the perturbation and concomitant conditions of the system that can only be fully understood through deep-reflection self-assessment and discovery.

Martha Rogers[17] and Margaret Newman[18] corroborate this view of suffering. Rogers's theory suggests that suffering is a manifestation of the inseparable and multidimensional human-environmental energy field that continues to evolve in nonlinear and increasingly diverse patterns that form the very substance and focus of nursing as a discipline. According to Rogers, these manifestations have neither inherent positive nor negative valence but are assessed and valued individually within the lifeworld of the individual. Suffering, then, is a pattern that has created dis-ease or constraint in the system. Consistent with van Hooft's beliefs about the nature of suffering, Newman offers that current suffering is a composite of "information enfolded from the past and information which will enfold in the future," an embodied wholeness that continually expands to create meaning and possibilities for wholeness and healing.[19(p39)] This adds to our understanding of suffering as an opportunity for growth and evolving universal consciousness through ongoing interpretation and reinterpretation across all spheres of experience.

Parse[20] adds that interpretation is a process of human becoming through individually valuing and freely choosing from multiple possibilities in order to become more organizationally coherent. Thus, suffering as a process is continually emergent as the system strives toward meaning making and adaptation in order to create the right relationship to ensure its ongoing growth and telos. Aligned with Nietzsche's beliefs that suffering is critical to the process of becoming fully human,[21] Parse suggests that it is systems dis-ease that creates suffering, which in turn provides the impetus for growth and transformation. At times, meaning is elusive and suffering continues; at others there is resolution and understanding. Thus, suffering provides opportunity and momentum for growth, healing, and change.

Suffering or dis-ease is alleviated through the creation of right relationship which occurs across levels of scale within the human-environmental whole system.[14,22] Physical suffering can often be relieved through reducing inflammation and easing the friction or relationship between tissues. Facilitating the repair of interpersonal relationships can heal and reestablish connections that are broken through disagreement and misunderstandings. Right relationships are facilitated and supported by processes described by Watson[23] in her theory of caring and historically have been implemented at the person, family, and community levels of scale. Thus, the relief of suffering is cultivated over time and through relationships that encourage exploration and meaning making so that the system continues with purpose and growth.

As we consider the two case exemplars presented in this chapter, we can more fully appreciate the nature and expression of personal and planetary suffering. As Matt's life patterns have evolved over time, he currently ascribes a negative valence to his experiences, perceiving dis-ease across multiple aspects of his life. This evaluation is prompted by enfolded experiences of partial resolution of some of the manifestations that he considers particularly troublesome and ongoing lack of resolution of others. A local stress (viral infection) has created more distal systems expression (frustrations, questioned purpose and meaning), further contributing to his degree of suffering and further entrenching suffering as the behavioral patterning of the system. Resolution of Matt's suffering will require self-appraisal and examination of the meaning of his suffering and dis-ease created by the many symptoms he is experiencing as well as the dis-ease that occurs through losses associated with hearing and ability to find purpose through music.

Planetary suffering is similarly dis-ease manifested within an inanimate system created over time through enfolding/unfolding of inputs and experiences. The level of suffering can be evaluated through the planetary expressions that threaten Earth's very existence and ongoing stability and will be relieved as the system makes meaning of its suffering and evolves in a way that ensures telos through caring-healing relationships with all systems' elements.

Reducing the Impact of Suffering: An Integrative Nursing Approach

The principles of integrative nursing (Box 17.1), informed by the theoretical perspectives of CSS and nursing theories, can be used to frame nursing practice and provide specific strategies that can be employed to ameliorate suffering and improve overall systems well-being.[4]

Box 17.1 Integrative Nursing Principles

1. Human beings are whole systems inseparable from and influenced by environments.
2. Human beings have an innate capacity for healing and well-being.
3. Integrative nursing is person centered and relationship based.
4. Nature has healing and restorative properties that contribute to health and well-being.
5. Integrative nursing is informed by evidence and uses a full range of conventional and integrative approaches, employing the least intensive intervention possible depending on the need and context.
6. Integrative nursing focuses on the health and well-being of caregivers as well as those they serve.

The first principle of integrative nursing, "human beings are whole systems inseparable from and influenced by environments," highlights the interconnected nature of human beings and all systems. The body, mind, and spirit of humans are inextricably linked and thus human suffering impacts every aspect of personhood. Humans are also shaped and influenced by their environments, which is why attentiveness to the social, environmental, and behavioral determinants of health is critical. If this principle holds true, our environment is similarly shaped by its inhabitants and patterns of behavior; human activity becomes a planetary determinant of health and well-being. Therefore, to reduce planetary suffering, we must be equally vigilant about the environmental conditions as well as the human behaviors that shape them.

The second principle of integrative nursing, "human beings have the innate capacity for health and well-being," is based on the understanding that the body has the innate capacity for healing and restoration on many levels. When the integrity of the skin is damaged by a cut, scrape, or deeper wound, the body automatically goes into a process of inflammation, cell proliferation, and ultimately cellular repair. It is indeed a compelling example of the body's innate capacity to heal. There are other examples of physical healing. While neurons do not divide and are not capable of mitosis after injury, surviving nerve cells reorganize and establish new neural connections.[24]

The mind also has the capacity to help humans heal. The brain has a property called neuroplasticity and is capable of changes in structure and function. Changes can occur as a result of experiences as well as purely internal mental activity, our thoughts.[25] Positive emotions flood our brains with dopamine and serotonin, enhance immune system functioning, diminish the inflammatory response to stress, and change the scope and boundaries of the brain.[26] And people have the capacity to heal from deep grief, loss, and suffering as well as psychological, emotional, and spiritual traumas. People who have experienced the death of a loved one rarely describe themselves as recovering or "getting over it." They do describe healing from a profound loss that is often characterized as a journey toward wholeness.

Similarly, natural systems have the capacity to repair and regenerate. As Speck and Speck[27] suggest, our planet has a powerful capacity to heal itself. When oil spills occur, marshes and wetlands produce increasing numbers of oil-consuming microbes, speeding the oil degradation and reducing environmental suffering.[28] Forest regrowth following devastating fires has similarly been documented. Low-intensity fires restore nutrients to soil; nonnative grasses are eradicated, making way for growth of native plants, which in turn provide food sources for birds and animals.[29]

The third principle emphasizes that integrative nursing is person centered and relationship based. Humans have an innate need for connection and intimacy. Relationships that are healthy and mutual are core to healing and the alleviation of suffering. Allowing ourselves to love and be loved opens up our vulnerability to both experiencing and healing from suffering. Relationships are also central to alleviating suffering of our inanimate environment. Relationships between flora and fauna are critical to environmental healing. Birds drop seeds that ultimately help in reforestation. Similarly, human-environmental relationships facilitate both suffering and healing. Planetary suffering can be eased when human beings appreciate their essential relationship to their surrounding world and begin to walk softly upon the earth.

The fourth principle of integrative nursing is that nature has healing and restorative properties that contribute to health and well-being, reinforcing the reciprocity and centrality of the human-environmental relationship. According to the biophilia hypothesis, human beings are innately drawn to nature and the natural world, and nature has properties that are healing and restorative.[30,31] Systematic literature reviews support the growing evidence that being in nature is associated with reduction in blood pressure as well as reduced heart rate and respiratory distress/shortness of breath, with preliminary evidence pointing to changes in biological markers associated with the stress response and changes in neurological activity and brain activation.[32,33] Spending time in nature not only reduces human suffering; ultimately, these nature-based experiences invite a radical shift in our being, knowing, and doing wherein we begin to see the planet as self, without which we as a species cease to exist.[34]

The fifth principle of integrative nursing focuses on the importance of using a full range of conventional and integrative approaches in our healing practices, employing the least intensive intervention possible depending on the need and context. Without a doubt, there are times that pharmacological and technological interventions are necessary to preserve life and restore health. However, often nonpharmacological approaches can be highly effective in reducing stress and suffering that are associated with pain,[35,36] anxiety and depression,[37,38] nausea,[39] and fatigue.[40]

Similarly, strategies to reduce planetary suffering vary in intensity from attitudinal shifts and awareness of the threats to planetary well-being to conscious acts to reduce personal and institutional carbon footprints. And, when faced with crisis-level symptoms of planetary suffering (e.g., major greenhouse gases at the highest levels for the past 800,000 years, loss of more than 50% of the vertebrate population in 45 years, and changes in climate/weather patterns over the past 10 years), integrative nurses are called to intervene through public/professional education, political action, and advocacy by partnering with organizations including the United Nations and Clinicians for Planetary Health (https://planetaryhealthalliance.org/clinicians-for-planetary-health) and the Alliance of Nurses for a Healthy Environment (https://envirn.org/about/).[41–43]

The sixth principle of integrative nursing addresses the importance of self-care and attention to the stress associated with both professional and lay caregiving roles. While this principle focuses on caregivers attending to their own self-care, it also calls for organizations to attend to workforce needs by creating systems that nurture and sustain caregiver as well as patient well-being. Caregiver suffering has been well documented in light of the past 2 years with the severe acute respiratory syndrome-coronavirus 2 (SARS-CoV-2) pandemic.[44] The exhaustion and suffering of our health care workforce is in the news daily with attendant shortages across human, financial, and materials resourcing. The National Academy of Medicine has launched a clinician well-being initiative that highlights the critical need for self-care along with systems change.[45] Failure to address system issues that contribute to stress and burnout will compromise any efforts made to address the well-being of the health care workforce.

Education and practice standards for all health care providers now feature self-care skills as a critical component of a caregiver's toolkit. Further, quality and safety standards increasingly require health care systems to demonstrate attention to a culture that sustains and supports workforce well-being and an environment that nurtures both patients and caregivers. Quinn[22] notes that the way of the healer requires cultivation of self—actively living-walking a path of self-healing and self-caring that recognizes vulnerabilities and suffering in not only others but also self. When extended beyond the local caregiver, healing and compassionate relief of suffering require attention to the whole of our being—to the planet.

Matt's Plan of Care

At the individual and family level of care, integrative nurses use caring/healing relationships, individualized person-centered care, and evidence-informed traditional and emerging therapeutics to promote health and well-being and alleviate both acute and chronic suffering. Matt's health care team included an integrative mental health advanced practice registered nurse (APRN), a primary care provider, and a psychiatrist. As Matt reflected on the plan of care he created with his integrative mental health APRN, he noted that while antipsychotic drugs work wonders for his hallucinations and stop delusions, they don't touch the other symptoms that contribute to his deep suffering.

He is very invested in his self-care plan that includes music, journaling, intense aerobic exercise, outdoor activities, and mindfulness. He has noticed that anger, rigid thinking, and a lack of nuance and spectrum in his life are precursors to schizophrenic symptoms. If he can become aware of his thought processes soon enough, he can often prevent a psychotic episode from happening. Routine and structure are critical.

Recently, when he was experiencing a lot of paranoia and high anxiety, he took his dog for a mile-long walk on snowshoes. Matt's symptoms reduced dramatically. The combination of exercise, time in the woods, and being with an animal companion was enough to "reset my brain," noted Matt. When he found his way back to playing music, he described a powerful experience when he was playing with another musician: "As we began playing, the audience was enveloped in the music. The music flowed out of us like a river. I felt some of the deepest catharsis I had ever known. We played our hearts out."

While suffering in life is unavoidable, healing is possible. As Matt's story illustrates, healing is a journey toward wholeness that engages the body, mind, and spirit. His plan of care encompassed each of the six principles of integrative nursing. His care was whole-person focused, tapped into his innate capacity to heal, was person centered and relationship based, extensively incorporated nature, utilized both conventional and integrative interventions, and continually encouraged self-care and self-efficacy. Integrative nursing embraces an approach to the alleviation of suffering and healing that is both simple and complex and more accessible than is offered by a purely conventional medical model approach.

In summarizing this journey toward wholeness, Matt noted, "Life is not about grand gestures. Peace and serenity come from the small day-to-day tasks. Life is truly made up of these moments. I received great joy from splitting kindling today, knowing what a blessing it is to have a warm home. Need to stay grateful."

Earth's Plan of Care

Given the level of crisis and the degree of suffering that currently exist, reducing planetary suffering will require engagement across the six principles of integrative nursing. Integrative nurses realize that without intensive intervention, suffering and degradation of the physical conditions on the planet will continue to worsen. Potter[46] calls upon integrative nurses to first cultivate an active awareness of the interconnectedness of nature and our natural environment to human health and well-being (Principles 1 and 4). She claims that reducing planetary suffering will necessarily ease human suffering and improve health across populations: "We must recognize that we have to preserve nature as a source of our healing."[46]

Walking softly upon the earth as recommended by Indigenous populations worldwide to reduce our carbon footprint constitutes another approach to reverse the suffering created through human activity (Principles 2 and 3). Rosa et al.[34] call upon integrative nurses to engage in grassroot efforts to advocate and participate in recycling programs, transition to a diet that is plant based and locally sourced, select products and packaging that reduce impact on the planet, and model planetary self-care and stewardship. Reducing suffering through personal as well as professional commitment to a healthy planet is a critical first step on the path toward healing.

Using the full continuum of strategies to reduce planetary suffering (Principle 5), Schenk[47] reminds nursing to engage in active environmental stewardship that includes community and patient education, political and professional advocacy, and knowledge generation in order to reduce suffering and planetary dis-ease and disruption. Recognizing that nurses constitute the largest health care provider workforce globally and continue to enjoy public trust and confidence, Schenk and others encourage nurses to join citizen action groups that support community gardens, farmers markets, public transportation, and biking/walking corridors. Recognizing that health education extends beyond symptom management on a personal level, integrative nurses can engage in education about the benefits of a plant-based diet, reduced use of plastics and other nonrecyclable packaging, and chemical-free environments. As thought leaders and experts, nurses can ease planetary suffering and facilitate healing through political action and advocacy, weaving together the story of human and environmental well-being and raising awareness across all sectors of the population.

Professional Suffering: An Integrative Approach to Restoring Wholeness

While there has been increased attention to the suffering of the health care workforce during the SARS-CoV-2 pandemic, burnout and chronic, unremitting stress among nurses have been long documented.[48] According to a recent survey,[49] 90% of nurses are thinking about leaving the profession in the next year, citing reasons that go beyond the current pandemic. Seventy-one percent of nurses with more than 15 years of nursing experience are considering leaving as soon as possible or within the next few months. Issues cited include high patient-to-nurse staffing ratios; increased workload due to ancillary staff shortages, forcing nurses to procure supplies, clean units, and attend to clerical details; inefficient operational workflows; poor communication; and administrative burdens. Poor processes, inefficient operational workflows, and administrative burden are key drivers of stress and burnout. Jenna's story (Case Exemplar 17.3) is one that is familiar to many and her suffering is a shared experience across the profession.

Case Exemplar 17.3

Professional Suffering

During the COVID-19 pandemic, Jenna decided to work as a travel nurse. While she had left the ICU environment 6 months previously to return to school, the need for nurses was so great that she decided that she would go where she was needed the most. This brought her to COVID ICUs in multiple large cities across the United States.

Early in the pandemic, there were few drugs and no clear treatment protocols to care for desperately sick patients. "It was like flying the plane blind," Jenna recalled. To make matters even worse, patients were cut off from family members due to the infectious nature of the virus. This meant that nurses needed to provide extensive emotional, social, and spiritual support as well as manage all the technical and technological aspects of care. Jenna noted that all the nurses were required to give 110% every day, and most days, that was not enough. The level of death, despair, and suffering was unlike anything Jenna had experienced.

After 8 months, Jenna described herself as being anxious, depressed, and in a state of deep mental anguish. In other words, she, herself, was suffering.

A Systems Response to Suffering Informed by Integrative Nursing

Effective leadership is a critical strategy for addressing the pervasive suffering of nurses. Leaders must foster an environment where nurses feel heard, supported, and valued. Integrative nursing embraces leadership competencies that focus on systems thinking and can be applied to complex situations such as the pandemic and dysfunctional processes and inefficiencies that exacerbate stress and burnout. Six whole-systems leadership competencies integral to creating a systems response to improve the environment of care within which nurses work include

- deep listening,
- awareness of systems,
- awareness of self,
- seeking diverse perspectives,
- suspending certainty and embracing uncertainty, and
- taking adaptive action.[50]

Integrative nurse leaders deeply listen so that they truly understand issues and engage staff in generating meaningful and effective options. They think from a systems perspective and recognize that getting at the root cause of issues is critical rather than adopting superficial fixes that lack meaning and sustainability. Integrative nurse leaders are keenly focused on self-awareness, recognizing that awareness of motivations, feelings, and beliefs enables leaders to make effective decisions. Integrative nurse leaders seek diverse perspectives, recognizing that conflicting points of view can sharpen thinking and lead to innovative options. Suspending certainty and embracing uncertainty enable leaders to see beyond habitual lenses to get a broader and potentially more accurate view of organizational issues. Taking adaptive action involves continuous learning, taking time to recognize patterns, and balancing an inclusive, deep listening approach with a bias toward action.

The nursing leadership in Jenna's hospital began with an organizational assessment to identify the systems issues that were creating stress, burnout, and suffering across their nursing staff and units. Through a combination of surveys, focus group interviews, unit observations, and individual interviews, they found that supporting individual well-being initiatives among the nursing staff, reducing patient-to-staff ratios, improving the physical environment (e.g., exposure to natural lighting, reducing clutter, providing quiet spaces), and ensuring adequate time off were priority systemic changes needed to reduce the suffering and improve well-being among the staff. They met with staff and unit leaders to develop implementation plans and redesign the care environment to address these needed modifications and make lasting systemic change that would result in improved caregiver experiences and well-being while reducing turnover and burnout.

With these changes, Jenna felt personally encouraged to engage in self-assessment and to begin her own healing journey to well-being. She explored lifestyle factors including diet and nutrition, movement, sleep, and thoughts and emotions. She determined that with scheduling modifications she could engage in additional exercise, improve her rest and sleep habits, and engage in meaningful activities in her community. She felt empowered by leadership to express these needs through staff/leadership shared governance and by advocating for scheduling that permitted a lifestyle that resulted in joy and fulfillment rather than stress and suffering.

Conclusion

Integrative nursing is a way of being, knowing, and doing that advances a whole-health perspective to optimize well-being. Integrative nurses use evidence-informed strategies to support whole-person, whole-system, and planetary healing.[4] The three case exemplars illustrate very different manifestations of suffering, yet the six principles of integrative nursing provided practical and unambiguous guidance that can both shape and direct care at the level of the patient and planet as well as organizational and systems change necessary to create pathways that reduce suffering and support healing. Whether caring for patients or facilitating healing through political action and advocacy, integrative nursing provides a framework that can inform action.

References

1. American Nurses Association. *Code of Ethics for Nurses*. American Nurses Publishing; 2015.
2. American Nurses Association. *The Scope and Standards of Practice*. 4th ed. American Nurses Publishing; 2021.
3. Stilwell P, Hudon A, Meldrum K, Pagé MG, Wideman TH. What is pain-related suffering? Conceptual critiques, key attributes, and outstanding questions. *J Pain*. 2022;23(5):729–738.doi:10.1016/j.jpain.2021.11.005
4. Voss ME, Sandquist L, Otremba K, Kreitzer MJ. Integrative nursing: a framework for whole-person mental health care. *Creative Nursing*. 2023;29(1):1–19.
5. Definition of suffering. *Merriam-Webster Dictionary*. Updated May 2022. Accessed May 1, 2022. https://www.merriam-webster.com/dictionary/suffering
6. Cassell EJ. The nature of suffering. In: Youngner SJ, Arnold RM, eds. *The Oxford Handbook of Ethics at the End of Life*. Oxford University Press; 2016:221. Accessed April 28, 2022. https://DOI:10.1093/oxfordhb/9780199974412.013.17
7. Bueno-Gomez N. Conceptualizing suffering and pain. *Ethics Humanit Med*. 2017;12(7):1–11. Accessed April 10, 2022. doi:10.1186/s13010-017-0049-5
8. Pesut B, Wright D, Thorne S, et al. What's suffering got to do with it? A qualitative study of suffering in the context of Medical Assistance in Dying (MAID). *BMC Palliat Care*. 2021;20(174):2–15. Accessed April 12, 2022. https://doi.org/10.1186/s12904-021-00869-1
9. Siler S, Borneman T, Ferrell B. Pain and suffering. *Semin Oncol Nurs*. 2019;35(3):310–314. Accessed April 1, 2022.https://doi:10.1016/j.soncn.2019.04.013
10. VanderWeele TJ. Suffering and response: directions in empirical research. *Soc Sci Med*. 2019;224:58–66. Accessed April 5, 2022. https://doi.org/10.1016/j.socscimed.2019.01.041.
11. Cassell E, Rich B. Intractable end-of-life suffering and the ethics of palliative sedation. *Pain Med*. 2010;11(3):435–438.
12. Van Hooft S. Suffering and the goals of medicine. *Med Health Care Philos*. 1998;1:125–131.
13. Van Hooft S. The suffering body. *Health*. 2000;4(2):179–195. Accessed April 5, 2022. https://doi.org/10.1177/136345930000400203
14. Koithan M. Concepts and principles of integrative nursing. In: Kreitzer MJ, Koithan M, eds. *Integrative Nursing*. 2nd ed. Oxford University Press; 2019:4–5.
15. Complex systems science: where does it come from and where is it going to? Updated January 2018. Accessed January 22, 2018. http://www.necsi.edu/research/overview/ccs15.html
16. Koithan M, Bell IR, Niemeyer K, Pincus D. A complex systems science perspective for whole systems of CAM research. *Forschende Komplementarmedizin und Klassische Naturheilkunde*. 2012;19(Suppl. 1):7–14.
17. Rogers M. Nursing: a science of unitary human beings. In: Riehl-Sisca JP, ed. *Conceptual Models for Nursing Practice*. 3rd ed. Appleton & Lange; 1989:181–182.
18. Newman M. *Transforming Presence: The Difference That Nursing Makes*. FA Davis; 2008.
19. Newman MA. Newman's theory of health as praxis. *Nurs Sci Q*. 1990;3(1):37–41. Accessed April 22, 2022. https://doi:10.1177/089431849000300109.
20. Parse R. *Illuminations: The Human Becoming Theory in Practice and Research*. National League for Nursing; 1999.
21. Foa Dienstag J. Schopenhauer vs Nietzsche: the meaning of suffering. IAI News. Published April 30, 2021. Accessed May 24, 2022. https://iai.tv/articles/schopenhauer-vs-nietzsche-the-meaning-of-suffering-auid-1801
22. Quinn JF. The way of the healer. In: Kreitzer MJ, Koithan M, eds. *Integrative Nursing*. 2nd ed. Oxford University Press; 2019:46.
23. Watson, J. *Caring Science as Sacred Science*. Rev ed. Lotus Library; 2021.

24. Pfisterer U, Khodosevich K. Neuronal survival in the brain: neuron type-specific mechanisms. *Cell Death Dis.* 2017;8(3):e2643. Accessed May 25, 2022. https://doi:10.1038/cddis.2017.64

25. Dahl CJ, Wilson-Mendenhall CD, Davidson RJ. The plasticity of well-being: a training-based framework for the cultivation of human flourishing. *Proc Natl Acad Sci U S A.* 2020;117(51):32197–32206. Accessed May 12, 2022. https://doi:10.1073/pnas.2014859117

26. Fredrickson BL, Joiner T. Reflections on positive emotions and upward spirals. *Perspect Psychol Sci.* 2018;13(2):194–199. Accessed May 12, 2022. https://doi:10.1177/1745691617692106

27. Speck O, Speck T. An overview of bioinspired and biomimetic self-repairing materials. *Biomimetics (Basel).* 2019;4(1):26. Accessed May 28, 2022. https://doi:10.3390/biomimetics4010026

28. Pete AJ, Bharti B, Benton MG. Nano-enhanced bioremediation for oil spills: a review. *ACS EST Engg.* 2021;1(6):928–946. Accessed May 28, 2022. https://doi.org/10.1021/acsestengg.0c00217

29. Cagle A. What happens after wildfire sweeps through forest. Sierra Club. Published March 30, 2022. Accessed May 1, 2022. https://www.sierraclub.org/sierra/what-happens-after-wildfire-sweeps-through-forest

30. Barbiero G, Berto R. Biophilia as evolutionary adaptation: an onto- and phylogenetic framework for biophilic design. *Front Psychol.* 2021;12:700–709. Accessed May 12, 2022. https://doi:10.3389/fpsyg.2021.700709

31. Lumber R, Richardson M, Sheffield D. Beyond knowing nature: contact, emotion, compassion, meaning, and beauty are pathways to nature connection. *PLoS One.* 2017;12(5):e0177186. Accessed May 12, 2022. https://doi:10.1371/journal.pone.0177186

32. Jimenez MP, DeVille NV, Elliott EG, et al. Associations between nature exposure and health: a review of the evidence. *Int J Environ Res Public Health.* 2021;18(9):4790. Accessed May 12, 2022. https://doi:10.3390/ijerph18094790

33. Shuda Q, Bougoulias ME, Kass R. Effect of nature exposure on perceived and physiologic stress: a systematic review. *Complement Ther Med.* 2020;53:1025134. Accessed May 12, 2022. https://doi:10.1016/j.ctim.2020.102514

34. Rosa W, Upvall M, Andrus V. Integrative nursing and planetary health. In: Kreitzer MJ, Koithan M, eds. *Integrative Nursing.* 2nd ed. Oxford University Press; 2019:60.

35. Tang SK, Tse MMY, Leung SF, Fotis T. The effectiveness, suitability, and sustainability of non-pharmacological methods of managing pain in community-dwelling older adults: a systematic review. *BMC Public Health.* 2019;19(1):1488. Accessed May 12, 2022. https://doi:10.1186/s12889-019-7831-9

36. Hargett JL, Criswell AC. Non-pharmacological interventions for acute pain management in patients with opioid abuse or opioid tolerance: a scoping review protocol. *JBI Database System Rev Implement Rep.* 2019;17(7):1283–1289. Accessed May 12, 2022. https://doi:10.11124/JBISRIR-2017-003878

37. Davis SP, Bolin LP, Crane PB, Crandell J. Non-pharmacological Interventions for anxiety and depression in adults with inflammatory bowel disease: a systematic review and meta-analysis. *Front Psychol.* 2020;11:538741. Accessed May 12, 2022. https://doi:10.3389/fpsyg.2020.538741

38. Zhang X, Zhou G, Chen N, Zhang Y, Gu Z. Effect of non-pharmacological interventions on anxiety, depression, sleep quality, and pain after orthopedic surgery: a protocol for systematic review and network meta-analysis. *Medicine (Baltimore).* 2021;100(44):e27645. Accessed May 12, 2022. https://doi:10.1097/MD.0000000000027645

39. Hamdy G, Alagizy H, Said O, Shehata M. Efficacy of non pharmacological technique on chemotherapy induced nausea, vomiting and retching among breast cancer patients.

IOSR-JNHS. 2017;6(5):60–72. Accessed May 12, 2022. https://doi:10.9790/1959-060 5056072

40. Ho LYW, Ng SSM. Non-pharmacological interventions for fatigue in older adults: a systematic review and meta-analysis. *Age Ageing*. 2020;49(3):341–351. Accessed May 12, 2022. https://doi:10.1093/ageing/afaa019

41. Whitmee S, Haines A, Beyrer C, et al. Safeguarding human health in the Anthropocene epoch: report of the Rockefeller Foundation–Lancet Commission on planetary health. *Lancet*. 2015;386(10007):1973–2028. Accessed April 13, 2022. https://doi.org/10.1016/S0140-6736(15)60901-1

42. Schenk EC, Potter TM, Cook C, Huffling K, Rosa WE. Nurses promoting inclusive, safe, resilient, and sustainable cities and communities: taking action on COVID-19, systemic racism, and climate change. *Am J Nurs*. 2021;121(7):66–69. Accessed May 28, 2022. https://doi:10.1097/01.NAJ.0000758540.26343.2e

43. Rosa WE, Catton H, Davidson PM, et al. Nurses and midwives as global partners to achieve the sustainable development goals in the Anthropocene. *J Nurs Scholarsh*. 2021;53(5):552–560. Accessed May 28, 2022. https://doi:10.1111/jnu.12672

44. Young E, Milligan K, Henze M, Johnson S, Weyman K. Caregiver burnout, gaps in care, and COVID-19: effects on families of youth with autism and intellectual disability. *Can Fam Physician*. 2021;67(7):506–508. Accessed April 10, 2022. https://doi.org/10.46747/cfp.6707506

45. Committee on Systems Approaches to Improve Patient Care by Supporting Clinician Well-Being. *Taking Action Against Clinician Burnout: A Systems Approach to Professional Well-Being*. National Academies of Sciences, Engineering, and Medicine; 2019. https://doi.org/10.17226/25521

46. Potter T. Planetary Health: An Integrative Approach to the Great Transition. Oral presentation at International Integrative Nursing Symposium. April 2022. Online.

47. Schenk E. Environmental Stewardship in Healthcare: A Nursing Perspective. Oral presentation at the Butterfield Upstream Keynote Lecture Series. April 2022. Spokane, WA.

48. Henshall C, Davey Z, Jackson D. Nursing resilience interventions—a way forward in challenging healthcare territories. *J Clin Nurs*. 2020;29(19–20):3597–3599. Accessed May 29, 2022. https://doi:10.1111/jocn.15276

49. Siwicki B. Report: 90% of nurses considering leaving the profession in the next year. Healthcare IT News. Published March 24, 2022. Accessed May 12, 2022. https://www.healthcareitnews.com/news/report-90-nurses-considering-leaving-profession-next-year.

50. Kreitzer MJ. Whole systems leadership and healing. In: Kreitzer MJ, Koithan M, eds. *Integrative Nursing*. 2nd ed. Oxford University Press; 2019.

18

"What Is the Nature of Suffering and What Are the Goals of Nursing?"

Betty R. Ferrell and William E. Rosa

The second edition of this book on suffering and the goals of nursing adds both breadth and depth to the conversation we began with the publication of the first edition in 2008.[1] Our first edition was prompted by our observation that nurses are the largest health care profession—comprising an estimated 59% of the health care workforce worldwide and spending the highest proportion of direct patient-facing time at any point along a given disease trajectory.[2] Ultimately, nurses are the most likely clinicians to be present across all settings for patients who are suffering and their families. From the labor ward to hospice, from the trauma center to home care, the art and science of nursing becomes known through the nurse's abilities to give comfort; demonstrate empathy, caring, and compassion; and deliver high-quality, evidence-based care in a manner that humanizes patients and fosters trusting relationships. Nurses are sojourners with those who suffer in all circumstances, both in spaces where well-being is nurtured and sustained and in places where dignity is degraded or threatened. The skills and capacities needed for nurses to identify suffering, sit with it, allow for it, and meet people wherever they may be with whatever emotions they may be feeling is a practice calling for constant growth and development.

Yet the description, scope, and value of nurses' roles and responsibilities in responding to suffering are often misunderstood or ignored altogether by interprofessional partners, health systems leadership, and the public at large. It may be quite difficult for nurses—be they clinicians, researchers, educators, advocates, and/or administrators—to articulate (or even understand) the many inner dimensions and textures of being a first responder to suffering. This current volume aims to provide a substantive reflection on these gaps at the intersection of the authors' expertise, the best available evidence, and set against the backdrop of emergent social discourse. In this way, we hope to support nurses in identifying their own opportunities to better ameliorate suffering while offering an expanded vision of the highest potential of the nursing profession to provide person-centered and holistic care for both individuals and the human collective amid the unpredictability of the living-dying continuum.

Suffering: An Evolving Concept

In the years since the release of the first edition, nurses have witnessed immense suffering in patients with serious illness across all ages and diseases, as well as among

Betty R. Ferrell and William E. Rosa, *"What Is the Nature of Suffering and What Are the Goals of Nursing?"* In: *The Nature of Suffering and the Goals of Nursing*. Second Edition. Edited by: William E. Rosa and Betty R. Ferrell, Oxford University Press.
© Oxford University Press 2023. DOI: 10.1093/oso/9780197667934.003.0018

patients' loved ones, communities, and the bereaved. Citizens and countries of the world have seen how their interdependence, characterized by either solidarity or indifference, influences the extent to which suffering is manifested and perpetuated. Rapidly spreading communicable diseases—such as the Ebola outbreak in West Africa (2014–2016) and the COVID-19 pandemic—have added elements of fear, panic, worry, and mass loss and grief to how people from every walk of life understand, explain, cope with, process, and respond to suffering. Armed conflict, the climate crisis, and other humanitarian and public health emergencies have become unavoidable realities that directly inform how the sick suffer, how the healthy remain well, and the extent to which nurses can fulfill their professional roles and simultaneously honor multiple loyalties to patients, employers, and their own moral compass.[3]

Of utmost importance is the elevated societal urgency to dismantle all forms of racism and casteism and to reconstruct equitable health and social care systems based on the threads of inclusion and justice. These goals will only be accomplished through a strategic recentering of marginalized and systematically disenfranchised groups and concerted investments to address the social determinants of health at all levels. There are morally unjust disparities not only in how people access health care services but also in how and why they suffer during illness.

A key exemplar is the global burden of suffering. The Lancet Commission on Global Access to Palliative Care and Pain Relief coined the term "serious health-related suffering" based on 20 health conditions that are widely recognized as causing substantial physical and psychological distress.[4] The commission stated that suffering is "health-related when it is associated with illness or injury of any kind" and it is "serious when it cannot be relieved without professional intervention and when it compromises physical, social, spiritual, and/or emotional functioning."[(p1392)] They estimated that more than 61 million people worldwide experience serious health-related suffering, the vast majority of whom live in low- and middle-income countries with no or extremely limited access to palliative care services or palliative care medicines (e.g., opioids for pain and symptom management).[4] Indeed, nearly 90% of the global palliative care need is unmet, with people in the poorest countries experiencing needless suffering without the policy protections, infrastructure, interventions, or training for health professionals to provide the physical, psychosocial, or spiritual care required.[5] In this case, the evidence shows that (1) people suffer merely because they live in poor countries and (2) people know the relief of suffering because of their proximity to wealth.

Beyond the travesties imposed by global divides of the rich and poor, suffering is deeply embedded in the social fabric, woven by legacies of white supremacy, colonialism, patriarchy, hetero- and cisnormativity, and other deliberate misappropriations and violations of power. For example, the malignancies of all forms of racism—individual, interpersonal, systemic, structural—inform unacceptably disparate pain, end-of-life, and other clinical outcomes for Black, Indigenous, and all persons of color.[6-8] Homophobia, transphobia, and other forms of violence and discrimination against minoritized sexual and gender identity persons lead to higher rates of social isolation, suicide, and substance abuse among lesbian, gay, bisexual, transgender, and queer/questioning (LGBTQ+) people when compared to non-LGBTQ+ groups.[9-12] The list goes on of those whose suffering is underassessed, undertreated, or silenced: older people, incarcerated persons, persons experiencing homelessness, persons with mental or physical disabilities, and many others. The bias and exclusion of these groups call us to question what we think we know about intergenerational suffering, suffering from toxic and chronic stressors, and the burdens faced by people with intersectional and multiple minoritized identities. Furthermore, it holds nurses and the broader health workforce accountable for uncovering and responding to the meaning and significance of historical narratives, social structures, and the pervasive "isms" that mediate and moderate suffering.

As the social consciousness continues to awaken to the seemingly endless ways injustice both predicts and exacerbates suffering, it is no longer acceptable or feasible to only provide nursing care for the person before us. A broader and more refined scope of nursing's contributions, and obligations, is needed. Indeed, when we care for this person and respond to their suffering in this moment, we are—in essence—caring for the consequences of a legacy and a history (e.g., the social determinants of health) alongside the symptoms and emotional burdens of how the current illness is being experienced. The contributing authors of this text remind us again and again that suffering is both driven and mitigated not only by the inner lifeworld of the patient but also by the situational, environmental, and relational covariates of society and the health system. When we care for one, we care for a community. There can be no doubt that the amount of suffering in the world and the toll it takes on all of us is significant. But so is the gift and calling that is nursing.

Nursing: An Evolving Duty to Care

In the mid-19th century, nursing scholars began to recognize the role of nursing beyond the physical care of bathing patients, managing wounds, and delivering other medically prescribed treatments. Nurse theorists began defining professional nursing and describing the intimate relationship between nurses and those they served, commencing a scholarly and scientific journey into the influence of psychosocial support, therapeutic presence, deep listening, and bearing witness to suffering. Nursing leaders began to push the profession beyond a goal of restoring function, increasing oral intake, or healing physical injuries toward a new vision in which expert nursing care also meant being fully present and available, listening to the voices of suffering, recognizing those aspects of patients' lives that will not be fixed or cured, and providing comfort through our very intimate bond as nurses with patients and their loved ones.

The caring theorists offered language to explain the power of "being with" rather than "doing to" and of "allowing for" over "fixing" or "changing" the circumstances that arise during the nurse-patient encounter.[13] Holistic and integrative nursing scholars have opened our awareness to use all ways of knowing—the personal, empirical, sociopolitical, ethical, and aesthetic—and develop comfort with 'not knowing' in order to engage patients and effectively respond to suffering.[14,15] Other recent approaches, such as nurse coaching, have created communication and relationship-building tools to ground the art of nursing in replicable and cohesive competencies.[16] These paradigm shifts have each helped move nurses beyond assistant or technician roles toward becoming experts in facilitating healing and alleviating suffering for the human condition. These elements of "being with" and "allowing for," of using all ways of knowing at our disposal, and of using evidence-informed communication skills to express empathy and inclusion are fundamental to the professional nursing obligation to care for those who are suffering.

As this narrative of nurses as a caring presence in suffering was first emerging, noted nurse scholars Kahn and Steeves wrote about the basic tenets of suffering through a nursing lens.[17] They described nurses as "witnesses and moral agents" and they identified four ways that nurses witness suffering through firsthand observations, through serving a ceremonial role, as expert witnesses, and as visionaries. These roles enable nurses to speak for those who are suffering and advocate for their care—core to the professional practice of nursing. Kahn and Steeves also describe the tenets of suffering (Box 18.1).[17]

These tenets provide a roadmap for nurses to step into the potential discomfort of being with suffering. When examined closely, Kahn and Steeves show that knowing and responding to suffering is an iterative and lifelong process. Their tenets remind nurses that no aspect of suffering can be presumed or taken for granted and that each human experience is only known through time, caring, intention, and an appreciation for the countless variables that factor into the suffering equation. Kahn and Prefer Steeves' explicit mention of assumptions invites pause in how nurses carry their own implicit biases or opinions when meeting the suffering patient and encourages introspection about ways they might interrupt the sometimes-unconscious cycle of transference and countertransference during patient engagement. These tenets give hope that while the sources of suffering are innumerable—and may be ultimately unknowable—there is also a basic structure to suffering and a larger process at play that includes both the nurse's capacity to care and the patient's coping skills and relational supports.

Kahn and Prefer Steeves' roadmap also reminds us of the importance of that broader and more refined scope extending beyond the current nurse-patient encounter and encompassing the sources of suffering that may pre-date this moment, the expressions of suffering that may be arising within this moment, and the implications of suffering

---

Box 18.1 Tenets of Suffering as Described by Kahn and Steeves[17]

- Suffering is a private, lived experience of a whole person, unique to each individual.
- Suffering results when the most important aspects of a person's identity are threatened or lost.
- Because suffering depends on the meaning of an event or loss for the individual, it cannot be assumed present or absent in any given clinical condition.
- Suffering also can be viewed as an experience of lost personal meaning.
- Possible sources of suffering are innumerable.
- We recognize certain kinds of experiences as forms of suffering; we acknowledge these forms as experiences that will lead to suffering for many who experience them.
- As a fundamental human experience, suffering has a basic structure.
- The experience of suffering involves the person in a larger process that includes the person's own coping with suffering and the caring of others.
- The caring environment in which the processes of suffering occur can influence a person's suffering positively and negatively.

for the patient and their loved ones that may reach long beyond this moment. Watson called this phenomenon the "transpersonal caring moment"—recognizing that both nurse and patient come to this present encounter with a lifetime of history and past experiences that inform their perceptions and responses right now.[18] Additionally, the remnants of this current encounter will stay with the nurse and patient for the remainder of their lives and will continue to have an impact on their self-perceptions and perceptions of others. Whether the nurse is caring or devoid of caring, their demonstration will long live in the minds and memories of their patient. The former may be remembered as life-giving or healing (i.e., biogenic), while the latter may be viewed as harmful (i.e., biocidic).

These early contributions to defining suffering from a nursing vision and recognizing the role of nursing in responding to suffering are reflected in Case Exemplar 18.1.

Case Exemplar 18.1

Mayola is a 59-year-old African American woman seen in a public hospital outpatient clinic for a painful draining wound on her breast, today diagnosed as stage 4 breast cancer. Mayola is alone, now being seen by Regina, a nurse practitioner who is attempting to discuss treatment options and care with Mayola, who is greatly distressed, sobbing, clutching her purse, rocking in her chair, and repeating, "Oh Jesus, no, no, Oh Jesus …" Regina recognizes the extreme distress, closes and sets aside her laptop and consent forms, and sits next to Mayola. Regina gently touches Mayola's hand but maintains space and lowers her head and listens to Mayola's chants until Mayola finally becomes silent, but her crying increases. Regina says, "I can't imagine what it must be like to hear the words you have heard today—that you have cancer." Mayola sobs, saying, "Just like my mother." As Mayola repeats these words, her face appears to contort and her sobs seem to extend to deep expressions of grief. Regina remains silent as Mayola shares the story of her mother who had breast cancer when Mayola was a child and received no care in the southern United States, where there was no hospital for Black people in their area. Regina listens and assures Mayola that she will receive care, but Mayola then moves from deep distress and grief to a sense of panic as she begins to recognize how her own life is about to change. Mayola tells Regina that she is a single parent and her oldest son, James, the first of the family to attend college, depends on her for financial and emotional support. She can't miss work; this is all that matters. Regina listens, assures Mayola that the care team will be there for her and her son, and suggests that she return later in the week with her son to discuss plans for care. Regina asks if Mayola has a picture of her son, what he is studying in school, and also who is available to support Mayola. Regina also asks Mayola if she can assist her with transportation to get home today and if she would like a call from the clinic social worker to learn more about her needs. As Mayola prepares to leave, Regina notices that she is holding a small cross in her hand. Regina places her hand on Mayola's, assuring her that she will be there for her during each step ahead, and pauses for a moment of silence before she assists her in leaving.

Regina, an undoubtedly very busy nurse overwhelmed by the realities of current practice, has lived into the words echoed by Kahn and Steeves.[17] She has offered her presence, resisted the urge to offer solutions or silence the suffering, and begun a relationship with Mayola that will greatly impact her experience in the months ahead.

The Nature of Suffering and the Goals of Nursing: An Evolving Dynamic

The first edition of *The Nature of Suffering and the Goals of Nursing* concluded with the creation of 10 fundamental tenets of the nature of suffering and the goals of nursing.[1] These tenets began our attempts to understand the nature of suffering from the vision of nursing and our place as nurses to intimately accompany those who suffer. This second edition brings many other voices: the authors of this book include nurses from a wide range of clinical areas, and yet all share the common ground of nursing. While synthesizing the contributing authors' perspectives in this current volume, we revisit these tenets and expand upon them to provide additional context for nurses to feel confident in their response to suffering while coming to a place of understanding of those deeper personal and existential questions that are ultimately unknowable, are unanswerable, or may cause distressing thoughts and feelings for both the patient and the nurse as a witness. An updated list of the tenets of suffering can be found in Box 18.2.

Nurses not only build relationships with patients in their care but also, as they become more expert in their practice, build a relationship with the very essence of suffering over time. Nurses will likely learn to anticipate suffering, readily identifying the missed clinical opportunities or other circumstances that will lead to a patient's distress or dis-ease. Although there will be countless cases when a nurse might feel that the patient's suffering is not sufficiently alleviated, consistent reflection on relevant individual and system-level factors may be helpful to create environments that can bear the weight of suffering and empower nurses to sustain themselves.

At the individual level, nurses may seek to better know their own experiences of suffering, which can range from their own past traumas and losses to the moral distress and moral suffering confronted in their work (see Chapter 16). Nurses' unaddressed suffering may diminish their capacity to bear witness and remain present for their patients' suffering. It may also abate their own sense of well-being; cause harm to their psychosocial, mental, and emotional health; and preclude opportunities for joy, meaning, and purpose in their nursing role. The opportunity to know how we respond to seeing and processing suffering is part of building a sustainable nursing career. Individual reflection could be kept private, discussed with colleagues as a debriefing mechanism, or talked about with the support of a counselor or therapist. Any approach that intuitively helps the nurse to feel seen, heard, acknowledged, and validated may be helpful. Some examples for reflection might include:

- Am I aware of any sadness, grief, anxiety, or worry I feel related to my work? If I needed help, support, or assistance to manage my suffering, would I be able to ask for it?

Box 18.2 Tenets of Suffering

1. Suffering is described as a loss of control, which creates insecurity. Suffering people often feel helpless and trapped, unable to escape their circumstances.

2. In most instances, suffering is associated with loss. The loss may be of a relationship, some aspect of the self, identity, or the physical body. The loss may be evident only in the mind of the sufferer, but it nonetheless leaves a person feeling diminished and with a sense of brokenness.

3. Suffering is intensely personal, informed significantly by the meaning that the sufferer makes of their experience.

4. One's experience of suffering cannot be separated from the environmental context, which may include their social determinants of health, their home and relational dynamics with family or other relationships, their past experiences of trauma and/ or marginalization, and their perceptions of health systems and clinicians, among other multi-level factors.

5. Suffering is accompanied by a range of intense thoughts and emotions including sadness, anguish, fear, abandonment, despair, worry, demoralization, regret, and myriad other thoughts and emotions.

6. Suffering can be deeply linked to a recognition of one's own mortality. When threatened by serious illness, people may fear the end of life. Fears about end of life may be characterized by worry about pain or physical distress, questions about one's legacy and relationships, and uncertainty about an afterlife, among other concerns. Conversely, for others, living with serious illness may cause a yearning for death as an end to suffering.

7. Suffering often involves asking the question "Why?" Illness or loss may be seen as untimely and undeserved. Suffering people seek to find meaning and answers for that which is unknowable.

8. Suffering is often associated with a sense of separation from the world. Individuals may express intense loneliness and yearn for connection with others while also feeling intense distress about dependency on others.

9. Suffering is often accompanied by spiritual or existential distress. Regardless of the presence or absence of religious affiliation, individuals experiencing illness may feel a sense of hopelessness. When life is threatened, there may be a self-evaluation of what has been lived and what remains undone. Becoming weak, feeling vulnerable, and facing mortality may cause one to reevaluate their relationship with a higher being or worldview.

10. Suffering is not synonymous with pain but is closely associated with it. Physical pain is closely related to psychological, social, and spiritual/existential distress. Pain that persists without meaning becomes suffering.

11. Suffering occurs when the individual feels voiceless. This may occur when the person is mute to give words to their experience or when their "screams" are unheard.

12. There is no singular antidote to suffering. Suffering does not need to be fixed, changed, or altered. The one suffering often seeks to be seen, heard, acknowledged, validated, and fully expressed. Suffering that is deemed unbearable by the sufferer will likely call for a range of physical, emotional, psychological, and spiritual/existential responses. These responses may be required from nurses, interprofessional partners, and health systems.

13. Experiences of individual healing and wholeness are possible in the face of suffering, even in the absence of cure or resolution. Suffering does not inherently diminish the opportunities for the sufferer to know joy, love, and connection.

14. Suffering occurs in the context of all physical and mental illness, in the process of aging, and in the final phases of living and dying. There is no hierarchy or quantification of suffering when living in the face of illness. Each expression of suffering can be valued as an opportunity to remain present, listen more deeply, provide comfort, and ensure dignity.

15. Suffering may have collateral and/or sustained effects on those who bear witness, including families, communities, caregivers, and nurses.

- How do I respond to my own suffering at the end of a stressful day?
- How do I process the suffering I see on a daily basis? Where do I put it?
- How do I attend to my own sadness or unresolved feelings after a patient dies?
- What are the hardest parts of seeing people suffer? What parts are in my control and what parts are not?
- Does my suffering matter? Why or why not?

System-level changes are required to support nurses in their work and nurture environments that provide whole-person care not only for patients but also for nurses. Systems that do not prioritize the human experience are likely to become blind to the suffering of all involved and without the tools needed to respond to it. Reflecting on the current state of the system in which we work can bring about the courage to make necessary change at all levels so that nurses can fulfill their duty to care for patients who are suffering. Some of these reflections may include:

- Is my system attuned to the needs, experiences, and history of the local communities we serve? How can we improve these critical relationships to inform health system practices?
- Do system priorities and values explicitly mention the commitment to ensuring dignified care for patients and their loved ones? Is there a way to prioritize these aspects of health care delivery?
- Is nurses' duty to care respected, honored, and celebrated by the system at large? What changes are needed to amplify nurses' roles, responsibilities, and needs?
- Are there pathways to communicate openly, honestly, and transparently with leadership about how to improve nursing care for patients?
- How does the system invest in sustaining the well-being and addressing the suffering of staff?

Conclusion

In concluding this volume, we would be remiss if we did not acknowledge the suffering of nurses that has been exacerbated by the COVID-19 pandemic, other global humanitarian crises, and continued health system deficits since the release of the first edition. Nurses' mental, emotional, and physical well-being have been compromised in countless ways and yet they continue to walk alongside patients and their loved ones as the most trusted of health professionals. Without question, tremendous healing will be needed in the years ahead, not only for our colleagues and the broader nursing profession but also for health systems at large.

The work of nursing will continue to be both rewarding and challenging in ways that only nurses can understand. This truth is at the root of our joy, our purpose, and our suffering. While the nature of suffering may continue to be ultimately unknowable, the goals of nursing will forever be intertwined with the duty to bear witness and respond compassionately to the unfolding journey of those in our care.

References

1. Ferrell BR, Coyle N, eds. *The Nature of Suffering and the Goals of Nursing.* Oxford University Press; 2008.
2. World Health Organization. State of the world's nursing: investing in education, jobs and leadership. Published 2020. Accessed July 3, 2022. https://www.who.int/publications/i/item/9789240003279
3. Rosa WE, Grant L, Knaul FM, et al. The value of alleviating suffering and dignifying death in war and humanitarian crises. *Lancet.* 2022;399(10334):1447–1450. doi:10.1016/S0140-6736(22)00534-7
4. Knaul FM, Farmer PE, Krakauer EL, et al. Alleviating the access abyss in palliative care and pain relief-an imperative of universal health coverage: the Lancet Commission report [published correction appears in Lancet. Mar 9, 2018]. *Lancet.* 2018;391(10128):1391–1454. doi:10.1016/S0140-6736(17)32513-8
5. Connor S. Global atlas of palliative care. 2nd ed. Published 2020. Accessed July 3, 2022. https://cdn.who.int/media/docs/default-source/integrated-health-services-(ihs)/csy/palliative-care/whpca_global_atlas_p5_digital_final.pdf?sfvrsn=1b54423a_3
6. Kara M, Foster S, Cantrell K. Racial disparities in the provision of pediatric psychosocial end-of-life services: a systematic review [published online ahead of print, May 18, 2022]. *J Palliat Med.* 2022;25(10):1510–1517. doi:10.1089/jpm.2021.0476
7. Jones T, Luth EA, Lin SY, Brody AA. Advance care planning, palliative care, and end-of-life care interventions for racial and ethnic underrepresented groups: a systematic review. *J Pain Symptom Manage.* 2021;62(3):e248–e260. doi:10.1016/j.jpainsymman.2021.04.025
8. Estrada LV, Agarwal M, Stone PW. Racial/ethnic disparities in nursing home end-of-life care: a systematic review. *J Am Med Dir Assoc.* 2021;22(2):279–290.e1. doi:10.1016/j.jamda.2020.12.005
9. Harding R, Epiphaniou E, Chidgey-Clark J. Needs, experiences, and preferences of sexual minorities for end-of-life care and palliative care: a systematic review. *J Palliat Med.* 2012;15(5):602–611. doi:10.1089/jpm.2011.0279
10. Haviland K, Burrows Walters C, Newman S. Barriers to palliative care in sexual and gender minority patients with cancer: a scoping review of the literature. *Health Soc Care Community.* 2021;29(2):305–318. doi:10.1111/hsc.13126
11. McDermott E, Nelson R, Weeks H. The politics of LGBT+ health inequality: conclusions from a UK scoping review [published online ahead of print, Jan 19, 2021]. *Int J Environ Res Public Health.* 2021;18(2):826. doi:10.3390/ijerph18020826

12. The National Academies of Sciences, Engineering, & Medicine. Understanding the well-being of LGBTQI+ populations. Published 2020. Accessed July 3, 2022. https://nap.nation alacademies.org/catalog/25877/understanding-the-well-being-of-lgbtqi-populations

13. Rosa W, Horton-Deutsch S, Watson J, eds. *A Handbook for Caring Science: Expanding the Paradigm*. Springer; 2019.

14. Helming MAB, Shields DA, Avino KM, Rosa WE, eds. *Holistic Nursing: A Handbook for Practice*. 8th ed. Jones & Bartlett Learning; 2022.

15. Kreitzer MJ, Koithan M, eds. *Integrative Nursing*. 2nd ed. Oxford University Press; 2019.

16. Southard ME, Dossey BM, Bark L, Schaub BG, eds. *The Art & Science of Nurse Coaching: The Provider's Guide to Coaching Scope & Competencies*. American Nurses Association; 2021.

17. Kahn DL, Steeves RH An understanding of suffering grounded in clinical practice and research. In Ferrell BR, ed. *Suffering*. Sudbury, MA: Hones & Bartlett; 1996:3–28.

18. Watson J. *Unitary Caring Science: Philosophy and Praxis of Nursing*. University Press of Colorado; 2018.

Index

For the benefit of digital users, indexed terms that span two pages (e.g., 52–53) may, on occasion, appear on only one of those pages.

Tables, figures, and boxes are indicated by *t*, *f*, and *b* following the page number